To David Bull,

who made this book possible

and Lara Noel Borowski

who taught us about living and dying

Acknowledgments

Many people have helped us write this book. Among the most important are the first 1,000 participants of the Stanford University Chronic Disease Self-Management study. These have been followed by hundreds of thousands of other workshop participants in more than 25 countries and as many languages. All of these people, along with our wonderful workshop Leaders, have told us what information they needed and helped us make adjustments as we went along. All of you have informed this new edition.

There are also many professionals who have assisted us: Sonia Alvarez, MA, MPH, Lara Borowski, MPH, Lynn Beatie, PT, MPT, MHA, Roberto Benzo, MD, Bonnie Bruce, RD, DrPH, Ann Constance, MA, RD, CDE, Nazanin Dashtara, MPH, Laurie Doyle, MPH, Robin Edelman, MS, RD, CDE, Chaplain Bruce Feldstein, MD, Karen Freimark, MEd, Margo Harris, MPH, Peg Harrison, MSW, Margaret Haynes, MPA, Mary Hobbs, MPH, Susan Kayman, PhD, Marty Klein, PhD, Patricia League, RN, John Lynch, PhD, David McCulloch, MD, Cynthia McRae, PhD, Elaine McMahon, MS, RN, Nancy Moline, RN, MEd, CDE, Cheryl Owen, RN, Katy Plant, MPH, Denise Portello, MPH, RD, Catherine Regan, PhD, Richard Seidel, PhD, Joyce Tanaka, RN, MSN, CDE, Sandra Wilson, PhD, Michelle Wong, MPH, MPP. To all of you, your help has been gratefully received.

There are also many friends, leaders, and trainers who have given us wonderful advice and added richness to our thinking: Nancy Brannigan, María Hernández-Marin, Lynne Newcombe, Jim Phillips, Jean Thompson.

A special thanks to Gloria Samuel, who kept us all on track. We would also like to thank our T-Trainers, Master Trainers, and Leaders. There are now thousands of you. You have made many suggestions that have helped us with this new edition.

We would also like to thank the publishers for permission to adapt sections from *The Healthy Mind, Healthy Body Handbook* (also published as *The Mind & Body Health Handbook*) by David Sobel, MD and Robert Ornstein, PhD (published by DRx).

Finally, thanks to David Bull to whom this book is dedicated. David was our first publisher and had faith in this project that allowed us to proceed. Without him, there may never have been a book. His son Jim has continued the family tradition with support and encouragement for this fourth edition.

If you would like to learn more about our continuing research, online internet programs, trainings, and materials see our website: http:// patienteducation.stanford.edu.

We are continually revising and improving this book. If you have any suggestions or comments that will make the book better, please send them to self-management@stanford.edu.

Contents

Disclaimer

This book is not intended to replace common sense, professional medical or psychological advice. You should seek and get appropriate professional evaluation and treatment for problems—especially unusual, unexplained, severe, or persistent symptoms. Many symptoms and diseases require and benefit from specific medical or psychological evaluation and treatment. Don't deny yourself proper professional care.

- If your symptoms or problems persist beyond a reasonable period despite using self-care recommendations, you should consult a health professional. What is a reasonable period will vary; if you're not sure and you're feeling anxious, consult a health care professional.

- If you receive professional advice in conflict with this book, you should rely upon the guidance provided by your health care professional. He or she is likely to be able to take your specific situation, history and needs into consideration.

- If you are having thoughts of harming yourself in any way, please seek professional care immediately.

This book is as accurate as its publisher and authors can make it, but we cannot guarantee that it will work for you in every case. The authors and publisher disclaim any and all liability for any claims or injuries that you may believe arose from following the recommendations set forth in this book. This book is only a guide; your common sense, good judgment, and partnership with health professionals are also needed.

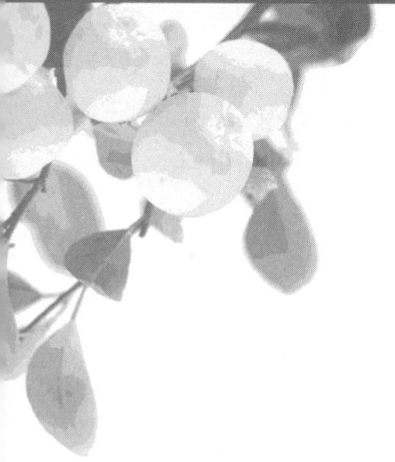

CHAPTER 1

Overview of Self-Management

Nobody wants to have a chronic long-term illness. Unfortunately, most of us will experience two or more of these conditions during our lives. This book has been written to help people with chronic illness explore healthy ways to live with a physical or mental condition. This may seem like a strange concept. How can you have an illness and live a healthy life? To answer this, we need to look at what happens with most chronic health problems. These diseases, be they heart disease, diabetes, depression, liver disease, bipolar disorder, emphysema, or any one of a host of others, cause most people to experience fatigue as well as to lose physical strength and endurance. In addition, they may cause emotional distress, such as frustration, anger, anxiety, or a sense of helplessness. Health is soundness of body and mind, and a healthy life is one that seeks that soundness. Therefore, a healthy way to live with a chronic illness is to work at overcoming the physical, mental, and emotional problems caused by the condition. The challenge is to learn how to function at your best regardless of the difficulties life presents. The goal is to achieve the things you want to do and to get pleasure from life. That is what this book is all about.

Before we go any further, let's talk about how to use this book. Throughout this book you will find information to help you learn and practice self-management skills. This is not a textbook; you might think of it as a workbook. You do not need to read every word in every chapter. Instead, read the first two chapters and then use the table of contents to find the information you need. Feel free to skip around and to take notes right in the book. This will help you learn the skills you need in order to follow your individual path.

You will not find any miracles or cures in these pages. Rather, you will find hundreds of tips and ideas to make your life easier. This advice comes from physicians and other health professionals, as well as people like you who have learned to positively manage their chronic health problems. Please note that we said "positively manage." There is no way to avoid managing a chronic condition. If you choose to do nothing, that is one way of managing. If you only take medication, that is another management style. If you choose to be a positive self-manager and undergo all the best treatments that health care professionals have to offer, and to be proactive in your own day-to-day management, you will live a healthier life.

In this chapter we discuss chronic illness in general as well as point out the most common problems. In addition, we give some guidance on the self-management skills that are unique to particular conditions. You will soon see that the problems and skills have much more in common than you might think, no matter what the health problem may be. This is good news in that most people have more than one chronic condition. Therefore, learning the common life skills allows you to successfully manage your life, not just a single condition. The rest of the book gives you the tools needed to become a great manager of both your chronic conditions and all the other aspects of your life.

What Exactly Is a Chronic Health Condition?

Health problems can be characterized as either "acute" or "chronic." Acute health problems usually begin suddenly, have a single cause, are often easily diagnosed, last a short time, and get better with medication, surgery, rest, and time. Most people with acute illnesses are cured and return to normal health. There is usually relatively little uncertainty for the patient or the doctor; both usually know what to expect. The illness typically follows a cycle of getting worse for a while, carefully treating or observing the symptoms, and then getting better. Finally, the care of acute illness depends on the body's ability to heal itself and sometimes on a health professional's knowledge and experience in finding and administering the correct treatment.

Appendicitis is an example of an acute illness. It typically begins rapidly, signaled by nausea and pain in the abdomen. The diagnosis of appendicitis, once established by examination,

Table 1.1 **Differences Between Acute and Chronic Disease**

	Acute Disease	**Chronic Disease (long-term)**
Beginning	Usually rapid	Slow
Cause	Usually one, identifiable	Often uncertain, especially early on
Duration	Short	Usually for life
Diagnosis	Commonly accurate	Sometimes difficult
Tests	Give good answers	Often of limited value
Role of professional	Select and conduct treatment	Teacher and partner
Role of patient	To follow orders	Partner of health professionals, responsible for daily management

leads to surgery for removal of the inflamed appendix. There follows a period of recovery and then a return to normal health.

Chronic illnesses are different (see Table 1.1). They usually begin slowly and proceed slowly. For example, a person may slowly develop blockage of the arteries over decades and then might have a heart attack or a stroke. Arthritis generally starts with brief annoying twinges that gradually increase. Unlike acute disease, chronic illnesses usually have multiple causes that vary over time. These causes may include heredity, lifestyle (smoking, lack of exercise, poor diet, stress, and so on), and exposure to environmental factors such as secondhand smoke or air pollution and to physiological factors such as low levels of thyroid hormone or changes in brain chemistry that may cause depression.

The combination of many causes and unknown factors can be frustrating for those of us who want quick answers. It is difficult for both the doctor and the patient when clear answers aren't available. In some cases, even when diagnosis is rapid, as in the case of a stroke or heart attack, the long-term effects may be hard to predict. The lack of a regular or predictable pattern is a major characteristic of most chronic illnesses.

Unlike acute disease, where full recovery is expected, chronic illness usually leads to more symptoms and loss of physical or mental functioning. With chronic illness many people assume that the symptoms they are experiencing are due to the disease itself. While the disease can certainly cause pain, shortness of breath, fatigue, and the like, it is not the only cause. Each of these symptoms can contribute to the other symptoms. What's more, the symptoms can feed on each other. For example, depression causes fatigue, pain causes physical limitations, and these can lead poor sleep and more fatigue. The interactions of these symptoms make the condition worse. It becomes a *vicious cycle* that only gets worse unless we find a way to break the cycle (see Figure 1.1 on the next page).

Throughout this book we examine ways of breaking the cycle and getting away from the problems of physical and emotional helplessness.

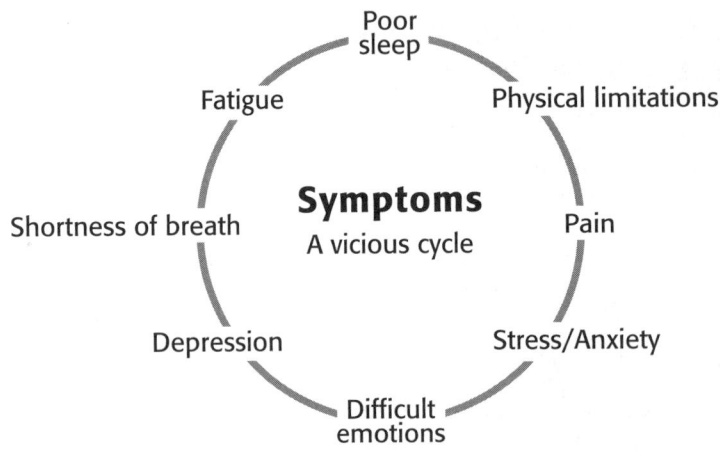

Figure 1.1 **The Vicious Cycle of Symptoms**

What Causes a Chronic Disease?

To answer this question, we need to understand how the body operates. As you know, cells are the building blocks of tissues and organs: the heart, lungs, brain, blood, blood vessels, bones, and muscles—in fact, everything in the body. For a cell to remain alive and function normally, three things must happen: it must be nourished, receive oxygen, and get rid of waste products. If anything goes wrong with any of these three functions, the cell becomes diseased. If cells are diseased, the organ or tissue suffers. If this happens you may experience limitations in your ability to be active in daily life. The differences among chronic diseases depend on which cells and organs are affected and the processes by which the disruption occurs. For example, during a stroke, a blood vessel in the brain becomes blocked or bursts. Oxygen and nutrition are cut off for part of the brain supplied by that artery. As a result, the part of your body controlled by the damaged brain cells, such an arm, a leg, or a portion of your face, loses function.

If you have heart disease, heart attacks occur when the vessels supplying blood to the heart muscle become blocked. This is called a coronary thrombosis. When this happens, oxygen is cut off, the heart muscle is injured, and pain results. After the injury the heart may be less effective in supplying the rest of your body with oxygen-carrying blood. Because the heart is pumping blood less efficiently through the body, fluid accumulates in tissues, and you may experience shortness of breath and fatigue.

With diseases of the lungs, either there is a problem getting oxygen to the lungs, as with bronchitis or asthma, or the lungs cannot effectively transfer oxygen to the blood, as with emphysema. In both cases the body is deprived of oxygen.

In diabetes, the pancreas does not produce enough insulin or produces insulin that cannot be used efficiently by the body. Without this insulin the body's cells are not able to use the glucose (sugar) in the blood for energy.

In liver and kidney disease, the cells of these organs do not work properly, making it difficult for the body to get rid of waste products.

The basic consequences of these diseases are similar: loss of function due to a reduction in oxygen, accumulation of waste products, or inability of the body to use glucose for energy.

Loss of function also occurs in arthritis, but for other reasons. In osteoarthritis, cartilage (the cushioning material found on the ends of bones and as the "disks" between the vertebrae of the back) becomes worn, frayed, or displaced, causing pain. We often do not know exactly why the cartilage cells begin to weaken or die. But the results are pain and disability.

Most mental illnesses are caused by imbalances in chemicals and structural changes in the brain. Too much or too little of these chemical neurotransmitters can affect our moods, thoughts, and behaviors. Treatment of such conditions as depression, bipolar disorder, and schizophrenia often includes restoring chemical balance with medications as well as changes in the environment or self-care practices to support effective coping.

Different Diseases, Similar Symptoms

Because chronic illness starts with a malfunction at the cellular level, we may not notice the disease until it intrudes in our life by causing symptoms or declares itself through an abnormal test result.

Although the biological causes of chronic illnesses differ, the problems they cause for people are similar. For example, most people with chronic conditions suffer fatigue and loss of energy. Sleeping problems are common. In one case there is pain, while in another case there is trouble breathing. Disability, to some extent, is a part of chronic disease. It may be the inability to use your hands well because of arthritis or stroke or difficulty in walking due to shortness of breath, stroke, arthritis, or diabetes. Sometimes disability is caused by a lack of energy, extreme fatigue, or change in mood.

Depression can be both the reflection of a chronic or recurrent imbalance in brain chemicals and "feeling down" or "feeling blue" that results from having other chronic illnesses. It is hard to maintain a cheerful disposition when your condition causes annoying problems that are unlikely

to go away. Along with the depression come fear and concern for the future. Will I be able to remain independent? If I can't care for myself, who will care for me? Will I get worse? How bad will it get? Both disability and depression may bring loss of self-esteem.

Because there are similarities among chronic illnesses, the essential management tasks and skills you need to learn in order to live with different chronic illnesses are also similar.

Perhaps the most important skill of all is learning to respond to your illness on an ongoing basis to solve day-to-day problems. After all, you live with your condition 24 hours a day; your health care provider sees you only a tiny portion of this time. This means that *you* must manage your condition. Table 1.2 on page 7 illustrates some of the self-management problems caused by chronic conditions.

From this brief introduction you can see that chronic illnesses have more in common than first meets the eye. In this book we talk about managing these illnesses. For most of the book, however, we will talk more about the

Self-Management Skills

- Problem solving and responding as your disease gets better and worse

- Maintaining a healthy lifestyle with regular exercise, healthy eating, sound sleep habits, and stress management

- Managing common symptoms

- Making decisions about when to seek medical help and what treatments to try

- Working effectively with your health care team

- Using medications safely and effectively while minimizing side effects

- Finding and using community resources

- Talking about your illness with family and friends

- Adapting social activities

Table 1.2 **Self-Management Problems for Common Chronic Conditions**

Chronic Condition	Possible Problems Caused by Chronic Conditions				
	Pain	Fatigue	Shortness of Breath	Physical Function	Difficult Emotions
Anxiety/Panic Disorder		✔	✔	✔	✔
Arthritis	✔	✔		✔	✔
Asthma and Lung Disease		✔	✔	✔	✔
Cancer	✔	✔	✔	✔	✔
Chronic Heartburn and Acid Reflux	✔				✔
Chronic Pain	✔	✔		✔	✔
Congestive Heart Failure		✔	✔		✔
Depression		✔		✔	✔
Diabetes	✔	✔		✔	✔
Heart Disease	✔	✔	✔	✔	✔
Hepatitis	✔	✔			✔
High Blood Pressure					✔
HIV Disease (AIDS)	✔	✔	✔	✔	✔
Inflammatory Bowel Disease	✔				✔
Irritable Bowel Syndrome	✔				✔
Kidney Stones	✔				
Multiple Sclerosis	✔	✔		✔	✔
Parkinson's Disease	✔	✔		✔	✔
Peptic Ulcer Disease	✔				✔
Renal Failure		✔			✔
Stroke		✔		✔	✔

management tasks common across many illnesses. If you have more than one health problem, you need not be confused about how to start. The approaches that work for heart disease will also help with lung disease, arthritis, depression, or a stroke. Start with the problem or condition that bothers you most. Table 1.3 on pages 8 and 9 outlines some of the management skills that may be needed to deal with disease-specific problems. Some of these skills are also discussed later in the book in the chapters dealing with specific diseases.

Same Disease, Different Response

Arthur suffers from severe arthritis. He is in pain most of the time and can't sleep. He took early retirement because of his arthritis and now, at age 55, he spends his days sitting at home bored. He avoids most physical activity because of the pain, weakness, and shortness of breath. He has become very irritable. Most people, including his family, don't enjoy his company. It even seems too much trouble when the grandchildren he adores come to visit.

Isabel, age 66, also suffers from severe arthritis. Every day she manages to walk several blocks to the local library or the park. When the pain is severe, she practices relaxation techniques and tries to distract herself. She works several hours a week as a volunteer at a local hospital. She also loves going to see her young grandchildren and even manages to take care of them for a while when her daughter has to run errands. Her husband is amazed at how much zest she has for life.

Arthur and Isabel both live with the same condition with similar physical problems. Yet their abilities to function and enjoy life are very different. Why? The difference lies largely in their attitudes toward the disease and their lives. Arthur has allowed his life and physical capacities to wither. Isabel has learned to take an active role in managing her chronic illness. Even though she has limitations, she controls her life instead of letting the illness control it.

Attitude cannot cure chronic illness. But a positive attitude and certain self-management skills can make it much easier to live with. Much research now shows that the experience of pain, discomfort, and disability can be modified by circumstances, beliefs, mood, and the attention we pay to symptoms. For example, with arthritis of the knee, a person's degree of depression has been found to be a better predictor of how disabled, limited, and uncomfortable the person will be than the evidence of physical damage to the knee on X-rays. What goes on in a person's mind is at least as important as what is going on in the person's body.

In other words, why is it that two people with similar chronic conditions can function in their lives so differently? One may be able to minimize the effect of symptoms, while the other is extremely disabled. One may focus on healthy living, while the other is completely concentrated on the disease. One of the keys in shaping the impact of any disease is how effective and engaged the person is in self-management.

Table 1.3 **Management Skills for Dealing with Chronic Conditions**

	Management Skills							
Chronic Condition	Pain Management	Fatigue Management	Breathing Techniques	Relaxation and Managing Emotions	Nutrition	Exercise	Medications	Other Management Tools
Anxiety/Panic Disorder		✔	✔	✔	✔	✔	✔	• Behavioral techniques to decondition triggers
Arthritis	✔	✔		✔	✔	✔	✔	• Use of assistive devices • Appropriate use of joints • Use of cold/heat • Pacing of activities
Asthma and Lung Disease		✔	✔	✔		✔	✔	• Use of inhalers and peak flow meters • Avoid triggers
Cancer	✔	✔		✔	✔	✔	✔	• Varies with site of the cancer • Managing effects of surgery, radiation, and chemotherapy
Chronic Pain	✔	✔		✔		✔	✔	• Pacing of activities • Specific exercises • Use of pain management techniques
Congestive Heart Failure		✔	✔	✔	✔	✔	✔	• Monitoring of daily weight • Sodium/salt restriction
Depression		✔		✔	✔	✔	✔	• Engaging in pleasant activities • Exposure to light (phototherapy)
Diabetes	✔	✔		✔	✔	✔	✔	• Home blood glucose monitoring • Insulin injection • Foot care • Regular eye (retinal) exams
Heartburn and Acid Reflux					✔		✔	• Avoid stomach irritants (e.g., coffee, alcohol, aspirin, nonsteroidal anti-inflammatory medications) • Elevation of bed

Management Skills								
Chronic Condition	Pain Management	Fatigue Management	Breathing Techniques	Relaxation and Managing Emotions	Nutrition	Exercise	Medications	Other Management Tools
Heart Disease	✔	✔	✔	✔	✔	✔	✔	• Know and watch for warning signs of heart attack
Hepatitis	✔	✔		✔	✔		✔	• Avoid use of alcohol, IV drugs, medications toxic to liver • Preventing spread of infection (e.g., for hepatitis B and C, safer sex practices, hygiene)
High Blood Pressure				✔	✔	✔	✔	• Home blood pressure monitoring • Sodium/salt restriction
HIV Disease (AIDS)	✔	✔	✔	✔	✔	✔	✔	• Preventing spread of infection (e.g., safer sex practices, hygiene) • Watch for signs of early infection • Avoid IV drugs
Inflammatory Bowel Disease	✔			✔	✔		✔	
Irritable Bowel Syndrome	✔			✔	✔		✔	
Kidney Stones	✔				✔		✔	• Maintain fluid intake • Avoid calcium or oxalates, depending on type of stones
Multiple Sclerosis	✔	✔		✔	✔	✔	✔	• Management of incontinence • Management of mobility
Parkinson's Disease		✔		✔	✔	✔	✔	• Mobility
Peptic Ulcer Disease	✔			✔	✔	✔	✔	• Avoid stomach irritants (e.g., coffee, alcohol, aspirin, nonsteroidal anti-inflammatory medications) and early infection
Renal Failure		✔		✔	✔		✔	• Dialysis
Stroke		✔		✔		✔	✔	• Use of assistive devices

Understanding the Chronic Illness Path

The first responsibility of any chronic condition self-manager is to understand the disease. This means more than learning about what causes the illness, what symptoms it may cause, and what you can do. It also means observing how the disease and its treatment affect you. An illness is different for each person, and with experience you and your family will become experts at determining the effects of the disease and its treatment. In fact, you are the only person who lives with your health problem every minute of every day. Therefore, observing how it affects you and making accurate reports to your health care providers are essential parts of being a good manager. Most chronic illnesses go up and down in intensity. They do not follow a steady path. Let's look at an example.

John, Sandra, and Mary all have a blood pressure of 160/100, which is too high.

Mary tells her doctor that she sometimes forgets her medications and is not getting much exercise. She is also overweight. Her doctor talks with her, and together they work out a plan to help her remember her medications, to start an exercise program, and to cut down on the amount of food she eats.

John says he is taking his medications, exercising, and eating well. The doctor decides to change his medications, as what he is currently taking is probably not working.

Sandra does not want to take medication. She is doing everything she can to lower her blood pressure: eating well, losing weight, and exercising. Unfortunately, though her blood pressure has improved a bit, it is not good enough. The doctor talks to her about the dangers of high blood pressure and advises starting a medication. In the end Sandra decides that this might be best.

The successful management of high blood pressure varied for each of these patients but depended on each one's communicating his or her unique situation, experiences, and preferences to the doctor. In other words, effective control of the illness involved an observant patient communicating openly with the health care provider.

When you develop a chronic illness, you become more aware of your body. Minor symptoms that were ignored may now cause concerns. For example, is this chest pain a signal of a heart attack? Is this pain in my knee a sign that the arthritis has gotten worse? There are no simple reassuring answers. Nor is there a fail-safe way of sorting out serious signals from minor temporary symptoms that can be ignored.

It is helpful to know and understand the natural rhythms of your chronic illness. In general, symptoms should be checked out with your doctor if they are unusual, severe, or persistent or if they occur after starting a new medication or treatment plan.

Throughout this book we give some specific examples of what actions to take if you experience certain symptoms. But this is where your partnership with your health care provider becomes critical. Self-management does not mean going it alone. Get help or advice when you are concerned or uncertain.

From what has just been said, self-management may seem like a simple enough concept.

Both at home and in the business world, managers direct the show. They don't do everything themselves; they work with others, including consultants, to get the job done. What makes them managers is that they are responsible for making decisions and making sure that their decisions are carried out.

As the manager of your illness, your job is much the same. You gather information and hire a consultant or team of consultants consisting of your physician and other health professionals. Once they have given you their best advice, it is up to you to follow through. All chronic illnesses need day-to-day management. We have all noticed that some people with severe physical problems get on well while others with lesser problems seem to give up on life. The difference often lies in their management style.

Managing a chronic illness, like managing a family or a business, is a complex undertaking. There are many twists, turns, and midcourse corrections. By learning self-management skills, you can ease the problems of living with your condition.

The key to success in any undertaking is, first, deciding what you want to do; second, deciding how you are going to do it; and, finally, learning a set of skills and practicing them until they have been mastered. Success in chronic disease self-management is the same. In fact, mastering such skills is one of the most important tasks of life.

We will describe hundreds of skills and tools to help relieve the problems caused by chronic illness. We do not expect you to use all of them. Pick and choose. Experiment. Set your own goals. *What you do may not be as important as the sense of confidence and control that comes from successfully doing something you want to do.* We have learned that knowing the skills is not enough. We need a way of incorporating these skills into our daily lives. Whenever we try a new skill, the first attempts may be clumsy, slow, and show few results. It is easier to return to old ways than to continue trying to master new and sometimes difficult tasks. The best way to master new skills is through practice and evaluation of the results.

Self-Management Skills

What you do about something is largely determined by how you think about it. For example, if you think that having a chronic illness is like falling into a deep pit, you may have a hard time motivating yourself to crawl out, or you may even think the task is impossible. The thoughts you have can greatly determine what happens to you and how you handle your health problems.

Some of the most successful self-managers are people who think of their illness as a path. This path, like any path, goes up and down. Sometimes it is flat and smooth. At other times the way is rough. To negotiate this path one has to use many strategies. Sometimes you can go fast; other times you must slow down. There are obstacles to negotiate.

Good self-managers are people who have learned three types of skills to negotiate this path:

- **Skills needed to deal with the illness.** Any illness requires that you do new things. These may include taking medicine, using an inhaler, or using oxygen. It means more frequent interactions with your doctor and the health care system. Sometimes there are new exercises or a new diet. Even diseases such as cancer require self-management. Chemotherapy, radiation, and surgery can all be made easier through good day-to-day self-management. All of these constitute the work you must do just to manage your illness.

- **Skills needed to continue your normal life.** Just because you have a chronic illness does not mean that life does not go on. There are still chores to do, friendships to maintain, jobs to perform, and family relationships to continue. Things that you once took for granted can become much more complicated in the face of chronic illness. You may need to learn new skills or adapt the way you do things in order to maintain the things you need and want to do.

- **Skills needed to deal with emotions.** When you are diagnosed as having a chronic illness, your future changes, and with this come changes in plans and changes in emotions. Many of the new emotions are negative. They may include anger ("Why me? It's not fair"), fear ("I am afraid of becoming dependent on others"), depression ("I can't do anything anymore, so what's the use?"), frustration ("No matter what I do, it doesn't make any difference. I can't do what I want to do"), or isolation ("No one understands, no one wants to be around someone who is sick"). Negotiating the path of chronic illness, then, also means learning skills to work with these negative emotions. We will teach you some skills to manage these emotions.

With this as background, you can think of self-management as the use of skills to manage the work of living with your illness, continuing your daily activities, and dealing with emotions brought about by chronic illness.

Final Points to Ponder

- **You are not to blame.** Chronic diseases are caused by a combination of genetic, biological, environmental, and psychological factors. For example, stress alone does not cause most chronic illnesses. Mind matters, but mind cannot always triumph over matter. If you fail to recover, it is not because of lack of right mental attitude. There are many things you can control that will help you cope with chronic illness. Remember, you are not responsible for causing the disease or failing to cure it, but you are responsible for taking action to manage your illness.

- **Don't do it alone.** One of the side effects of chronic illness is a feeling of isolation. As supportive as friends and family members may be, they often cannot understand what you are experiencing as you struggle to cope with a chronic illness. Chances are, however, that there are others who know firsthand what it is like to live with a chronic condition just like yours. Connecting with other people with similar conditions can reduce your sense of isolation, help you understand what to expect based on a fellow patient's perspective, offer practical tips on how to manage symptoms and feelings on a day-to-day basis, give you the opportunity to help others cope with their illness, help you appreciate your strengths and realize that things could be worse, and inspire you to take a more active role in managing your illness by seeing others coping successfully. Support can come from reading a book or a newsletter about how someone lives with a chronic illness. Or it can come from talking with others on the telephone, in support groups, or even linking online through computer and electronic support groups.

- **You're more than your disease.** When you have a chronic disease, too often the center of attention becomes your disease. But you are more than your disease—more than a "heart patient" or "lung patient." And life is more than trips to the doctor and managing symptoms. It is essential to cultivate areas of your life that you enjoy. Small daily pleasures can help balance the other parts in which you have to manage uncomfortable symptoms or emotions. Find ways to enjoy nature by growing a plant or watching a sunset, or indulge in the pleasure of human touch or a tasty meal, or celebrate companionship with family or friends. Finding ways to introduce moments of pleasure is vital to chronic disease self-management. Focus on your abilities and strengths rather than disabilities and problems. Helping others is one way to increase your own sense of what you can do instead of focusing on what you can't. Celebrate small improvements. If chronic illness teaches anything, it is to live each moment more fully. Within the true limits of whatever disease you have, there are ways to enhance your function, sense of control, and enjoyment of life.

- **Illness can be an opportunity.** Illness, even with its pain and disability, can enrich our lives. It can make us reevaluate what is really important, shift priorities, and move in exciting new directions that we may never have considered before.

  Jill has breast cancer. Since her diagnosis, she lives more fully than ever: "I was a housewife, lost and aimless after my children grew up and left home. One of the first things I did after the diagnosis was go and teach myself to swim with my head in the water. I had always kept it above, too scared to put my whole self in. That had been the story of my life. Now I do whatever I want. I don't think about how much time there is, just what I want to do with mine. Surprisingly, I feel less afraid of living."

A heart attack sometimes makes people decide to slow down. They would rather have more time to deepen relationships with family and friends. A chronic disease that restricts movement may lead some to think again about unused intellectual talents. Meg learned a new language and found an overseas pen pal; Fred dared write the novel he always thought he was "too stupid" to write. Though chronic illness may close some doors, you can choose to open new ones.

Suggested Further Reading

Cousins, Norman. *Anatomy of an Illness as Perceived by the Patient.* New York: Norton, 2005.

Gruman, Jessie. *AfterShock. What to Do When the Doctor Gives You—or Someone You Love—a Devastating Diagnosis.* New York: Walker, 2010. See also Gruman's Web site, which offers a selection of further resources: http://www.aftershockbook.com/

Selak, Joy H., and Steven M. Overman. *You Don't Look Sick: Living Well with Invisible Chronic Illness.* Binghamton, N.Y.: Haworth Medical Press, 2005.

Sobel, David, and Robert Ornstein. *The Healthy Mind, Healthy Body Handbook.* Los Altos, Calif.: DRX, 1996.

Sobel, David, and Robert Ornstein. *Healthy Pleasures,* 2nd ed. Reading, Mass.: Addison-Wesley, 1997.

Sobel, David, and Robert Ornstein. *Mind and Body Health Handbook: How to Use Your Mind and Body to Relieve Stress, Overcome Illness, and Enjoy Healthy Pleasures,* 2nd ed. Los Altos, Calif.: DRX, 1998.

Weil, Andrew. *Healthy Aging: A Lifelong Guide to Your Physical and Spiritual Well-Being.* New York: Knopf, 2005.

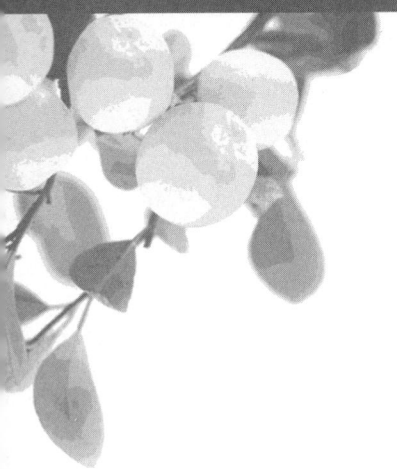

CHAPTER 2

Becoming an Active Self-Manager

IT IS IMPOSSIBLE TO HAVE a chronic condition without being a self-manager. Some people manage by withdrawing from life. They stay in bed or socialize less. The disease becomes the center of their existence. Other people with the same condition and symptoms somehow manage to get on with life. They may have to change some of the things they do or the way that things get done. Nevertheless, life continues to be full and active. The difference between these two extremes is not the illness but rather how the person with a chronic condition decides to manage the illness. Please note the word *decides*. Self-management is always a decision: a decision to be active or a decision to do nothing, a decision to seek help or a decision to suffer in silence. This book will help you with these decisions.

Like any skill, active self-management must be learned and practiced. This chapter will start you on your way by presenting the three most important self-management tools: problem solving, decision making, and action planning. Remember: you are the manager.

15

Like the manager of an organization or a household, you must do all of the following things:

1. Decide what you want to accomplish.
2. Look for various ways to accomplish this goal.
3. Draft a short-term action plan or agreement with yourself.
4. Carry out your action plan.
5. Check the results.
6. Make changes as needed.
7. Reward yourself for your success.

Problem Solving

Problems sometimes start with a general uneasiness. Let's say you are unhappy but not sure why. Upon closer examination, you find that you miss contact with some relatives who live far away. With the problem identified, you decide to take a trip to visit these relatives. You know what you want to accomplish, but now you need to make a list of ways to solve the problem.

In the past you have always driven, but you now find driving tiring, so you seek other ways of travel. You consider leaving at noon instead of early in the morning and making the trip in two days instead of one. You consider asking a friend along to share the driving. There is also a train that stops within 20 miles of your destination, or you might fly. You decide to take the train.

The trip still seems overwhelming, as there is so much to do to prepare. You decide to write down all the steps necessary to make the trip a reality. These include finding a good time to go, buying a ticket, figuring out how to handle luggage, seeing if you can make it up and down the stairs to get on the train, wondering if you can walk on a moving train to get food or go to the bathroom, and figuring out how you will get to the station. Each of these steps can be an action plan.

To start making your action plan, you promise yourself that this week you will call and find out just how much the railroad can help. You also decide to start taking a short walk each day, including walking up and down a few steps so that you will be steadier on your feet. You then carry out your action plan by calling the railroad and starting your walking program.

A week later you check the results. Looking back at all the steps to be accomplished, you see that a single call answered many questions. The railroad can help people who have mobility problems and has ways of dealing with many of your concerns. However, you are still worried about walking. Even though you are walking better, you are still unsteady. You make a change in your plan by asking a physical therapist about this, and he suggests using a cane or walking stick. Although you don't like using it, you realize that a cane will give you the extra security needed on a moving train.

You have just engaged in problem solving to achieve your goal to take a trip. Now let's review the specific steps in problem solving.

Steps in Problem Solving

1. **Identify the problem.** This is the first and most important step in problem solving— and usually the most difficult step as well. You may know, for example, that stairs are a problem, but it will take a little more effort

to determine that the real problem is fear of falling.

2. **List ideas to solve the problem.** You may be able to come up with a good list yourself, but you may sometimes want to call on your consultants. These can be friends, family, members of your health care team, or community resources. One note about using consultants: these folks cannot help you if you do not describe the problem well. For example, there is a big difference between saying that you can't walk because your feet hurt and saying that your feet hurt because you cannot find walking shoes that fit properly.

3. **Pick an idea to try.** As you try something new, remember that new activities are usually difficult. Be sure to give your potential solution a fair chance before deciding it won't work.

4. **Check the results** after you've given your idea a fair trial. If all goes well, your problem will be solved.

5. If you still have the problem, pick another idea from your list and try again.

6. **Use other resources** (your consultants) for more ideas if you still do not have a solution.

7. Finally, if you have gone through all of the steps until all ideas have been exhausted and the problem is still unsolved, you may have to accept that your problem may not be solvable right now. This is sometimes hard to do. The fact that a problem can't be solved right now doesn't mean that it won't be solvable later or that other problems cannot be solved. Even if your path is blocked, there are probably alternative paths. Don't give up. Keep going.

Problem-Solving Steps

1. Identify the problem.
2. List ideas to solve the problem.
3. Select one method to try.
4. Check the results.
5. Pick another idea if the first didn't work.
6. Use other resources.
7. Accept that the problem may not be solvable now.

Living with Uncertainty

Living with uncertainty is one of the hardest self-management tasks. It is something that most of us cannot avoid. Uncertainty is also one of the causes of emotional ups and downs. The diagnosis of a chronic condition takes away some of our sense of security and control. It can be frightening. We are following our life path, and suddenly we are forced to detour to a different, unwanted path. And even as we work with health professionals and start new treatments, this uncertainty continues. Of course, we all have an uncertain future, but most people do not think about this. When we have a chronic condition, however, this becomes an important part of our lives. We are uncertain about our future health, and perhaps about our ability to continue to do the things we want, need, and like to do. Many people find it very challenging to make decisions while accepting uncertainty.

Making Decisions: Weighing the Pros and Cons

Making decisions is an important tool in our self-management toolbox. There are some steps that are a little like problem solving to help us make decisions.

1. **Identify the options.** For example, you may have to make a decision about getting help in the house or continuing to do all the work yourself. Sometimes the options are to change a behavior or to not change at all.

2. **Identify what you want.** It may be important for you to continue your life as normally as possible, to have more time with your family, or not have to shovel the walkways, cut the grass, or clean the house. Sometimes identifying your deepest, most important values (like spending time with family) helps set priorities and increase your motivation to change.

3. **Write down pros and cons for each option.** List as many items as you can for each side. Don't forget the emotional and social effects.

4. **Rate each item on the list** on a 5-point scale with 0 indicating "not at all important" and 5 indicating "extremely important."

5. **Add up the ratings for each column** and compare them. The column with the higher total should give you your decision. If the totals are close or you are still not sure, skip to the next step.

6. **Apply the "gut test."** For example, does going back to work part-time feel right to you? If so, you have probably reached a decision. If not, the way you feel should probably win out over the math.

Decision-Making Example

Should I get help in the house?

Pro	Rating	Con	Rating
I'll have more time	4	It's expensive	3
I'll be less tired	4	It's hard to find good help	1
I'll have a clean house	3	They won't do things my way	2
		I don't want a stranger in the house	1
Total	11		7

Add up the points for the pro and con lists. The decision in this example would be to get help because the pro score (11) is significantly higher than the con score (7). If this feels right in your gut, you have the answer.

Now it's your turn! Try making a decision using the following chart. It's OK to write in your book.

Decision to be made

Pro	Rating	Con	Rating
Total			

The key to successful problem solving and decision making is taking action. We will talk about this next.

Taking Action

You have looked at a problem or made a difficult decision. Knowing what to do is not enough. It is time to do something, to take action. We suggest that you start by doing one thing at a time.

Goal Setting

Before you can take action, you must decide what you want to do first. You must be realistic and specific when stating your goal. Think of all the things you would like to do. One self-manager wanted to climb 20 steps to her daughter's home so that she could join her family for a holiday meal. Another wanted to overcome anxiety and attend social events. Still another wanted to continue to ride his motorcycle but could no longer lift his 1,000-pound bike when it was laying on the ground.

One of the problems with goals is that they often seem like dreams. They are so far off, big, or difficult that we are overwhelmed and don't even try to accomplish them. We'll tackle this problem next. For now, take a few minutes and write your goals below (add more lines if you need to).

Goals

_____

_____

_____

_____

Put a star (★) next to the goal you would like to work on first.

Don't reject a goal until you have thought about alternatives. Sometimes we reject alternatives without knowing much about them. In the earlier example, our traveler was able to make a list of alternative travel arrangements and then chose the train.

There are many ways to reach any specific goal. For example, our self-manager who wanted to climb 20 steps could start off with a slow walking program, could start to climb a few steps each day, or could look into having the family gathering at a different place. The man who wanted to attend social events could start with going on very short outings, asking a friend to go along to help, using distraction techniques when feeling anxious, or talking to the health care team about therapy or medication. Our motorcycle rider could buy a lighter motorcycle, use a sidecar, put "training wheels" on his bike, buy a three-wheeled motorcycle, or give up riding.

As you can see, there are many options for reaching each goal. The job here is to list the options and then choose one or two to try out.

Sometimes it is hard to think of all the options yourself. If you are having problems, it is time to use a consultant. Share your goal with family, friends, and health professionals. You can call community organizations such as the American Heart Association or the National Multiple Sclerosis Society. You can use the Internet. Don't ask what you should do. Rather, ask for suggestions. It is always good to have a list of options.

A note of caution: many options are never seriously considered because you assume they don't exist or are unworkable. Never make this assumption until you have thoroughly investigated the option. One woman we know had lived in the same town all her life and felt that she knew all about the community resources. When she was having problems with her health insurance, a friend from another city suggested contacting an insurance counselor. However, the woman dismissed this suggestion because she was certain that this service did not exist in her town. It was only when, months later, the friend came to visit and called the Area Agency on Aging (which exists in most counties in the United States) that the woman learned that there were three insurance counseling services nearby. Our motorcycle rider thought that training wheels on a Harley was a crazy idea but investigated. He added 15 years to his riding life using training wheels. In short, never assume anything. Assumptions are major self-management enemies.

Write the list of options for your main goal here. Then put a star (★) next to the two or three options on which you would like to work.

Options

_____

_____

_____

_____

Making Short-Term Plans: Action Planning

Once a decision has been made, we have a pretty good idea of where we are going. However, this goal may be overwhelming. How will I ever move, how will I ever be able to paint again, how will I ever by able to _____ (you fill in the blank)? The secret is to not try to do everything at once. Instead, look at what you can realistically expect to accomplish within *the next week*. We call this an action plan: something that is short-term, is doable, and sets you on the road toward your goal. The action plan should be about something you want to do or accomplish. It is a tool to help you do what you wish. Do not make action plans to please your friends, family, or doctor.

Action plans are probably your most important self-management tool. Most of us can do things to make us healthier but fail to do them. For example, most people with chronic illness can walk—some just across the room, others for half a block. Most can walk several blocks, and some can walk a mile or more. However, few people have a systematic exercise program.

An action plan helps us do the things we know we should do, but we should start with what we *want* to do. Let's go through all the steps for making a realistic action plan.

First, decide what you will do this week. For a step climber, this might be climbing three steps on four consecutive days. The man who wants to continue riding his motorcycle might spend half an hour on two days researching lighter motorcycles and motorcycle training wheels.

Make very sure that your plans are "action-specific"; that is, rather than just deciding "to lose weight" (which is not an action but the result of an action), you will "replace soda with tea."

Next, make a specific plan. Deciding what you want to do is worthless without a plan to do it. The plan should answer all of the following questions:

- Exactly **what** are you going to do? Are you going to walk, how will you eat less, what distraction technique will you practice?

- **How much** will you do? This question is answered with something like time, distance, portions, or repetitions. Will you walk one block, walk for 15 minutes, eat half portions at lunch and dinner, practice relaxation exercises for 15 minutes?

- **When** will you do this? Again, this must be specific: before lunch, in the shower, upon coming home from work. Connecting a new activity with an old habit is a good way to make sure it gets done. Consider what comes right before your action plan that could trigger the new behavior. For example, brushing your teeth reminds you to take your medication. Another trick is to do your new activity before an old favorite activity such as reading the paper or watching a favorite TV program.

- **How often** will you do the activity? This is a bit tricky. We would all like to do things every day, but that is not always possible. It is usually best to decide to do an activity three or four times a week to give yourself "wiggle room" if something comes up. If you do more, so much the better. However, if you are like most people, you will feel less pressure if you can do your activity three or four times a week and still feel successful. (Note that taking medications is an exception. This must be done exactly as directed by your doctor.)

There are some general guidelines for writing your action plan that may help. First, start where you are or start slowly. If you can walk for only one minute, start your walking program by walking one minute once every hour or two, not by trying to walk a block. If you have never done any exercise, start with a few minutes of warm-up. A total of 5 or 10 minutes is enough. If you want to lose weight, set a goal based on your existing eating behaviors, such as having half portions. For example, "losing a pound this week" is not an action plan because it does not involve a specific action; "not eating after dinner for 4 days this week," by contrast, would be a fine action plan.

Second, give yourself some time off. All people have days when they don't feel like doing anything. That is a good reason for saying that you will do something three times a week instead of every day.

Third, once you've made your action plan, ask yourself the following question: "On a scale of 0 to 10, with 0 being totally unsure and 10 being totally certain, how sure am I that I can complete this entire plan?"

If your answer is 7 or above, this is probably a realistic action plan. If your answer is below 7, you should look again at your action plan. Ask yourself why you are unsure. What problems do you foresee? Then see if you can either solve the problems or change your plan to make yourself more confident of success.

Once you have made a plan you are happy with, write it down and post it where you will see it every day. Thinking through an action plan is one thing. Writing it down makes it more likely you will take action. Keep track of how you are doing and the problems you encounter. (A blank action plan form is provided at the end of this chapter. You may wish to make photocopies of it to use weekly.)

Success Improves Health

The benefits of change go beyond the pay-offs of adopting healthier habits. Obviously, you will feel better when you exercise, eat well, keep regular sleeping hours, stop smoking, and take time to relax. But regardless of the behavior that's altered, there's evidence that the feelings of self-confidence and control over your life that come from making any successful change improve your health.

As we age or develop a chronic illness, physical abilities and self-image may decline. For many people, it is discouraging to find that they can't do what they used to do or want to do. By changing and improving one area of your life, whether it is boosting your physical fitness or learning a new skill, you regain a sense of optimism and vitality. By focusing on what you can do rather than what you can't do, you're more likely to lead a more positive and happier life.

Basics of a Successful Action Plan

- It is something *you* want to do.

- It is achievable (something you can expect to be able to accomplish that week).

- It is action-specific.

- It answers the questions *What? How much? When?* and *How often?*

- You are sure that you will complete your entire plan at a level of 7 or higher on a scale from 0 = not at all sure to 10 = absolutely sure.

Carrying Out Your Action Plan

If the action plan is well written and realistically achievable, completing it is generally pretty easy. Ask family or friends to check with you on how you are doing. Having to report your progress is good motivation. Keep track of your daily activities while carrying out your plan. Many good managers have lists of what they want to accomplish. Check things off as they are completed. This will give you guidance on how realistic your planning was and will also be useful in making future plans. Make daily notes, even of the things you don't understand at the time. Later these notes may be useful in establishing a pattern to use for problem solving.

For example, our stair-climbing friend never did her climbing. Each day she had a different problem: not enough time, being tired, the weather being too cold, and so on. When she looked back at her notes, she began to realize that the real problem was her fear of falling with no one around to help her. She then decided to use a cane while climbing stairs and to do it when a friend or neighbor was around.

Checking the Results

At the end of each week, see if you completed your action plan and if you are any nearer to accomplishing your goal. Are you able to walk farther? Have you lost weight? Are you less anxious? Taking stock is important. You may not see progress day by day, but you should see a little progress each week. At the end of each week, check on how well you have fulfilled your action plan. If you are having problems, this is the time to use your problem-solving skills.

Making Midcourse Corrections (Back to Problem Solving)

When you are trying to overcome obstacles, the first plan is not always the most workable plan. If something doesn't work, don't give up. Try something else; modify your short-term plans so that your steps are easier, give yourself more time to accomplish difficult tasks, choose new steps toward your goal, or check with your consultants for advice and assistance. If you are not sure how to go about this, go back and read page 16.

How People Change

Thousands of studies have been done to learn how people change—or why they don't change. Here's what we have learned:

- Most people change by themselves, when they are ready. While physicians, counselors, spouses, and self-help groups coax, persuade, nag, and otherwise try to assist people to change their lifestyle and habits, most people do so without much help from others.

- Change is not an all-or-nothing process. It happens in stages. Most of us think of change as occurring one step at a time: each step is an improvement over the one before it. Although a few people do make changes this way, it is rare. More than 95% of people who successfully quit smoking do so only after a series of setbacks and relapses.

- In most cases, change resembles a spiral more than a straight line, with people reverting to previous stages before proceeding further ("two steps forward, one step back"). So relapses are not failures but setbacks, which are an integral part of change. And dealing with relapse is frequently a helpful way for people to learn how to maintain change. Relapsing provides feedback about what doesn't work.

- Efficient self-change depends on doing the right things at the right time. There's evidence that people who are given strategies inappropriate to their particular stage are less successful in changing than people who receive no assistance at all. For example, making an elaborate written plan of action when you really haven't decided you want to change is a prescription for failure. You're likely to get bored, discouraged, or frustrated before you even start.

- Confidence in your ability to change is the key ingredient for success. Your belief in your own ability to succeed predicts whether you will attempt change in the first place, whether you will persist if you relapse, and whether you will ultimately be successful in making the change.

Rewarding Yourself

The best part of being a good self-manager is the reward that comes from accomplishing your goals and living a fuller and more comfortable life. However, don't wait until your goal is reached; rather, reward yourself frequently for your short-term successes. For example, decide that you won't read the paper until after you exercise. Thus reading the paper becomes your reward. One self-manager buys only one or two pieces of fruit at a time and walks the half-mile to the supermarket every day or two to get more fruit. Another self-manager who stopped smoking used the money he would have spent on cigarettes to have his house professionally cleaned, and there was even enough left over to go to a baseball game with a friend. Rewards don't have to be fancy, expensive, or fattening. There are many healthy pleasures that can add enjoyment to your life.

One last note: not all goals are achievable. Chronic illness may mean having to give up some options. If this is true for you, don't dwell too much on what you can't do. Rather, start working on another goal you would like to accomplish. One self-manager we know who uses a wheelchair talks about the 90% of things he *can* do. He devotes his life to developing this 90% to the fullest.

Tools for Becoming a Self-Manager

Now that you understand the meaning of self-management, you are ready to begin learning to use the tools that will make you a successful one. Most self-management skills are similar for all diseases. Chapters 15 through 18 contain information on some of the more common chronic illnesses. If your illness is not covered, we apologize. If we had included everything, you would not be able to carry this book. We talk about medications and their uses in Chapter 13. The rest of the book is devoted to tools of the trade. These include exercise, nutrition, symptom management, preventing falls, communication, making decisions about the future, finding resources and information about advance directives for health care, and sex and intimacy.

My Action Plan

In writing your action plan, be sure it includes all of the following:

1.   What you are going to do (a specific action)
2.   How much you are going to do (time, distance, portions, repetitions, etc.)
3.   When you are going to do it (time of the day, day of the week)
4.   How often or how many days a week you are going to do it

Example: This week, I will walk (what) around the block (how much) before lunch (when) three times (how many).

This week I will _____ (what)

_____ (how much)

_____ (when)

_____ (how often)

How sure are you? (0 = not at all sure; 10 = absolutely sure) _____

Comments

Monday _____

Tuesday _____

Wednesday _____

Thursday _____

Friday _____

Saturday _____

Sunday _____

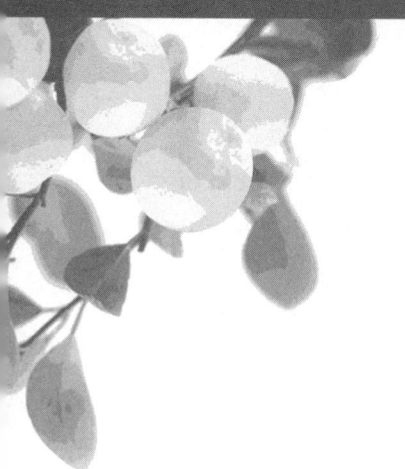

CHAPTER 3

Finding Resources

Aᴍᴀᴊᴏʀ ᴘᴀʀᴛ ᴏꜰ ʙᴇᴄᴏᴍɪɴɢ a self-manager is knowing when you need help and how to find help. When you seek help, you are not a victim of your condition. You are a good self-manager. Start by evaluating your condition—what you can do and what you want to do. You may find that there is a difference between what you can do and what you want to do (or have done). If so, it may be time to get help so that you can do the things that are most important to you.

As we begin to look for help, most of us start by asking family or friends. Sometimes this can be difficult. We are afraid that others will see us as weak. Sometimes our pride gets in the way. The truth is that most people want to be helpful but do not know how. Your job is to tell them what you need. Finding the right words to ask for help is discussed in Chapter 9. Unfortunately, some people either do not have family or close friends or cannot bring themselves to ask. Sometimes family or friends cannot offer all the help that is needed. Thankfully, we have another wonderful resource: our community.

Finding resources can be a little like a treasure hunt. As in a treasure hunt, creative thinking wins the game. Finding what you need may be as simple as looking in the telephone book and making a couple of phone calls or using the Internet. Other times it may take sleuthing. The community resource detective must find clues and follow them. Sometimes this means starting over when a clue leads to a dead end.

The first step is defining the problem and then deciding what you want. For example, suppose you find it difficult to prepare meals because standing for a long time is painful. After some thought, you decide that you want to continue cooking for yourself. You could do this if you could cook while sitting. Your treasure hunt is figuring out how to do this.

You look at kitchen stools and do not think this will work, so you decide that you need to redesign the kitchen. The hunt is on. Where can you find an architect or contractor who has experience in kitchen alterations for people with physical limitations? You need a starting point for your treasure hunt. The phone book has pages of ads and listings for architects and contractors. Some advertisers say they specialize in kitchens. None of the ads mention designing to accommodate physical limitations. So you must call and ask. After calling a few contractors, you come to realize that none are experienced in kitchens for the physically limited. Next you go to the Internet. You find a company that seems to be just what you need, but it is located more than 200 miles away.

Now what? You have a couple of choices. You can contact everyone listed until you find what you need. This could be time-consuming.

And even if you find someone suitable, you would still have to check references.

Who else might have the information you need? Maybe someone who works with people with physical disabilities would know. This opens a long list of possibilities: occupational and physical therapists, medical supply stores, the Center for Independent Living, and voluntary organizations such as the Arthritis Foundation. You decide to ask a friend who is a physical therapist.

He does not have the answer but says, "Gosh, Jack So-and-So just had his kitchen remodeled to accommodate his wheelchair." This is an excellent tip. Jack will almost certainly be able to give you the name of someone who does the kind of work you are seeking. He can also probably give you some ideas about the cost and hassle before you go any further. Unfortunately, though, Jack turns out to be not much help. Now what?

There are people in every community who are natural resources. These "naturals" or "connectors" seem to know everyone and everything about their community. They tend to be folks who have lived a long time in the community and have been closely involved in it. They are also natural problem solvers. The natural is the one that other people turn to for advice. This person always seems to be helpful. The natural could be a friend, a business associate, the mail carrier, your physician, your pet's veterinarian, the checker at the corner grocery, the pharmacist, a bus or taxi driver, the school secretary, a real estate agent, the Chamber of Commerce receptionist, or the librarian. All you need to do is think of this person as an information resource. Sometimes the natural will taste the thrill of the hunt and, like a modern-day Sherlock Holmes, announce that "the game is afoot!" and promptly join you in your search. You ask the postman, and he tells you about a contractor whose wife uses a wheelchair. He knows this because the guy just did a great job on his kitchen. You call the contractor and find everything you need.

Let's review the lessons from this example. The most important steps in finding the resources you need are these:

1. Identify the problem.

2. Identify what you want or need.

3. Look for resources in the phone book and on the Internet.

4. Ask friends, family, and neighbors for ideas.

5. Contact organizations that might deal with similar issues.

6. Identify and ask naturals.

One last note: the best sleuth follows several clues at the same time. This will save you lots of time and shorten the hunt. Watch out, though—once you get good at thinking about community resources creatively, you will become a natural in your own right!

Resources for Resources

When we need to find goods or services, there are certain resources we can call on. One resource often leads to another. The natural is one of those resources, but our community resource "detective's kit" needs a variety of other useful tools.

The phone book and Internet search engines are the most frequently used tools. These are particularly helpful if you are looking for someone to hire. For most searches, this is where to start.

Organizations and Referral Services

Almost all communities have one or more information and referral services. Sometimes these are related to a geographic area such as a city or county. Other times they are specific to an age group, such as the Area Agency on Aging. Sometimes they are specific to a condition such as disability or sickle cell disease. There are several types of agencies that operate these ser-

vices. Search under "United Way Information and Referral," "Senior Information and Referral" (or "Area Agency on Aging" or "Council on Aging"), and "information and referral." If you are using a phone book, be sure to check your county or city government listings. Once you have an information and referral telephone number, your searches will become much easier. These services maintain huge files of referral addresses and telephone numbers for just about any help you might need. Even if they don't have the answer you seek, they will almost always be able to refer you to another agency.

Voluntary agencies such as the American Heart Association and the American Cancer Society are great resources. There are similar organizations in most other countries. These agencies, funded by contributions from individuals and from corporate sponsors, provide up-to-date information about your health problem, as well as support and direct services to people with the illness. They also fund research intended to help people live better with their illness and to someday lead to a cure. For a small fee, you can become a member of one of these organizations, entitling you to receive regular bulletins by mail or e-mail. You do not, however, have to be a member to qualify for their services; they are here to serve you. Many of these organizations have wonderful Web sites. In our new world of cyberspace, you can live in rural North Dakota and get help on the Web from the Arthritis Foundation in Victoria, Australia.

There are other organizations in your community offering information and referral services along with direct services. These include the local chapter of AARP (formerly known as the American Association of Retired Persons), senior centers, community centers, and religious social service agencies. These organizations offer information, classes, recreational opportunities, nutrition programs, legal and tax help, and social programs. There is probably a senior center or community center close to you. Your city government office or local librarian will know where such resources are, and the calendar section of your newspaper will usually have information about programs these organizations offer.

Most religious groups offer information and social services to persons who need it, either directly through the place of worship or through organizations such as the Council of Churches, Catholic Diocese, or Jewish Family Services. To get help from religious organizations, start with the local place of worship, which will help you or refer you to someone who can help you. You usually need not be a member of the congregation or even of the religion to receive help.

Call your local hospital, clinic, or health insurance plan, and ask for the social service department. Your doctor will also be aware of the physical and mental health services available in the health care organizations he or she is affiliated with.

Libraries

Your public library is a particularly good resource if you are looking for information about your chronic condition. Even if you think you are an excellent library detective, it's a good idea to ask the reference librarian to make sure you haven't overlooked something. These people see volumes of material cross their desks constantly and are knowledgeable about the community (they're probably among the ranks of the local naturals). Even if you cannot get to the library, you can call or e-mail. Libraries are no longer just collections of books.

In addition to city or county libraries, there are other, more specialized health libraries. Ask your information and referral service if there is a health library in your community. Such libraries specialize in health-related resources, usually having a computerized database search service available along with the usual print, audiotape, and videotape materials. These libraries are usually maintained by nonprofit organizations and hospitals and will sometimes charge a small fee for use.

Universities and colleges also have libraries open to the public. By law, the regional "government documents" sections of these libraries must be open to the public at no charge. Government publications exist on just about any subject, and the health-related publications are particularly extensive. You can find everything from information on organic gardening to detailed nutritional recipes. The librarians are usually very helpful, and these publications represent "your tax dollars at work."

If you are fortunate enough to have a medical school in your community, you may be able to use its medical library. This, however, is a place to go to for information rather than to look for help with tasks. Naturally, you can expect to find a great deal of information about disease and treatment at a medical library. Unless you have special knowledge about medicine, however, the detailed information you find in a medical library can be confusing and even frightening. Use medical libraries with care.

Books

Books can be useful (indeed, you are reading a book now!). Many disease-related books contain reading and resource lists, either at the ends of chapters or at the back of the book. These lists can be very helpful. We identify some books as resources at the ends of many of the chapters in this book.

Newspapers and Magazines

Your local newspaper, especially if you live in a smaller community, can be an excellent resource. Be sure to look in the calendar of events. Even if you are not interested in a particular featured event, calling the contact telephone number may help you find what you are looking for. Look in other logical places for news stories that might also be of interest, especially the pages around the calendar section or, if you are looking for an exercise program for people with your health problem, for example, in the sports and fitness section.

Sometimes you can find clues in the classified section. Look under "announcements," "health," or any other heading that seems promising. Review the index of classified headings, which is usually printed at the front of the section near the rate information, to see which headings your newspaper uses.

There are a variety of general health magazines that can be useful, as well as some publications focusing on specific conditions such as diabetes or arthritis.

The Internet

Today most people have access to the Internet. Even if you are not an Internet user, you know an Internet user. Even if you do not have a computer, you can use one in your local library or ask a friend for help. The Internet is the fastest-growing source of information today. Information is being added every second of every day. The Internet offers information about health and anything else you can imagine. It also provides several ways in which you can interact with people all over the world. For example, someone who has Gaucher disease, a rare health condition, might find it difficult to find others with the same disease where she or he lives. The Internet can put the person in touch with a whole group of such people; it doesn't matter whether they are across the street or on the other side of the world.

The good thing about the Internet is that anyone can maintain a Web site, a Facebook or other social network page, a blog, or a group. That is also the bad thing about the Internet. There are virtually no controls over who is posting information or whether the information is accurate or even safe. This can mean that although there is a lot of information out there that might be very useful, it also means that you may encounter incorrect or even dangerous information. Therefore, you should never assume that information found on the Internet is entirely trustworthy. Approach information obtained online with skepticism and caution. Ask yourself, Is the author or sponsor of the Web site clearly identified? Is the author or source reputable? Is the information contrary to what everyone else seems to be saying about the subject? Does common sense support the information? What is the purpose of the Web site? Is someone trying to sell you something or win you over to a particular point of view?

One way to start analyzing the purpose of the Web site is to look at the URL (the address, starting with http://). The URL will usually look something like this:

http://patienteducation.stanford.edu/

At the end of the main part of a U.S.–based Web site's URL, you will most commonly see .edu, .org, .gov, or .com. This will give you a clue about the nature of the organization that owns the Web site. A college or university will have .edu, a nonprofit organization will have .org, a governmental agency will have .gov, and a commercial organization will have .com. As a general rule of thumb, .edu, .org, and .gov are fairly trustworthy sites, although a nonprofit organization can be formed to promote just about anything. A Web site with .com is trying to sell you a product or service or is selling advertising space on its site to others trying

to sell you something. This doesn't mean that a commercial Web site can't be a good one. On the contrary, there are many outstanding commercial sites dedicated to providing high-quality, trustworthy information. They are often able to cover the costs of providing this service only by selling advertising or by accepting grants from commercial firms. The URLs for some of our favorite reliable Web sites are listed at the end of this chapter.

The Internet and Social Networking Sites

Social networking sites and blogs are exploding on the Internet. Sites such as Facebook, MySpace, Foursquare, and Blogspot are currently very popular, but everything may change by the time this book is published. These sites enable the average person to communicate easily with others who want to listen (or read). Some sites, such as Facebook, require that users determine who will be allowed to read the thoughts they post on their page. Others, such as Blogspot, are more like personal journals that are open to anyone who finds them on the Internet.

Many such sites have been started by people living with particular health conditions, and the authors are eager to share their experiences. Some have discussion forums associated with them. The information and support offered can be valuable, but be cautious: some sites can be proposing unproven and dangerous ideas.

Discussion Groups on the Internet

Yahoo, Google, and other Web sites offer discussion groups for just about anything you can imagine. Anyone can start a discussion group about any subject. Groups are run by the people who start them. For any one health problem, you will probably find dozens of discussion groups. You can join them and the discussions if you wish, or just "lurk" (read without interacting). For the person with Gaucher disease, for example, a discussion group may allow her to connect to people who share her experiences. This may be her only opportunity to talk with someone else with her rare disease. For someone with bipolar disorder, it may be difficult to talk with someone face-to-face about his problems. To find discussion groups, go to the Google or Yahoo (or other) home page and search for a link to "groups."

Keep in mind that the Internet changes by the second. Our guidelines reflect conditions at the time this book was written. Things may have changed by the time you read this.

Becoming an effective resource detective is one of the jobs of a good self-manager. We hope that this chapter has given you some ideas about the process of finding resources in your community. Knowing how to search for resources will serve you better than being handed a list of resource agencies. If you find resources that you think we should add to future editions, kindly send them to self-management@stanford.edu.

Resources

- ☐ Association of Cancer Online Resources (ACOR): http://www.acor.org/
- ☐ CarePages: http://www.carepages.com/
- ☐ CaringBridge: http://www.caringbridge.org/
- ☐ Center for Advancing Health: http://www.cfah.org/
- ☐ Centers for Disease Control and Prevention (CDC): http://www.cdc.gov/
- ☐ HealthCentral: http://www.healthcentral.com/
- ☐ Mayo Clinic: http://www.mayoclinic.org/
- ☐ Memorial Sloan-Kettering Cancer Center: http://www.mskcc.org/
- ☐ National Cancer Institute: http://www.cancer.gov/
- ☐ National Institutes of Health (NIH): http://www.nih.gov/
- ☐ National Institutes of Health Office of Rare Diseases Research: http://www.rarediseases.info.nih.gov/
- ☐ National Library of Medicine: http://www.nlm.nih.gov/medlineplus/
- ☐ National Library of Medicine tutorial for evaluating Internet health information: http://www.www.nlm.nih.gov/medlineplus/evaluatinghealthinformation.html
- ☐ PatientsLikeMe: http://www.patientslikeme.com/
- ☐ Psych Central: http://www.psychcentral.com/
- ☐ QuackWatch: Your Guide to Quackery, Health Fraud, and Intelligent Decisions: http://www.quackwatch.org/
- ☐ Ratings of Health Web Sites: http://www.healthratings.org/
- ☐ U.S. Department of Health and Human Services (HHS): http://www.healthfinder.gov/
- ☐ WebMD: http://www.webmd.com/

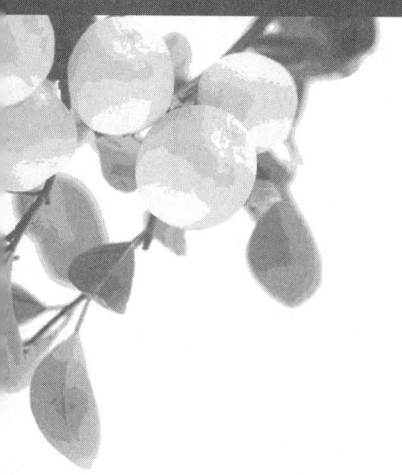

CHAPTER 4

Understanding and Managing Common Symptoms

CHRONIC ILLNESSES COME WITH SYMPTOMS. These are signals from the body that something unusual is happening. These symptoms may include fatigue, stress, shortness of breath, pain, itching, anger, depression, and sleep problems. Sometimes they cannot be seen by others, some are very difficult to describe, and we may not know when they will occur. Although some symptoms are common, the times when they occur and the ways in which they affect us are very personal. What's more, these symptoms can interact, which may worsen existing symptoms or even lead to new symptoms or problems.

Regardless of the causes of these symptoms, the ways in which we can manage them are often similar. These are our self-management tools. This chapter discusses several common symptoms, their causes, and some of the tools you can use to manage them. Additional cognitive tools—ways you can use your mind to help deal with many of these symptoms—are discussed in Chapter 5.

Dealing with Common Symptoms

Learning to manage symptoms is very similar to problem solving, discussed in Chapter 2. First, it is important to identify the symptom you are experiencing. Next, determine why you might be having the symptom now. This may sound like a simple process, but it is not always easy.

You can experience many different symptoms, and each symptom can have various causes and interact with other symptoms. The ways in which these symptoms affect one's life are also different. All of these factors can become very tangled, like the frayed threads of a cloth. To manage these symptoms, it is often helpful to figure out how to untangle the threads. One way to do this is to keep a daily diary or journal. This can be as simple as writing your symptoms on a calendar along with some notes about what you were doing before the symptom started or worsened, as shown in the example below. After a week or two, you may see a pattern. For example, you go out to dinner on Saturday evening and wake up in the night with stomach pain. Once you realize that when you go out, you overeat, you know to adjust what you order in the future. Or every time you go dancing, your feet hurt, but this does not occur when you walk. Could the shoes you wear account for the difference? Seeing patterns is for many people the first step in symptom self-management.

As you read through this chapter, you will note that many symptoms have the same causes. Also, one symptom may actually cause other symptoms. For example, pain may change the way you walk. This new way of walking may change your balance and cause a new pain or cause you to fall. As you gain a better understanding of the possible

Sample Calendar Journal

Mon.	Tue.	Wed.	Thur.	Fri.	Sat.	Sun.
Grocery shop	Babysit grandkids Pain P.M.	Tired	Water exercise Feel great	Little stiff Clean house	Dinner out Poor sleep	Tired

Mon.	Tue.	Wed.	Thur.	Fri.	Sat.	Sun.
Grocery shop	Babysit grandkids Pain P.M.	Tired	Water exercise Feel great	Clean house	Feel great	Feel great Dinner out Poor sleep

Using Different Symptom-Management Tools

■ **Choose a tool to try.** Be sure to give this method a fair trial. We recommend that you practice it for at least 2 weeks before deciding whether or not the tool is going to be helpful.

■ **Try some other tools, giving each a trial period.** It is important to try more than one tool because some tools may be more useful for certain symptoms or you may find that you simply prefer some techniques over others.

■ **Think about how and when you will use each tool.** For example, some of these tools may require more lifestyle changes than others. The best symptom managers learn to use a variety of techniques. These depend on your condition and what you want and need to do each day.

■ **Place some cues in your environment to remind you to practice these techniques.** Both practice and consistency are important for mastering new skills. For example, place stickers or notes where you'll see them, such as on your mirror, near the phone, in your office, on your computer, or on the car's dashboard. Change the notes from time to time so that you'll continue to notice them.

■ **Try linking the practice of each new tool with some other established daily behavior or activity.** For example, practice relaxation as part of your cooldown from exercise. Also, ask a friend or family member to remind you to practice each day; he or she may even wish to participate.

causes of your symptoms, you will be able to identify better ways to deal with them. You may also find ways to prevent or lessen certain symptoms.

Let's look at what you can do to lessen some of the more common symptoms experienced by people with particular chronic conditions.

Common Symptoms

These common symptoms are discussed in this chapter on the pages shown below.

■ Fatigue (p. 38)

■ Pain or Physical Discomfort (p. 39)

■ Shortness of Breath (p. 43)

■ Sleep Problems (p.46)

■ Depression (p. 50)

■ Anger (p. 56)

■ Stress (p. 58)

■ Memory Problems (p. 62)

■ Itching (p. 62)

■ Urinary Incontinence (p. 64)

Fatigue

A chronic condition can drain your energy. Fatigue is a very real problem for many people. It is not, as some might say, "all in the mind." Fatigue can keep you from doing things you'd like to do. It is often misunderstood by people who do not have a chronic illness. After all, others cannot usually see your fatigue. Unfortunately, spouses, family members, and friends sometimes do not understand the unpredictable way in which the fatigue associated with your condition can affect you. They may think that you are just not interested in certain activities or that you want to be alone. Sometimes you may not even know why you feel this way.

To be able to manage fatigue, it is important to understand that your fatigue may be related to several factors, such as these:

- **The disease itself.** No matter what illness or illnesses you have, whatever you do demands more energy. When a chronic illness is present, the body uses energy less efficiently. This is because the energy that could be going to everyday activities is being used to help heal the body. Your body may release chemical signals to conserve energy and make you rest more. Some chronic conditions are also associated with anemia (low blood hemoglobin), which can contribute to fatigue.

- **Inactivity.** Muscles that are not used regularly become deconditioned and less efficient at doing what they are supposed to do. The heart, which is made of muscle tissue, can also become deconditioned. When this happens, the ability of the heart to

pump blood, which carries necessary nutrients and oxygen to other parts of the body, is decreased. When muscles do not receive these necessary nutrients and oxygen, they cannot function properly. Deconditioned muscles tire more easily than muscles in good condition.

- **Poor nutrition.** Food is our basic source of energy. If the fuel we take in is of inferior quality, is not consumed in the appropriate quantities, or is improperly digested, fatigue can result. Rarely are vitamin deficiencies a cause of fatigue. For some people, weight results in fatigue. Extra weight causes an increase in the amount of energy needed to perform daily activities. Being underweight can also cause problems associated with fatigue. This is especially true for individuals with chronic obstructive pulmonary disease (COPD). Many people with COPD experience weight loss because of a change in their eating habits and therefore have increased fatigue.

- **Not enough rest.** For a variety of reasons, there are times when we do not get enough sleep or do not sleep well. This can also result in fatigue. We will discuss how to manage sleep problems in more detail later in this chapter.

- **Emotions.** Stress, anxiety, fear, and depression can also cause fatigue. Most people are aware of the connection between stress and feeling tired, but fewer are aware of the fact that fatigue is a major symptom of depression.

■ **Medications.** Some medications can cause fatigue. If you think your fatigue is medication-related, talk to your doctor. Sometimes medications or the dose can be changed.

If fatigue is a problem, start by trying to determine the cause. Again, a journal may be helpful. And start with the easiest things that are within your control to improve. Are you eating healthy foods? Are you exercising? Are you getting enough good-quality sleep? Are you effectively managing stress? If you answer no to any of these questions, you may be well on your way to finding one or more of the reasons for your fatigue.

The important thing to remember about your fatigue is that *it may be caused by things other than your illness.* Therefore, to combat and prevent fatigue, you must address the possible causes of your fatigue. This may mean trying a variety of self-management tools.

If your fatigue is the result of not eating well, such as eating too much junk food or drinking too much alcohol, then the solution is to eat better-quality foods in the proper quantities or to drink less alcohol. For others, the problem may be a decreased interest in food, leading to a lack of calories and subsequent weight loss. Chapter 11 discusses some of the problems associated with eating and provides tips for healthy eating.

People often say they can't exercise because they feel fatigued. Believing this creates a vicious cycle: people are fatigued because of a lack of exercise, and they don't exercise because of the fatigue. Believe it or not, motivating yourself to do a little exercise might be the answer. You don't have to run a marathon. The important thing is to get outdoors and take a short walk. If this is not possible, walk around your house or try some gentle chair exercises. See Chapter 6 for more information on getting started on an exercise program.

If emotions are causing your fatigue, rest will probably not help. In fact, it may make you feel worse, especially if your fatigue is a sign of depression. We will talk about how to deal with depression a little later in this chapter. If you feel that your fatigue may be related to stress, read the section on managing stress on pages 60–61.

Pain or Physical Discomfort

Pain or physical discomfort is a problem shared by many people with chronic illness. As with most symptoms of chronic illness, pain or discomfort can have many causes. The following are some of the most common causes.

■ **The disease itself.** Pain can come from inflammation, damage in or around joints and tissues, insufficient blood supply to muscles or organs, or irritated nerves, to name just a few sources.

■ **Tense muscles.** When something hurts, the muscles in that area become tense. This is your body's natural reaction to pain—to try to protect the damaged area. Stress can also cause you to tense your muscles. Tense muscles can cause soreness or pain.

■ **Muscle deconditioning.** With chronic disease, it is common to become less active, leading to a weakening of the muscles, or muscle deconditioning. When a muscle is weak, it tends to complain anytime it is used. This is why even the slightest activity can sometimes lead to pain and stiffness.

- **Lack of sleep or poor-quality sleep.** Pain often interferes with the ability to get either enough sleep or good-quality sleep. But poor sleep can also make pain worse and lessen your ability to cope with it.

- **Stress, anxiety, and emotions such as depression, anger, fear, and frustration.** These are all normal responses to living with a chronic condition, and they can affect your pain or discomfort. When we are stressed, angry, afraid, or depressed, everything, including the pain, seems worse.

- **Medications.** The medicine you are taking can sometimes cause abdominal or other discomfort, pain, weakness, or changes in your thinking. If you suspect that medications are the cause, talk with your doctor.

Controlling the "Pain Gates"

Research suggests that we are not helpless in the face of pain. The brain can regulate the flow of pain messages by sending electrical and chemical signals that open and close "pain gates" along nerve pathways.

For example, the brain can release powerful opiate-like chemicals—such as endorphins—that can effectively block pain. When people are very seriously injured, they sometimes experience little pain while they are focused on survival. How you focus your attention, your mood, and the way you view your situation can open or close the pain gates. The techniques in Chapter 5 can be helpful.

A Word About Chronic Pain

Chronic pain is pain that extends over months or years and is often difficult to explain. Most experts now believe that almost all unexplained chronic pain is caused by some type of physical problem: damaged or inflamed nerves, blood vessels, muscles, or other tissues. These underlying physical problems simply can't be pinpointed. It's not "all in your head."

Your day-to-day pain level is based on how your mind and body respond to pain. For example, the body quickly attempts to limit the movement of the damaged area. This causes muscle tension, which can cause more pain. Chronic pain often leads to inactivity. Muscles often become weakened and may then hurt with the slightest use.

Feelings of anxiety, anger, frustration, and loss of control also amplify the experience of pain. This doesn't mean that the pain is not real; it just means that emotions can make a painful situation worse.

Here are four examples of ways in which the mind and body interact:

- **Inactivity.** Because of the pain, you tend to avoid physical activity, which in turn causes you to lose strength and flexibility. The weaker and more out of condition you become, the more frustrated and depressed you feel. These negative emotions can open the pain gates and cause pain levels to rise.

- **Overdoing.** You may be determined to prove that you can still be active, so you overexert. This increases the pain and leads to more inactivity, more depression, and more pain.

Keep a Pain Diary

To get a clear understanding of how your moods, activities, and conditions affect your pain, keep a pain diary. Begin by recording your activities and pain levels 3 times a day, at regular intervals.

1. Record the date and time.
2. Describe the situation or activity (watching TV, doing housework, arguing, and so on).
3. Rate the physical sensation of pain on a scale from 0 (no pain) to 10 (worst pain).
4. Describe the pain sensation (for example, "deep aching pain in left lower back").
5. Rate the emotional distress of pain on a scale from 0 (no distress) to 10 (terribly distressed).
6. Describe the type of emotional distress (for example, "felt very angry" or "needed to cry").
7. Describe what you did, if anything, to alleviate the discomfort (took medication, had a massage, did a relaxation exercise, took a walk, and so on) and its effect.

Look for patterns. For example, is the pain worse after sitting for a long time? Is it less when you are engaged in a favorite hobby?

How much you notice pain may vary according to your mood, fatigue, and muscle tension. It's important to distinguish between physical pain sensations (physical stabbing, burning, and aching sensations) and emotional pain distress (the accompanying anger, anxiety, frustration, or sadness). This is useful because even if your physical pain cannot be reduced, you may feel better about the pain and experience less distress, anxiety, helplessness, and despair.

■ **Misunderstanding.** Your friends, family, boss, and coworkers may not understand that you are suffering and may dismiss your pain as "not real." This evokes more anger or depression.

■ **Overprotection.** Friends, family, and coworkers coddle you and make excuses for you. This can lead you to feel and act more dependent and disabled.

Fortunately, this downward spiral of mind-body interaction can be interrupted. Being told you have to learn to live with pain doesn't have to be the end of the road. It can be a new beginning. You can learn techniques such as the following:

■ To redirect your attention to control pain

■ To challenge negative thoughts that support pain

■ To cultivate more positive emotions

■ To slowly increase your activity and recondition yourself

Tools for Managing Pain

There are many tools for managing pain. Just as one cannot build a house with one tool, one often needs several tools to manage pain.

Exercise

Exercise and physical activity can be excellent pain relievers. The benefits of exercise as well as tips for starting an exercise program are discussed in Chapters 6 through 8. If you are not able to do the things you want and need to do because of physical limitations, a physical therapist may be helpful.

Mind-made medicine

You can also use your mind to manage pain through relaxation, imagery, visualization, and distraction (see Chapter 5). Positive thinking is another powerful way to challenge pain. Learn how to monitor and challenge negative thinking or self-talk. If you find yourself waking up in pain and saying, "I'm going to be miserable all day; I won't get anything done," tell yourself instead, "I've got some pain this morning, so I'll start with some relaxation and stretching exercises. Then I'll do some of the less demanding things I want to get done today." You will find more about positive thinking in Chapter 5.

Ice, heat, and massage

For pain in a local area such as the back or knee, the application of heat, cold, and massage have all been found to be helpful. These three tools work by stimulating the skin and other tissues surrounding the painful area, which increases the blood flow to these areas or blocks transmission of pain in nerve fibers.

Apply heat by using a heating pad or by taking a warm bath or shower (with the water flow directed at the painful area). You can make a substitute heating pad by placing rice or dry beans in a sock, knotting the top of the sock, and heating it in a microwave oven for 3 to 4 minutes. Before use, be sure to test the heat so as not to burn yourself. Do not use popcorn! Some people, however, prefer cold for soothing pain,

especially if there is inflammation. A bag of frozen peas or corn makes an inexpensive, reusable cold pack. Whether using heat or cold, place a towel between the source and skin. Also, limit the application to 15 or 20 minutes at a time (longer can burn or freeze the skin).

Massage is one of the oldest forms of pain management. Hippocrates (c. 460–380 B.C.) said, "Physicians must be experienced in many things, but assuredly also in the rubbing that can bind a joint that is loose and loosen a joint that is too hard." Self-massage is a simple procedure that can be performed with little practice or preparation. It stimulates the skin, underlying tissues, and muscles by rubbing with a little applied pressure. Some people like to use a mentholated cream with self-massage because it gives a cooling effect.

Massage, while relatively simple, is not appropriate for all cases of pain. Do not use self-massage for a "hot joint" (one that is red, swollen, and hot to the touch) or an infected area or if you are suffering from phlebitis, thrombophlebitis, or skin eruptions.

Medications

Acute pain usually responds to painkilling drugs, from mild over-the-counter analgesics for headaches to powerful narcotic medications for postoperative and cancer pain. Some medications can open up blood vessels in the heart or muscles that can relieve pain. Some types of chronic pain and arthritis respond well to anti-inflammatory medications. Surprisingly, some medications originally used to treat depression have been found to relieve pain in lower doses without problems of addiction. Narcotic medications are rarely suitable for chronic pain, as they can become less effective over time and require increasing doses. They can also interfere with breathing, balance, and sleep and cause disturbances in mood and the ability to think clearly. Sometimes injections of a local anesthetic or a surgical procedure can block pain signals from a painful area. This provides temporary or sometimes lasting relief from chronic pain.

Two final notes

■ If you have pain medication in the house, keep it in a place that will not be accessible to young people or visitors. The most common source of prescription drugs abused today in schools is the family medicine cabinet.

■ If you or someone you care for is nearing the end of life (estimated to have six months or less to live) and pain is a problem, consider asking for palliative or hospice care. Hospice units are staffed by special teams of health professionals who are experts in relieving end-of-life pain while allowing the patient to remain alert. At this point in life, addiction is not a concern; comfort is.

If pain continues to be a major influence in your life, discuss with your doctor your options, including referral to a pain management clinic.

Shortness of Breath

Shortness of breath, like so many other symptoms, can have several causes, all of which prevent your body from getting the oxygen it needs. (Before reading further in this section, you may wish to turn to Chapter 15, which discusses normal lung functioning as well as changes that take place in the lungs with chronic lung disease. Chapter 16 talks about heart disease, which can also cause shortness of breath.)

Excess weight can cause shortness of breath because added weight increases the amount of energy you use and therefore the quantity of oxygen you need. Weight also increases the workload for the heart. Thus if excess weight is coupled with chronic lung or heart disease, there is added difficulty in supplying the body with the oxygen it needs.

Deconditioning of muscles can also lead to shortness of breath. This deconditioning can affect the breathing muscles as well as other muscles in your body. When muscles become deconditioned, they are less efficient at doing what they are supposed to do. They require more energy (and oxygen) to perform activities. In the case of deconditioned breathing muscles, the problem is complicated. If the breathing muscles are not strong, it becomes harder to cough and clear mucus from the lungs. When there is mucus in the lungs, there is less space for fresh air.

Just as there are many causes of shortness of breath, there are many things you can do to manage this problem.

When you feel short of breath, don't stop what you are doing or hurry up to finish, but slow down. If shortness of breath continues, stop for a few minutes. If you are still short of breath, take medication if prescribed by your provider.

Shortness of breath can be frightening, and this fear can cause two additional problems. First, when you are afraid, you release hormones such as epinephrine. This causes more shortness of breath. Second, you may stop activity for fear that this will hurt you. If this happens, you will never build up the endurance necessary to help your breathing. The basic rule is to take things slowly and in steps.

Increase your activity gradually, generally by not more than 25% each week. Thus, if you are now able to garden comfortably for 20 minutes, next week increase it by a maximum of 5 minutes. Once you can garden comfortably for 25 minutes, you can again add a few more minutes.

Don't smoke, and—equally important—avoid smokers. This may sometimes be difficult because smoking friends may not realize how they are complicating your life. Your job is to tell them. Explain that their smoke is causing breathing problems for you and that you would appreciate it if they would not smoke when you are around. Also, make your house and especially your car "no smoking" zones. Ask people to smoke outside.

If mucus and secretions are a problem, drink plenty of fluids (unless your doctor has told you to limit what you drink). This will help thin the mucus and make it easier to cough up. Using a humidifier may also be helpful.

Use your medications and oxygen as prescribed. We often hear that drugs are harmful and should not be used. In many cases this is correct. However, when you have a chronic disease, drugs are often very helpful, even life savers. Don't skimp, cut down, or go without. Likewise, more is not better, so don't take more than the prescribed amount. If adjustments need to be made, let your health care provider make that decision.

Breathing Self-Management Tools

Here we'll discuss several tools that can help with better breathing; you will find more tools described in Chapter 15.

Diaphragmatic breathing ("belly breathing")

Diaphragmatic breathing is also called belly breathing because when you do it properly, the diaphragm descends into the abdomen. One of the problems that cause shortness of breath, especially for people with emphysema, chronic bronchitis, or asthma, is deconditioning of the diaphragm and chest breathing muscles. When deconditioning occurs, the lungs are not able to function properly. That is, they do not fill well, nor do they get rid of old air.

Most of us use mainly our upper lungs and chest for breathing. Because diaphragmatic or belly breathing goes deeper, it requires a little practice to learn to fully expand the lungs. This deep breathing strengthens the breathing muscles and makes them more efficient, so breathing is easier. These are the steps for diaphragmatic breathing:

1. Lie on your back with pillows under your head and knees.

2. Place one hand on your stomach (at the base of your breastbone) and the other hand on your upper chest.

3. Breathe in slowly through your nose, allowing your stomach to expand outward. Imagine that your lungs are filling

with fresh air. The hand on your stomach should move upward, and the hand on your chest should not move or should move only slightly.

4. Breathe out slowly, through pursed lips. At the same time, use your hand to gently push inward and upward on your abdomen.

5. Practice this technique for 10 to 15 minutes, three or four times a day, until it becomes automatic. If you begin to feel a little dizzy, rest or breathe out more slowly.

You can also practice diaphragmatic breathing while sitting in a chair:

1. Relax your shoulders, arms, hands, and chest. Do not grip the arms of the chair or your knees.

2. Put one hand on your abdomen and the other on your chest.

3. Breathe in through your nose, filling the area around your waist with air. Your chest hand should remain still and the hand on your abdomen should move.

4. Breathe out without force or effort.

Once you are comfortable with this technique, you can practice it almost anytime, while lying down, sitting, standing, or walking. Diaphragmatic breathing can help strengthen and improve the coordination and efficiency of the breathing muscles, as well as decrease the amount of energy needed to breathe. In addition, it can be used with any of the relaxation techniques that use the power of your mind to manage your symptoms (described in Chapter 5).

Pursed-lip breathing

A second technique, pursed-lip breathing, usually happens naturally for people who have problems emptying their lungs. It can also be used if you are short of breath or breathless.

1. Breathe in, and then purse your lips as if to blow across a flute or into a whistle.

2. Using diaphragmatic breathing, breathe out through pursed lips without any force.

3. Remember to relax the upper chest, shoulders, arms, and hands while breathing out. Check for tension. Breathing out should take longer than breathing in.

By mastering this technique while doing other activities, you will be better able to manage your shortness of breath.

The next two techniques may be helpful for removing secretions (mucus, phlegm).

Huffing

This technique combines one or two forced huffs (puffs of breath) with diaphragmatic breathing. It is useful for removing secretions from small airways.

1. Take in a breath as you would for diaphragmatic breathing.

2. Hold your breath for a moment.

3. Huff—keep your mouth open while squeezing your chest and abdominal muscles to force out the air (this is a little like panting).

4. If possible, do another huff before taking in another breath.

5. Take two or three diaphragmatic breaths.

6. Huff once or twice.

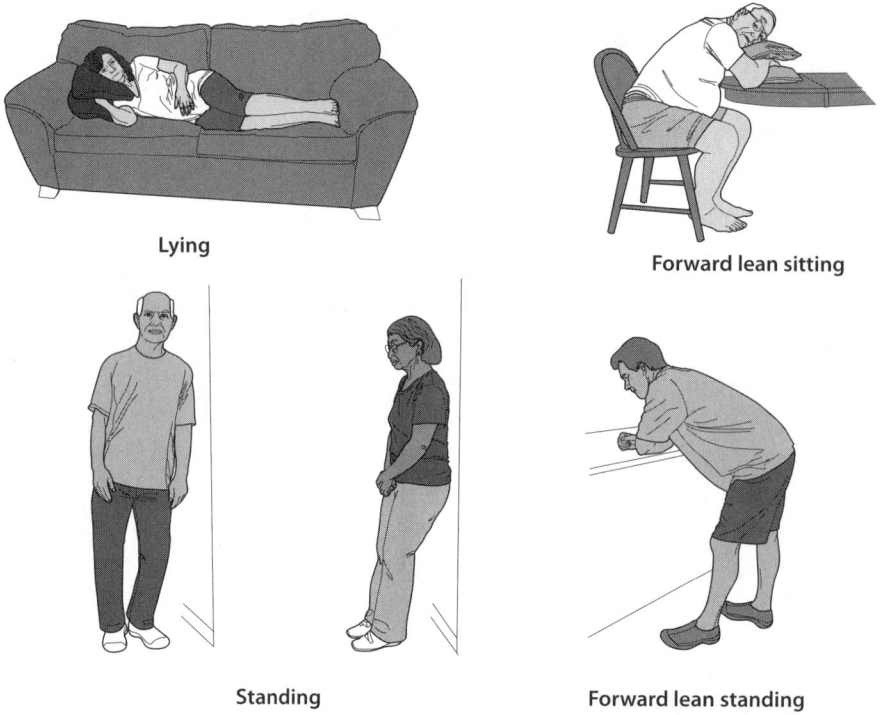

Lying

Forward lean sitting

Standing

Forward lean standing

Positions That Will Help If You Are Breathless or Short of Breath

Controlled cough

This helps remove secretions (phlegm) from larger airways.

1. Take in a full, slow diaphragmatic breath.
2. Keep shoulders and hands relaxed.
3. Hold the breath for a moment.
4. Cough (tighten the abdominal muscles to force the air out).

You can find more about controlled coughing in Chapter 15.

Note: If you have a bout of uncontrolled coughing, this may help:

- Avoid very dry air or steam.
- Swallow as soon as the bout starts.
- Sip water.
- Suck on lozenges or hard candy.
- Try diaphragmatic breathing, being sure to breathe in through your nose.

Sleep Problems

Sleep is a time during which the body can concentrate on healing. Little energy is required to maintain body functioning when we sleep. When we do not get enough sleep, we can experience a variety of other symptoms, such as fatigue, inability to concentrate, irritability, increased pain, and weight gain. Of course, this does not mean that all these symptoms are always caused by a lack of sleep. Remember, the symptoms associated with chronic disease can have many causes. Nevertheless, improving the quality of your sleep can help you manage many of these symptoms, regardless of the cause.

How Much Sleep Do You Need?

The amount of sleep needed varies from person to person. Most people do best with 7½ hours. Some feel refreshed with just 6, but others need 8 to 10 to function well. If you are alert, feel rested, and function well during the day, chances are you're getting enough sleep.

Sleep is a basic human need, like food and water. Getting less sleep one night is not a big problem. But if you get less sleep than you require night after night, your quality of life and mood may suffer.

Getting a Good Night's Sleep

The self-management techniques we offer here are clinically proven, with a 75% to 80% success rate. They are not "quick fixes" like sleep medications, but they'll give you more effective (and safer) results in the long run. Allow yourself at least 2 to 4 weeks to see some positive results and 10 to 12 weeks for long-term improvement.

Things to do before you get into bed

- **Get a comfortable bed** that allows for ease of movement and good body support. This usually means a good-quality, firm mattress that supports the spine and does not allow the body to stay in the middle of the bed. A bed board, made of ½- to ¾-inch (1 to 2 cm) plywood, can be placed between the mattress and the box spring to increase the firmness. Heated waterbeds, airbeds, or foam mattresses are helpful for some people with chronic pain because they support

weight evenly by conforming to the body's shape. If you are interested, try one out at a friend's home or a hotel for a few nights to decide if it is right for you. An electric blanket or mattress pad, set on low heat, or a wool mattress pad are also effective at providing heat while you sleep, especially on cool or damp nights. If you decide to use electric bedding, be sure to follow the instructions carefully to prevent getting burned.

- **Warm your hands and feet** with gloves or socks. For painful knees, it often helps to cut the toes off warm stockings and use the remainders as sleeves over the knees.

- **Find a comfortable sleeping position.** The best position depends on you and your condition. Sometimes the use of small pillows placed in the right places can relieve pain and discomfort. Experiment with different positions and the use of pillows. Also check with your health care provider for specific recommendations given your condition.

- **Elevate the head of the bed** 4 to 6 inches on wooden blocks to make breathing easier. This is especially helpful if you have heartburn or gastric reflux.

- **Keep the room at a comfortable temperature.** This can be either warm or cool. Each of us is different.

- **Use a vaporizer** if you live where the air is dry. Warm, moist air often makes breathing and sleeping easier.

- **Make your bedroom safe and comfortable.** Keep a lamp and telephone by your bed, within easy reach. If you use a cane, keep it by the bed where you will not trip over it.

This way you can use it when you get up during the night.

- **Keep eyeglasses by the bed** when you go to sleep. This way, if you need to get up in the middle of the night, you can easily put on your glasses and see where you are going!

Things to avoid before bedtime

- **Avoid eating.** You may feel sleepy after eating a big meal, but that is not an appropriate way to help you fall asleep and get a good night's sleep. Sleep is supposed to allow your body time to rest and recover, and when it is busy digesting food, this takes valuable time and attention away from the healing process. If you find that going to sleep feeling hungry keeps you awake, try drinking a glass of warm milk at bedtime.

- **Avoid alcohol.** You may think that that alcohol helps you sleep better because it makes you feel relaxed and sleepy, but in fact, alcohol disrupts your sleep cycle. Alcohol before bedtime can lead to shallow sleep and frequent awakenings throughout the night.

- **Avoid caffeine late in the day.** Caffeine is a stimulant, and it can keep you awake. Coffee, tea, colas and other sodas, and chocolate all contain caffeine, so go easy on them as evening approaches.

- **Avoid smoking to help you sleep.** Aside from the fact that smoking itself can cause complications and a worsening of your chronic disease, falling asleep with a lit cigarette can be a fire hazard. Furthermore, the nicotine contained in cigarettes is a stimulant.

- **Avoid diet pills.** Diet pills often contain stimulants, which may interfere with falling asleep and staying asleep.

- **Avoid sleeping pills.** Although the name "sleeping pills" sounds like the perfect solution for sleep problems, these remedies tend to become less effective over time. Also, many sleeping pills have a rebound effect—that is, if you stop taking them, it is more difficult to get to sleep. Thus, as they become less effective, you can have even more problems than you had when you first started taking the pills. All in all, it is best to use other approaches and to avoid using sleeping pills.

- **Avoid using a computer or watching TV** for about an hour before you go to bed. The light from computer and TV screens can disrupt your natural sleep rhythms.

- **Avoid diuretics (water pills) before bedtime.** You may want to take them in the morning so that your sleep is not interrupted by frequent trips to the bathroom. Unless your doctor has recommended otherwise, don't reduce the overall amount of fluids you drink, as these are important for your health. However, you may want to limit the amount you drink right before you go to bed.

How to develop a routine

- **Maintain a regular rest and sleep schedule.** Try to go to bed at the same time every night and get up at the same time every morning. If you wish to take a brief nap, take one in the afternoon, but do not take a nap after dinner. Stay awake until you are ready to go to bed.

- **Reset your sleep clock when necessary.** If your sleep schedule gets off track (for example, you go to bed at 4:00 A.M. and sleep until noon), you'll have to reset your internal sleep clock. To do so, try going to bed an hour earlier or later each day until you reach the hour you want to go to sleep. This may sound strange, but it seems to be the best way to reset your sleep clock.

- **Exercise at regular times each day.** Not only will the exercise help you obtain better-quality sleep, but it will also help set a regular pattern for your day. However, avoid exercising immediately before bedtime.

- **Get out in the sun every morning,** even if it is only for 15 or 20 minutes. This helps regularize your body clock and rhythms.

- **Do the same things every night before going to bed.** This can be anything from listening to the news to reading a chapter of a book to taking a warm bath. By developing and sticking to a "get ready for bed" routine, you will be telling your body that it's time to start winding down and relax.

- **Use your bedroom only for sleeping and sex.** If you find that you get into bed and you can't fall asleep, get out of bed and go into another room until you begin to feel sleepy again. Keep the lighting there low.

What to do when you can't get back to sleep

Many people can get to sleep without a problem but then wake up with the "early morning worries" and can't turn off their minds. Then they get more worried because they cannot go back to sleep once they have awakened. Keeping your mind occupied with pleasurable or interesting thoughts will ward off the worries and help you get back to sleep. For example, try a distraction technique such as quieting your mind by counting backward from 100 by threes or by naming a flower for every letter of the alphabet. The relaxation techniques described in Chapter 5 may also be helpful. If after a while you really can't sleep, get up and do something—read a book, wash your hair, play a game of solitaire (not on the computer). After 15 or 20 minutes, go back to bed.

It can also help to set a "worry time." Does a racing mind keep you awake? If it does, designate a "worry time" well before bedtime, during which you write down your problems and concerns, and then make a to-do list to get them off your mind. Then you can relax and sleep well at night, knowing that you can worry again during tomorrow's worry time.

Don't worry about not getting enough sleep. If your body needs sleep, you will sleep. Also, remember that people tend to need less sleep as they get older.

Sleep Apnea and Snoring

If you fall asleep "as soon as your head hits the pillow" or fall asleep regularly in front of the TV and are tired when you wake up in the morning, even after a full night's sleep, you may have a sleep disorder. People who have the most common sleep disorder, obstructive sleep apnea, often do not know it. When they are asked about their sleep, they respond, "I sleep just fine." Sometimes the only clue is that others complain about their loud snoring. Sleep specialists believe that obstructive sleep apnea is very common and alarmingly underdiagnosed.

With sleep apnea, the soft tissue in the throat or nose relaxes during sleep and blocks the airway, requiring extreme effort to breathe. The person struggles against the blockage for up to a minute, then wakes just long enough to gasp air, and falls back to sleep to start the cycle all over again. The person is rarely aware that he or she has awakened dozens of times during the night and does not get the deep sleep needed to restore the body's energy and help with the healing process. This, in turn, leads to more symptoms such as fatigue and pain.

Sleep apnea can be a serious or even life-threatening medical problem. It has been linked to heart disease and stroke and is thought to be the cause of death for many people who die in their sleep after a heart attack. Sleep experts suggest that people who are tired all the time in spite of a full night's sleep or who find that they need more sleep now than when they were younger should be evaluated for sleep apnea or other sleep disorders, especially if they (or their spouses) report snoring. You can find more about sleep apnea in Chapter 15.

Getting Professional Help

The majority of sleep problems can be solved with the techniques just mentioned, but there are times when you need professional assistance. When should you get help?

- If your insomnia persists for 6 months or is seriously affecting your daytime functioning (your job or your social relationships), despite faithfully following the self-help program described here

- If you have great difficulty staying awake during the day, especially if your daytime sleepiness causes or comes close to causing an accident

- If your sleep is disturbed by breathing difficulties, including loud snoring with long pauses, chest pain, heartburn, leg twitching, excessive pain, or other physical conditions

- If your difficulty sleeping is accompanied by depression, problems with alcohol, sleeping medications, or addictive drugs

Don't put off asking for help. Most sleep problems can be solved. Once they're gone, you'll enjoy a better night's sleep and better health.

Depression

Most people with a chronic illness sometimes feel depressed. As with pain, there are different degrees of depression. These can range from being occasionally sad or blue to serious clinical depression. Sometimes we do not know we are depressed. More often we may not want to admit it. How you handle depression makes the difference.

Depression and Bad Moods

Feeling sad sometimes is natural. "Normal" sadness is a temporary feeling, often linked to a specific event or loss. We sometimes use the word *depressed* to describe feeling sad or disappointed: "I'm really depressed about missing out visiting with my friends." In these circumstances we feel sad, but we can still relate to others and find joy in other areas of our lives.

Sometimes depression lasts longer, as when we lose a loved one or are diagnosed with a serious illness.

If your depressed or sad feelings are severe, long-lasting, and recurrent, you may be experiencing clinical depression. It drains the pleasure out of life, leaving you feeling hopeless, helpless, and worthless. With severe depression, feelings may become numb, and even crying brings no relief.

Depression affects everything: the way you think, the way you behave, the way you interact with others, and even the way your body functions.

What Causes Depression?

Depression is not caused by personal weakness, laziness, or lack of willpower. Heredity, your chronic illness, and your medications may all play a role in depression. The way you think, especially negative thoughts, can also produce and sustain a depressed mood. Negative thoughts can be automatic, recur endlessly, and are often not linked to any event or triggering cause. Certain feelings and emotions also contribute to depression.

- **Fear, anxiety, or uncertainty about the future.** Feelings that result from worries about finances, your disease or treatment, or concerns about your family can lead to depression. By facing these issues as soon as possible, both you and your family will will spend less time worrying and have more time to enjoy life. This can have a healing effect. We talk more about these issues and how to deal with them in Chapter 19.

- **Frustration.** Frustration can have many causes. You may find yourself thinking, "I just can't do what I want," "I feel so helpless," "I used to be able to do this myself," or "Why doesn't anyone understand me?" The longer you accept these feelings, the more alone and isolated you are likely to feel.

- **Loss of control over your life.** Many things can make you feel like you are losing control. These include having to rely on medications, having to see a doctor on a regular basis, or having to count on others to help you do things like bathing, dressing, and preparing meals. This feeling of loss of control can make you lose faith in yourself and your abilities. Even though you may not be able to do everything yourself, you can still be in charge. You are the coach for your team.

Not all depression behavior is negative. Sometimes unrealistic cheeriness will mask what the person is really feeling, and the wise observer will recognize the brittleness or phoniness of the mood. Refusal to accept offers of help, even in the face of obvious need for it, is a frequent symptom of unrecognized depression.

Depressed feelings can lead to such behaviors as withdrawal, isolation, and lack of physical activity. These behaviors can cycle back to create more depressed feelings. The paradox of depression-related behavior is that the more you engage in the behavior, the more likely it is that you will drive away the people who can support and comfort you. Most of our friends and family want to help us feel better, but often they don't really know what to do to help. As their efforts to comfort and reassure us are frustrated, they may at some point throw up their hands and quit trying. Then the depressed person winds up saying, "See, nobody cares."

This again reinforces the feelings of loss and loneliness.

All these factors, along with others, can contribute to an imbalance in the chemicals in your brain (neurotransmitters). This imbalance can result in changes in the way you think, feel, and act. Changing the way you think and behave can be a powerful and effective way of changing your brain chemistry, lightening depression, and improving an ordinary bad mood.

Am I Depressed?

Here is a quick test for depression: Ask yourself what you do to have fun. If you do not have a quick answer, consider the additional possible symptoms of depression listed here.

Consider your mood over the past two weeks. Which of the following have you experienced?

- **Little interest or pleasure in doing things.** Not enjoying life or other people may be a sign of depression. Symptoms include not wanting to talk to anyone, to go out, or to answer the phone or doorbell.

- **Feeling down, depressed, or hopeless.** Feeling persistently blue can be a symptom of depression.

- **Trouble falling or staying asleep or sleeping too much.** Awakening and being unable to return to sleep or sleeping too much and not wanting to get out of bed can signal a problem.

- **Feeling tired or having little energy.** Fatigue—feeling tired all the time—is often a clear-cut symptom of depression.

- **Poor appetite or overeating.** This change may range from a loss of interest in food to unusually erratic or excessive eating.

- **Feeling bad about yourself.** Have you felt that you are a failure or have let yourself or your family down? Have you had a feeling of worthlessness, a negative image of your body, or doubts about your own self-worth?

- **Trouble concentrating.** Have you found it hard to do such things as reading the newspaper or watching television?

- **Lethargy or restlessness.** Have you been moving or speaking so slowly that other people could have noticed? Or the opposite, have you been so fidgety or restless that you have been moving around a lot more than usual? Either can be a sign of depression.

- **Wishing yourself harm or worse.** Thoughts that you would be better off dead or of hurting yourself in some way are often the hallmark of severe depression.

Depressed people may also experience weight gain or loss, loss of interest in sex or intimacy, loss of interest in personal care and grooming, inability to make decisions, and more frequent accidents.

*If several of these symptoms seem to apply to you, please get some help from your doctor, good friends, a member of the clergy, a psychologist, or a social worker. Do not wait for these feelings to pass. If you are thinking about harming yourself or others, get help **now**. Don't let a tragedy happen to you and your loved ones.*

Fortunately, the treatments for depression, including antidepressant medications, counseling, and self-help, are highly effective in decreasing the frequency, length, and severity of depression. Depression, like other symptoms, can be managed.

How to Lighten Depression and Bad Moods

The most effective treatments for depression are medications, counseling, and self-help.

Medications

Antidepressant medications that help balance brain chemistry are highly effective. Most antidepressant medications take from several days to several weeks before they begin to work. Then they usually bring significant relief. Don't be discouraged if you don't feel better immediately. Stick with it. To get the maximum benefit you may need to take certain medications for 6 months or more.

Side effects are usually most noticeable in the first few weeks and then lessen or go away. If the side effects are not especially severe, continue to take your medication. As your body gets used to the medication, you will begin to feel better. It is important to remember to take your medication every day. If you stop the medication because you're feeling better (or worse), you may relapse. Antidepressant medications are not addictive, but talk with your doctor before stopping or changing the dose.

Counseling

Several types of psychotherapy can also be highly effective, relieving symptoms up to 60% to 70% of the time. As with medications, counseling rarely has an immediate effect. It may be weeks (or longer) before you see improvement. Therapy can be brief, usually involving one to two sessions a week for several months. By learning new skills for ways to think and relate, psychotherapy may also help reduce the risk of recurrent depression.

Self-help

Self-help can also be surprisingly effective. You can learn many successful psychotherapy techniques on your own. For mild to moderate depression or just to lift your mood, the self-help strategies discussed here can sometimes be very productive. One study showed that reading and practicing self-help advice improved depression in nearly 70% of patients.

These skills and strategies can be used alone or to supplement medications and counseling.

■ **Eliminate the negative.** First let's talk about what does not help depression or bad moods. Being alone and isolating yourself, crying a lot, getting angry and yelling, blaming your failure or bad mood on others, or using alcohol or other drugs usually leaves you feeling worse. Are you taking tranquilizers or narcotic painkillers such as Valium, Librium, Restoril, codeine, Vicodin, sleeping medications, or other "downers"? These drugs intensify depression or may cause depression as a side effect. However, do not stop taking the medication before first talking with your doctor, as there may be important reasons for continuing its use or you may experience withdrawal reactions.

Do you drink alcohol to feel better? Alcohol is also a downer. There is virtually no way to escape depression unless you unload these negative influences from your brain. For most people, one or two drinks in the evening is not a problem, but if your mind is not free of alcohol during most of the day, you are having trouble with this drug. Talk this over with your doctor or call Alcoholics Anonymous.

■ **Plan for pleasure.** When you are feeling blue or depressed, the tendency is to withdraw, isolate yourself, and restrict activities. That is, in fact, the wrong thing to do. Maintaining or increasing activities is one of the best antidotes for depression. Going for a walk, looking at a sunset, watching a funny movie, getting a massage, learning another language, taking a cooking class, or joining a social club can all help keep your spirits up and keep you from falling into a situation where you can get depressed.

But sometimes having fun isn't such an easy prescription. You may have to make a deliberate effort to plan pleasurable activities. Even if you don't feel like doing it, try to stick to the schedule. You may find that the nature walk, cup of tea, or half hour of listening to music will improve your mood despite your initial misgivings. Don't leave good things to chance. You might want to make up a schedule for your free time during the week and what you'd like to do with it.

If you are feeling hardly any emotion and the world seems devoid of color, make an effort to put some sensation back into your life. Go to a bookstore and look through your favorite section. Listen or dance to some upbeat music. Exercise or ask someone to give you a massage so you can reconnect with your body. Eat some spicy food. Treat yourself to a very hot bath, or try a cold shower. Go to a garden center and smell all the flowers.

Make plans and carry them out. Look to the future. Plant some young trees. Look

forward to your grandchildren's graduation from college even if your own kids are in high school. If you know that one time of the year is especially difficult, such as Christmas or a birthday, make specific plans for that period. Don't wait to see what happens. Be prepared.

■ **Take action.** Continue your daily activities. Get dressed every day, make your bed, get out of the house, go shopping, walk your dog. Plan and cook meals. Force yourself to do these things even if you don't feel like it. Taking action to solve the problems immediately facing you provides the surest relief from a bad mood. More important than what you change or how much you change are the confidence-building feelings that come from successfully changing something—anything! Taking action is the important thing. Incorporating some simple things into your life can boost your mood. You might decide to clean or reorganize a room, for instance, or a closet or even a desk drawer. Or get a new magazine subscription or call an old friend.

Be careful not to set yourself difficult goals or take on a lot of responsibility. Break large tasks into small ones, set some priorities, and do what you can as best you can. Learn some of the proven steps for taking successful action (see chapter 2). It may be wise when you are feeling depressed not to make big life decisions. For example, don't move to a new setting without first visiting for a few weeks and learning about the resources available to you in this new community. Moving can be a sign of withdrawal, and depression often intensifies when you are in a location away from friends and acquaintances. Besides, many troubles may move with you. At the same time, the support you may need to deal with your troubles may have been left behind.

■ **Socialize.** Join a group. Get involved in a church group, a book club, a community college class, a self-help class, or a senior nutrition program. If you can't get out, consider a group on the Internet. If you do this, be sure that the Internet group is moderated, that is, that someone is in charge to enforce the rules of the group. Don't isolate yourself. Try to seek out positive, optimistic people who can lighten your heavy feelings.

■ **Move your mood.** Physical activity lifts depression and negative moods. Depressed people often complain that they feel too tired to exercise. But the feelings of fatigue associated with depression are not due to physical exhaustion. Try to get at least 20 to 30 minutes a day of some type of exercise, from chair dancing to walking. If you can get yourself moving, you may find that you have more energy (see chapter 7).

■ **Think positive.** Many people tend to be excessively critical of themselves, especially when they're depressed. You may find yourself thinking groundless, untrue things about yourself.

As you challenge your automatic negative thoughts, begin to rescript the negative stories you tell yourself (see Chapter 5). For example, one of your underlying beliefs may be "Unless I do everything perfectly, I'm a failure." Perhaps this belief could be revised to "Success is doing the best that I can in any situation." Also, when you are depressed, it's easy to forget that anything nice has happened at all. Make a list of some of the good or positive events in your life.

■ **Do something for someone else.** Lending a helping hand to someone in need is one of the most effective ways to change a bad mood, but it is one of the least commonly used. Arrange to baby-sit for a friend, read a story to someone who is ill, or volunteer at a soup kitchen. When you're depressed, you may greet the advice of helping others with thoughts like "I've got enough troubles of my own. I don't need anyone else's." But if you can bring yourself to help someone else, even in a small way, you'll feel better about yourself. Feeling useful is good for self-esteem, and you will be temporarily distracted from your own problems. Helping others needier than yourself can help you appreciate your own assets and capabilities. By comparison, your problems and difficulties may not appear as overwhelming. Sometimes helping others is the surest way to help yourself.

Don't be discouraged if it takes some time to feel better. If these self-help strategies alone are not sufficient, seek help from your physician or a mental health professional. Often some "talk therapy" or the use of antidepressant medications (or both) can go a long way toward relieving depression. Seeking professional help and taking medications are not signs of weakness. They are signs of strength.

Anger

Anger is one of the most common responses to chronic illness. The uncertainty and unpredictability of living with a chronic disease may threaten your independence and control. At times you may find yourself asking, "Why me?" This is a normal response to chronic illness.

You may be angry with yourself, family, friends, health care providers, God, or the world in general. For example, you may be angry at yourself for not taking better care of yourself. You may be angry at your family and friends because they don't do things the way you want. Or you might be angry at your doctor because he or she cannot fix your problems. Sometimes your anger may be misplaced, as when you find yourself yelling at the cat or dog.

Sometimes the health condition itself causes anger. For example, a stroke or Alzheimer's disease can affect someone's emotions, leading the person to cry inappropriately or have temper flare-ups. Some people who are depressed or have anxiety disorders express their depression or anxiety through anger.

Aristotle (c. 384–322 B.C.) observed, "Anyone can get angry—that is easy— . . . but to do this to the right person, to the right extent, at the right time, with the right motive, and in the right way, that is not for everyone, nor is it easy."

The first step is recognizing or admitting that you are angry and identifying why or with whom. These are important steps to learning how to manage your anger effectively. This task also involves finding constructive ways to express your anger.

Defusing Anger

Research now suggests that people who vent their anger actually get angrier. But suppressing anger isn't the answer either. The angry feelings often smolder, only to flare up later. There are a couple of strategies you can use to reduce hostile feelings:

- You can raise your anger threshold—that is, allow fewer things to trigger your anger in the first place.

- You can choose how to react when you get angry—without either denying your feelings or giving in to the situation.

This sounds simple enough, but what gets in the way is our tendency to see anger as coming from outside ourselves—something over which we have little control. We see ourselves as helpless victims. We blame others and say, "You make me so angry!" We explode and then say, "I couldn't help it." We see friends as selfish and insensitive, bosses as snobs or bullies, friends as unappreciative. So it seems that our only choice is an outburst of hostility. But with a little practice, even a seasoned hothead can master a new repertoire of healthy and more effective responses.

There are several things you can do to help manage your anger.

Reason with yourself

How you interpret and explain a situation determines whether you will feel angry or not.

You can learn to defuse anger by pausing and questioning your anger-producing thoughts. If you change your thoughts, you can change your response. You can decide whether or not to get angry and then decide whether or not to act.

At the first sign of anger, count to three and ask yourself the following questions:

- **Is this really important enough to get angry about?** Maybe this incident isn't serious enough to merit the time and energy. Consider if the issue will likely make a big difference in your life.

- **Am I justified in getting angry?** You may also need to gather more information to really understand the situation to counteract jumping to conclusions or misinterpreting the intentions or actions of others.

- **Will getting angry make a difference?** More often than not, getting angry and losing your cool does not work and may even be punishing. Exploding or venting increases your angry feelings, puts a strain on your relationships, and potentially damages your health.

Cool off

Any technique that relaxes or distracts you—such as meditating or taking a long walk—can help you put out the fire within. Slow, deep breathing is one of the quickest and simplest ways to cool off (see page 129). When you notice anger building, take ten slow, relaxed breaths before responding. Sometimes withdrawing and buying some alone time can defuse the situation. Also, physical exercise provides a good natural outlet for stress and anger.

Verbalize without blame

One important technique is to learn how to communicate your anger out loud, preferably without blaming or offending others. This can be done by learning to use "I" (rather than "you") messages to express your feelings. (Refer to Chapter 9 for a discussion of "I" messages.) However, if you choose to express your anger verbally, know that many people will not be able to help you. Most of us are not very good at dealing with angry people. This is true even if the anger is justified. Therefore, you may also find it useful to seek counseling or join a support group. Voluntary organizations, such as the various heart, lung, liver, and diabetes associations and the Arthritis Foundation, may be useful resources in this area.

Modify your expectations

You may also find that you would benefit from modifying your expectations. You have done this throughout your life. For example, as a child you thought you could become anything—a fireman, a ballet dancer, a doctor, and so on. As you grew older, however, you reevaluated these expectations, along with your capabilities, talents, and interests. Based on this reevaluation, you modified your plans.

This same process can be used to deal with the effects of chronic illness on your life. For example, it may be unrealistic to expect that you will get "all better." However, it is realistic to expect that you can still do many pleasurable things. You have the ability to affect the progress of your illness by slowing your decline or preventing it from becoming worse. Changing your expectations can help you change your perspective. Instead of dwelling on the 10% of things you can no longer do, think about the 90% of things you can still do.

In short, anger is a normal response to having a chronic condition. Part of learning to manage the condition involves acknowledging this anger and finding constructive ways to deal with it.

Stress

Stress is a common problem. But what is stress? In the 1950s, the physiologist Hans Selye described stress as "the nonspecific response of the body to any demand made upon it." Others have expanded this definition to explain that the body adapts to demands, whether pleasant or unpleasant. For example, you may feel stress after experiencing negative events, such as the death of a loved one, or even joyful events such as the marriage of a child.

How Does Your Body Respond to Stress?

Your body is used to functioning at a certain level. When there is a need to change this level, your body must adjust to meet the demand. It reacts by preparing to take some action: Your heart rate increases, your blood pressure rises, your neck and shoulder muscles tense, your breathing becomes more rapid, your digestion slows, your mouth becomes dry, and you may begin sweating. These are signals of what we call stress.

Why does this happen? To take an action, your muscles need to be supplied with oxygen and energy. Your breathing increases in an effort to inhale as much oxygen as possible and to get rid of as much carbon dioxide as possible. Your heart rate increases to deliver the oxygen and nutrients to the muscles. Furthermore, body functions that are not immediately necessary, such as the digestion of food and the body's natural immune responses, are slowed down.

How long will these responses last? In general, they are present only until the stressful event passes. Your body then returns to its normal level of functioning. Sometimes, though, your body does not return to its former comfortable level. If the stress is present for any length of time, your body begins adapting to it. This chronic stress can contribute to the onset of some chronic conditions and can make the symptoms more difficult to manage.

Common Stressors

Regardless of the type of stressor, the changes in the body are the same. Stressors, however, are not completely independent of one another. In fact, one stressor can often lead to other stressors or even magnify the effects of existing stressors. Several stressors can also occur at the same time. For instance, shortness of breath can cause anxiety, frustration, inactivity, and loss of endurance. Let's examine some of the most common sources of stress.

Physical stressors

Physical stressors can range from something as pleasant as picking up your new grandchild to everyday grocery shopping or the physical symptoms of your chronic illness. What they have in common is that all of these stressors increase your body's demand for energy. If your body is not prepared to deal with this demand, the results may be anything from sore muscles to fatigue to a worsening of some disease symptoms.

Mental and emotional stressors

Mental and emotional stressors can also be either pleasant or uncomfortable. The joys you experience from seeing a child get married or meeting new friends may induce a similar stress response as feeling frustrated or worried because of your illness. Although this fact may seem surprising, the similarity comes from the way your brain perceives the stress.

Environmental stressors

Environmental stressors, too, can be both good and bad. They may be as varied as a sunny day, uneven sidewalks that make it difficult to walk, loud noises, bad weather, a snoring spouse, or secondhand smoke. Each creates a pleasurable or apprehensive excitement that triggers the stress response.

Isn't "Good Stress" a Contradiction?

As noted earlier, some types of stress can be good, such as a job promotion, a wedding, a vacation, a new friendship, or a new baby. These stressors make you feel happy but still cause the changes in your body that we have just discussed. Another example of a good stressor is exercise.

When you exercise or do any type of physical activity, there is a demand placed on the body. The heart has to work harder to deliver blood to the muscles; the lungs are working harder, and you breathe more rapidly to keep up with your muscles' demand for oxygen. Meanwhile, your muscles are working hard to keep up with the signals from your brain, which are telling them to keep moving.

As you maintain an exercise program for several weeks, you will begin to notice a change. What once seemed virtually impossible now becomes easier. Your body has adapted to this stress. There is less strain on your heart, lungs, and other muscles because they have become more efficient and you have become more fit. The same can happen with psychological stresses.

Many people become more resilient and stronger emotionally after experiencing emotional challenges to which they need to learn to adapt.

Recognizing When You Feel Stressed

Everyone has a certain need for stress. It helps your life run more efficiently. As long as you do not go past your body's breaking point, stress is helpful. You can tolerate more stress on some days than on others. But sometimes, if you are not aware of the different types of stress, you can go beyond your breaking point and feel that your life is out of control. Often it is difficult to recognize when you are under too much stress. The following are some of the warning signs:

■ Biting your nails, pulling your hair, tapping your foot, or other repetitive habits

■ Grinding your teeth or clenching your jaw

■ Tension in your head, neck, or shoulders

■ Feeling anxious, nervous, helpless, or irritable

■ Frequent accidents

■ Forgetting things you usually don't forget

■ Difficulty concentrating

■ Fatigue and exhaustion

Sometimes you can catch yourself when you are behaving or feeling stressed. If you do, take a few minutes to think about what it is that is making you feel tense. Take a few deep breaths and try to relax. Also, a quick body scan (described in Chapter 5) can help you recognize stress in your body. You will find additional good ideas for coping with stress in that chapter.

Let us now examine some tools for dealing with stress.

Dealing with Stress

Dealing effectively with stress need not be complicated. In fact, it can start with a simple three-step process:

1. **Identify your stressors by making a list.** Consider every area of your life: family, relationships, health, financial security, living environment, and so on.

2. **Sort your stressors.** For each stressor, ask yourself, Is it important or unimportant? and, Is it changeable or unchangeable? Then place each of your stressors in one of four categories:

   - Important and changeable
   - Important and unchangeable
   - Unimportant and changeable
   - Unimportant and unchangeable

   For example, needing to quit smoking is changeable and, for most people, important. Loss of a loved one or a job is important and unchangeable. The bad record of your favorite sports team, a traffic jam, or bad weather is unchangeable and may or may not be important. What really counts is what you think about each stressor.

3. **Match your strategy to each stressor.** Different strategies work for different stressors. Following are some strategies to help you be more effective in managing each type of problem.

   - **Important and changeable stressors.** These types of stressors are best managed by taking action to change the situation and to reduce the stress associated with

them. Useful problem-solving skills include planning and goal setting (see Chapter 2); imagery (page 77); positive, healthy thinking (page 75), effective communication (see Chapter 9), and seeking social support.

   - **Important and unchangeable stressors.** These stressors are often the most difficult to manage. They can make you feel helpless and hopeless. No matter what you do, you cannot make another person change, bring someone back from the dead, or delete traumatic experiences from your life. Even though you may not be able to change the situation, you may be able to use one or more of the following strategies:

1. Change the way you think about the problem. For example, think how much worse it could be, focus on the positive and practice gratitude (see page 86), deny or ignore the problem, distract yourself (see page 74), accept what you can't change.

2. Find some part of the problem that you can reclassify as changeable (you can't stop the hurricane, but you can take steps to rebuild).

3. Reassess how important the problem is in light of your overall life and priorities (maybe your neighbor's criticism isn't so important after all).

4. Change your emotional reactions to the situation and thereby reduce the stress (you can't change what happened, but you can help yourself feel

less distressed about it). Try writing or confiding your deepest thoughts and feelings (see page 87), seeking social support, helping others, enjoying your senses, relaxing, using imagery, enjoying humor, or exercising.

■ **Unimportant and changeable stressors.** If the stressor is unimportant, first try just letting it go. But if you can control it with relatively little effort, go ahead and deal with it. Solving small problems helps build your skills and confidence to tackle bigger ones. Use the same strategies as described for important and changeable problems.

■ **Unimportant and unchangeable stressors.** The best solution for these problems is to ignore them. Starting now, you are given permission to let go of unimportant concerns. These are common hassles, and everybody has their share of them. Don't let them bother you. You can distract yourself with humor, relaxation or imagery, or focusing on more pleasurable things.

Using Problem Solving

There are some situations that you recognize as stressful, such as being stuck in traffic, going on a trip, or preparing a meal. First, look at what it is about the particular situation that is stressful. Is it that you hate to be late? Are trips stressful because of uncertainty about your destination? Does meal preparation involve too many steps and demand too much energy?

Once you have determined what the problem is, begin looking for possible ways to reduce the stress. Can you leave earlier? Can you let someone else drive? Can you call someone at your destination and ask about wheelchair access, local mass transit, and other concerns? Can you prepare food in the morning? Can you take a short nap in the early afternoon?

After you have identified some possible solutions, select one to try the next time you are in the situation. Then evaluate the results. (This is the problem-solving approach that was discussed in Chapter 2.)

Managing the Stress

Whereas you can successfully manage some types of stress by modifying the situation, other types of stress seem to sneak up on you when you don't expect them. The approach to dealing with these types of stress also involves problem solving.

If you know that certain situations will be stressful, develop ways to deal with them before they happen. Try to rehearse, in your mind, what you will do when the situation arises so that you will be ready.

Certain chemicals you ingest can also increase stress. These include nicotine, alcohol, and caffeine. Some people smoke a cigarette, drink a glass of wine or beer, eat chocolate, or drink a cup of coffee to soothe their tension, but this may actually increase stress. Eliminating or cutting down on these stressors can help.

As noted earlier, other tools for dealing with stress include getting enough sleep, exercising, and eating well. Sometimes stress is so overwhelming that these tools are not enough. These are times when good self-managers turn to consultants such as counselors, social workers, psychologists, or psychiatrists.

In summary, stress, like every other symptom, has many causes and can therefore be managed in many different ways. It is up to you to examine the problem and try to find solutions that meet your needs and suit your lifestyle.

Memory Problems

Many people worry about changes in their memory, particularly as they age. Although all of us are sometimes forgetful, there are serious illnesses that cause memory loss, including Alzheimer's disease and other types of dementia. These are not a normal part of aging. Although symptoms can vary widely, the first problem many people notice is forgetfulness severe enough to affect their ability to function at home or at work or to enjoy lifelong hobbies. Alzheimer's and similar diseases may cause a person to become confused, get lost in familiar places, misplace things, or have trouble with language. The disease gets worse over time.

If you suspect that you or someone you know is experiencing symptoms, it is important to seek a diagnosis as soon as possible. There is currently no cure for dementia, but early detection allows you to get the maximum benefit from available treatments—treatments that may relieve some symptoms and help you maintain your independence longer. An early diagnosis allows you to take part in decisions about care, transportation, living options, and financial and legal matters. You can also start building a social network sooner and increase your chances of participating in clinical drug trials that help advance research.

If you are concerned about Alzheimer's or a similar condition, contact the Alzheimer's Association. Help is available 24 hours a day, 7 days a week. Contact information is provided at the end of this chapter.

Itching

Itching is one of the most difficult symptoms to understand. It is any sensation that causes an urge to scratch. Like other symptoms, it can have many different causes. Some of these we understand. When you get an insect bite or come in contact with poison ivy, your body releases histamines, which irritate nerve endings and cause itching. When the liver is damaged, it cannot remove bile products, and these are deposited in the skin, causing itching. In kidney disease, itching may be severe, but the exact cause is not clear. There are also other conditions, such as psoriasis, in which the causes of itching are not easily explained. We do know that other factors such as warmth, wool clothing, and stress can make itching worse. The following are some ways that may help you relieve your itching.

Moisture

Dry skin tends to be itchy; therefore, keep the skin moisturized by applying moisturizing creams several times a day. When you choose a moisturizer, be careful. Be sure to read the list of ingredients when buying a cream or lotion. Avoid products that contain alcohol or any other ingredient that ends in *-ol,* as they tend to dry the skin. In general, the greasier the product, the better it works as a moisturizer. Creams are better moisturizers than lotions, and products such as Vaseline, olive oil, and vegetable shortening are also very effective.

When taking a bath or shower, use warm water and soak for not less than 10 or more than 20 minutes. You also may want to add bath oil, baking soda, or "Sulzberger's household bath oil" to the water. To make this bath oil, stir 2 teaspoons of olive oil into a large glass of milk and add it to your bath. When you get out of the water, pat yourself dry immediately and apply your cream.

If your itching is caused by the release of histamines during an allergic reaction or from having had contact with an irritating substance, wash off the oils or offending agent, apply cold compresses, and take Benadryl or another antihistamine to help stop the reaction.

During cold weather it can be especially difficult to deal with itching because indoor heating tends to dry the skin. If this is a problem for you, the use of a humidifier might help. Also try to keep your home and office as cool as you can without being uncomfortable.

Clothing

The type of clothing you wear can also add to the itching sensations. Obviously, the best rule of thumb is to wear what is comfortable. This is usually clothing made from material that is not scratchy. Most people find that natural fibers such as cotton allow the skin to "breathe" better and are the least irritating to the skin.

Medications

Antihistamines will help if your itching is caused by the release of histamines. You can buy many of these products over the counter. They include triprolidine (Actifed), diphenhydramine (Benadryl), chlorpheniramine maleate (Chlor-Trimeton), cetirizine (Zyrtec), and loratidine (Claritin).

You can also buy creams that help soothe the nerve endings, such as Ben Gay and Vicks Vap-o-Rub. If you want an anti-itch cream, look for one that contains benzocaine, lidocaine, or pramoxine. However, be careful, because some people can have allergic reactions to these creams, especially benzocaine. Capsaicin creams may also help itching, although they will cause a burning sensation. Steroid creams that contain cortisone can also help control some types of itching. If you are confused about what over-the-counter products to buy, ask your doctor or pharmacist.

With the exception of moisturizing creams, no cream should be used on a long-term basis without talking to your doctor. If your itching continues with use of these over-the-counter products, you may want to talk to your doctor about trying the stronger prescription versions of these medications.

Stress

Anything that you can do to reduce the stress in your life will also help reduce the itching. We have already discussed some of the ways to deal with stress earlier in this chapter, and some additional techniques are described in Chapter 5.

Scratching

While our natural tendency is to scratch what itches, this really does not help, especially for chronic itching. Rather, it leads to a vicious cycle whereby the more you scratch, the more you tend to itch. Unfortunately, it is hard to resist scratching. However, you might try rubbing, pressing, or patting the skin when you feel the need to scratch. If you are not able to break this cycle yourself, consult a dermatologist, who may be able to help you find alternative ways to control the itching.

Itching is a common and undoubtedly very frustrating symptom for both patients and physicians to manage. If the self-management tips described here do not seem to help, it may be time to seek the help of a physician. Often he or she can prescribe medications that can help with some specific types of itching.

Urinary Incontinence: Loss of Bladder Control

Urinary incontinence means you have trouble controlling your bladder and accidentally leak urine. If you have trouble controlling your bladder, you are not alone. Many people are coping with this problem. Although urinary incontinence can occur in both men and women, it is more common in women. In many cases, incontinence can be controlled, if not cured outright.

It is common to experience incontinence during or after pregnancy or with menopause, aging, or weight gain. Activities that put increased pressure on the bladder, such as coughing, laughing, sneezing, and physical activity, can cause urine leakage. Incontinence can be related to changes in your hormones, weakening muscles or ligaments in the pelvic area, or the use of certain medications. Infections in the bladder can also cause temporary incontinence.

Urinary incontinence can affect your quality of life and lead to other health problems. Feeling embarrassed by urinary incontinence causes some people to avoid social activities or sex. Some people experience loss of confidence or depression as a result of incontinence. Leaked urine may also cause skin irritation and infections. The frequent urge to urinate can interfere with sound, restorative sleep. Slipping and falling on leaked urine when rushing to the bathroom can result in injury.

The good news is that there are many treatments that can control or even cure this condition. It may be reassuring to know that many of these are small things you can do at home. If none of the following solves the problem, talk to your doctor about other treatments. Don't be embarrassed. Your doctor has heard it all before.

There are three types of persistent or chronic loss of bladder control:

- **Stress incontinence** refers to small amounts of urine leaking out during exercise, coughing, laughing, sneezing, or other movements that squeeze the bladder. Kegel exercises (described under "Home Treatments") often improve this condition.

- **Urge incontinence**, or overactive bladder, happens when the need to urinate comes on so quickly that you don't have enough time to get to the toilet.

■ **Overflow incontinence** occurs when the bladder cannot empty completely.

Home Treatments

Small, effective changes to your lifestyle or behavior are the first treatments for urinary incontinence. For many people, these treatments effectively control or cure the problem.

Kegel exercises strengthen your pelvic floor muscles. This allows better control of your urine flow and prevents leaking. Learning Kegel exercises takes a bit of practice and patience. It may take a few weeks to feel an improvement in your symptoms.

Here is how to do Kegel exercises:

1. First, find the muscles that stop your urine. You can do this by repeatedly stopping your urine in midstream and starting again. Focus on the muscles that you feel squeezing around your urethra (opening for the urine) and anus (opening for your bowels).

2. Practice squeezing these muscles when you are not urinating. If your stomach or buttocks move, you're not using the right muscles.

3. Squeeze the muscles, hold for 3 seconds, and then relax for 3 seconds.

4. Repeat the exercise 10 to 15 times per session.

Complete at least 30 Kegel exercises every day. The wonderful thing about Kegels is that you can do them anywhere and anytime. No one will know what you are doing except you.

With urge incontinence, **retraining your bladder** may help.

■ Practice "double-voiding." Empty your bladder as much as possible, relax for a minute, and try to empty it again. This helps empty your bladder completely.

■ It sometimes helps to practice waiting a specified amount of time before urinating. This gradually retrains your bladder to require emptying less often.

■ Train yourself to urinate on a regular schedule, about every 2 to 4 hours during the day, whether or not you feel the urge. If you now need to urinate every 30 minutes, perhaps you can start by waiting to every 40 minutes and gradually work your way up to every 2 to 4 hours.

Consuming fewer beverages that stimulate the bladder and urine production, such as alcohol, coffee, tea, and other drinks that contain caffeine, can reduce your trips to the toilet.

If you carry extra weight, **losing weight** can reduce the pressure on your bladder. Studies show that a loss of just 10 percent of total body weight improves incontinence problems for many people.

Wearing absorbent pads or briefs does not cure incontinence but helps manage the condition.

Treatments and Medications

If changes in your lifestyle or behavior do not relieve your urinary incontinence, discuss with your doctor other treatments such as the use of medication, a pessary (a thin, flexible ring that can be worn inside the vagina to support the pelvic area), or, in some cases, surgery. You don't have to suffer in silence if you have urinary incontinence. Talk with your doctor.

In this chapter we have discussed common causes of some of the most common symptoms experienced by people with chronic conditions. In addition, we have described some tools that you can use to cope with your symptoms. Taking action to deal physically with your symptoms is necessary in coping with your illness on a day-to-day basis. But sometimes this just doesn't seem to be enough. There are times when you may wish to escape from your surroundings and just have "your time"—a time that allows you to clear your mind and gain a fresh perspective. The following chapter presents different ways to complement your physical-symptom management with thinking techniques—using the power of your mind—to help reduce and even prevent some of the symptoms you may experience.

Suggested Further Reading

Bourne, Edmund. *Coping with Anxiety: 10 Simple Ways to Relieve Anxiety, Fear, and Worry.* Oakland, Calif.: New Harbinger, 2003.

Carter, Les. *The Anger Trap: Free Yourself from the Frustrations That Sabotage Your Life.* San Francisco: Jossey-Bass, 2004.

Casarjian, Robin. *Forgiveness: A Bold Choice for a Peaceful Heart.* New York: Bantam Books, 1993.

Caudill, Margaret. *Managing Pain Before It Manages You,* 3rd ed. New York: Guilford Press, 2008.

David, Martha, Elizabeth Robbins Eshelman, and Matthew McKay. *The Relaxation and Stress Reduction Workbook.* Oakland, Calif.: New Harbinger, 2008.

DePaulo, J. Raymond, and Leslie Alan Horvitz. *Understanding Depression: What We Know and What You Can Do About It.* New York: Wiley, 2003.

Donoghue, Paul J., and Mary E. Siegel. *Sick and Tired of Feeling Sick and Tired: Living with Invisible Chronic Illness,* 2nd ed. New York: Norton, 2000.

Gordon, James S. *Unstuck: Your Guide to the Seven-Stage Journey Out of Depression.* New York: Penguin, 2008.

Hankins, Gary, and Carol Hankins. *Prescription for Anger,* 3rd ed. Newberg, Ore.: Barclay Press, 2000.

Hauri, Peter, and Shirley Linde. *No More Sleepless Nights.* New York: Wiley, 1993.

Jacobs, Gregg D. *Say Good Night to Insomnia.* New York: Holt, 2009.

Kabat-Zinn, Jon. *Full Catastrophe Living: Using the Wisdom of Your Body and Mind to Face Stress, Pain, and Illness.* New York: Delta, 2005.

Kabat-Zinn, Jon. *Mindfulness for Beginners: Reclaiming the Present Moment—and Your Life.* Louisville, Colo.: Sounds True, 2011.

Klein, Donald F., and Paul H. Wender. *Understanding Depression: A Complete Guide to Its Diagnosis and Treatment,* 2nd ed. New York: Oxford University Press, 2005.

Kleinke, Chris L. *Coping with Life Challenges,* 2nd ed. Pacific Grove, Calif.: Brooks/Cole, 2002.

McGonigal, Kelly. *The Willpower Instinct: How Self-Control Works, Why It Matters, and What You Can Do to Get More of It.* New York: Avery, 2011.

McKay, Matthew, Peter D. Rogers, and Judith McKay. *When Anger Hurts,* 2nd ed. Oakland, Calif.: New Harbinger, 2003.

Natelson, Benjamin H. *Facing and Fighting Fatigue: A Practical Approach*. New Haven, Conn.: Yale University Press, 1998.

Sobel, David, and Robert Ornstein. *The Healthy Mind, Healthy Body Handbook* (also published under the title *The Mind and Body Health Handbook*). Los Altos, Calif.: DRX, 1996.

Stahl, Bob, and Elisha Goldstein. *A Mindfulness-Based Stress Reduction Workbook*. Oakland, Calif.: New Harbinger, 2010.

Torburn, Leslie. *Stop the Stress Habit: Change Your Perceptions and Improve Your Health*. Bloomington, Indiana: iUniverse, 2008.

Turk, Dennis, and Justin Nash. "Chronic Pain: New Ways to Cope." In Daniel Goleman and Joel Gurin, eds., *Mind/Body Medicine*. New York: Consumer Reports Books, 1993.

Williams, Redford, and Virginia Williams. *Anger Kills: Seventeen Strategies for Controlling the Hostility That Can Harm Your Health*. New York: Random House, 1998.

Williams, Redford, and Virginia Williams. *Lifeskills: 8 Simple Ways to Build Stronger Relationships, Communicate More Clearly, and Improve Your Health*. New York: Three Rivers Press, 1998.

Other Resources

- ☐ American Chronic Pain Association: http://www.theacpa.org/

- ☐ National Sleep Foundation: http://www.sleepfoundation.org/

- ☐ The Alzheimer's Association's 24/7 Helpline provides information, referrals, and care consultation in 140 languages: (800) 272-3900; http://www.alz.org/

- ☐ National Association for Continence: http://www.nafc.org/

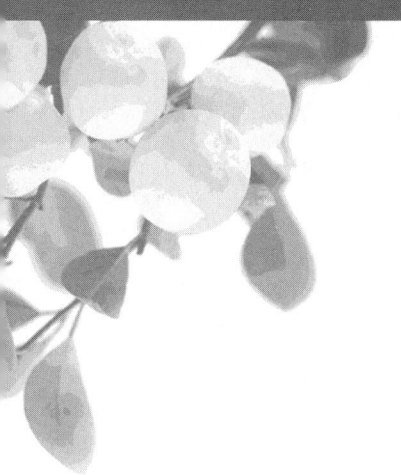

CHAPTER 5

Using Your Mind to Manage Symptoms

T HERE IS A STRONG LINK BETWEEN OUR THOUGHTS, attitudes, and emotions and our mental and physical health. One of our self-managers said, "It's not always mind over matter, but mind matters." Although thoughts and emotions do not directly cause our chronic conditions, they can influence our symptoms. Research has shown that thoughts and emotions trigger certain hormones or other chemicals that send messages throughout the body. These messages affect how our body functions; for example, thoughts and emotions can change our heart rate, blood pressure, breathing, blood sugar levels, muscle responses, immune response, concentration, the ability to get pregnant, and even our ability to fight off other illness.

All of us, at one time or another, have experienced the power of the mind and its effects on the body. Both pleasant and unpleasant thoughts and emotions can cause the body to react in different ways. Our heart rate and breathing can increase or slow down; we may experience sensations such as sweating (warm or cold), blushing, tears, and so on. Sometimes just a memory or an image can trigger these responses. For example, try this simple exercise: Imagine that you are holding a big, bright yellow lemon slice. You hold it close to your nose and smell its strong citrus aroma. Now you bite into the lemon. It's juicy! The juice fills your mouth and dribbles down your chin. Now you begin to suck on the lemon and its tart juice. What happens? The body responds. Your mouth puckers and starts to water. You may even smell the scent of the lemon. All of these reactions are triggered by the mind and its memory of your experience with a real lemon.

This example shows the power the mind has over the body. It also gives us a good reason to work to develop our mental abilities to help us manage our symptoms. With training and practice, we can learn to use the mind to relax the body, to reduce stress and anxiety, and to reduce the discomfort or unpleasantness caused by our physical and emotional symptoms. The mind can also greatly help relieve the pain and shortness of breath associated with various diseases and may even help a person depend less on some medications.

In this chapter we describe several ways in which you can begin to use your mind to manage symptoms. These are sometimes referred to as "thinking" or "cognitive" techniques because they involve the use of our thinking abilities to make changes in the body.

As you read, keep the following key principles in mind:

- **Symptoms have many causes**, which means there are many ways to manage most symptoms. If you understand the nature and causes of your symptoms, you will be able to manage them better.

- **Not all management techniques work for everyone.** It is up to you to experiment and find out what works best for you. Be flexible. This includes trying different techniques and checking the results to determine which management tool is most helpful for which symptoms and under what circumstances.

- **Learning new skills and gaining control of the situation take time.** Give yourself several weeks to practice before you decide if a new tool is working for you.

- **Don't give up too easily.** As with exercise and other new skills, using your mind to manage your health condition requires both practice and time before you notice the benefits. So even if you feel you are not accomplishing anything, don't give up. Be patient and keep on trying.

- **These techniques should not have negative effects.** If you become frightened, angry, or depressed when using one of these tools, do not continue to use it. Try another tool instead.

Relaxation Techniques

Many of us have heard and read about relaxation, yet some of us are still confused as to what relaxation is, its benefits, and how to do it.

Simply stated, relaxation involves using thinking techniques to reduce or eliminate tension from both the body and the mind. This usually results in improved sleep quality and less stress, pain, and shortness of breath. Relaxation is not a cure-all, but it can be an effective part of a treatment plan.

There are different types of relaxation techniques. Each has specific guidelines and uses. Some techniques are used mostly to achieve muscle relaxation, while others are aimed at reducing anxiety and emotional stress or diverting attention, all of which aid in symptom management.

The term *relaxation* means different things to different people. We can all identify things we do that help us relax. For example, we may walk, watch TV, listen to music, knit, or garden. These methods, however, are different from the techniques discussed in this chapter because they include some form of physical activity or require a stimulus such as music that is outside of the mind. The relaxation *tools* we are discussing here have us use our mind to help the body relax.

The goal of relaxation is to turn off the outside world so that the mind and body are at rest. This allows you to reduce the tensions that can increase the intensity or severity of symptoms.

Following are some guidelines to help you practice relaxation.

- **Pick a quiet place and time** when you will not be disturbed for at least 15 to 20 minutes. (If this seems too long, start with 5 minutes. By the way, in some homes the only quiet place is the bathroom. That is just fine.)

- **Try to practice the technique twice daily** and not less than 4 times a week.

- **Don't expect miracles.** Some of these techniques take practice. Sometimes it takes 3 to 4 weeks of consistent practice before you start to notice benefits.

- **Relaxation should be helpful.** At worst, you may find it boring, but if it is an unpleasant experience or makes you more nervous or anxious, you might switch to one of the other symptom management tools described in this chapter.

Relaxation Quick and Easy

Some types of relaxation are so easy, natural, and effective that people do not think of them as "relaxation techniques."

- Take a nap or a hot, soothing bath.

- Curl up and read or listen to a good book.

- Watch a funny movie.

- Make a paper airplane and sail it across the room.

- Get a massage.

- Enjoy an occasional glass of wine.

- Start a small garden or grow a beautiful plant indoors.

- Do some crafts such as knitting, pottery, or woodworking.

- Watch a favorite TV show.

- Read a poem or an inspirational saying.

- Go for a walk.

- Start a collection (coins, folk art, shells, or something in miniature).

- Listen to your favorite music.

- Sing around the house.

- Crumble paper into a ball and use a waste-basket as a basketball hoop.

- Look at water (ocean waves, a lake, or a fountain).

- Watch the clouds in the sky.

- Put your head down on your desk and close your eyes for 5 minutes.

- Rub your hands together until they're warm, and then cup them over your closed eyes.

- Vigorously shake your hands and arms for 10 seconds.

- Call up a friend or family member to chat.

- Smile and introduce yourself to someone new.

- Do something nice and unexpected for someone else.

- Play with a pet.

- Go to a vacation spot in your mind.

Relaxation Tools That Take 5 to 20 Minutes

These techniques take a bit longer but are quite effective.

Body scan

To relax muscles, you need to know how to scan your body and recognize where you are tense. Then you can release the tension. The first step is to become familiar with the difference between the feeling of tension and the feeling of relax-ation. This exercise will allow you to compare those feelings and, with practice, spot and release tension anywhere in your body. It is best done lying down on your back, but any comfortable position can be used. A body scan script can be found on page 73.

Relaxation response

In the early 1970s a physician named Herbert Benson studied what he calls the "relaxation response." According to Benson, our bodies have several natural states. One example is the "fight or flight" response experienced by people when faced with a great danger. The body becomes quite tense, which is followed by the body's natural ten-dency to relax; this is the relaxation response. As our lives become more and more hectic, our bod-ies tend to stay tense for long periods of time. We lose our ability to relax. The relaxation response helps change this.

Find a quiet place where there are few or no distractions. Find a comfortable position. You should be comfortable enough to remain in the same position for 20 minutes.

Choose a word, object, or pleasant feeling. For example, repeat a word or sound (such as the word *one*), gaze at a symbol (perhaps a flower), or concentrate on a feeling (such as peace).

Adopt a passive attitude. This is of the utmost importance. Empty all thoughts and distrac-tions from your mind. You may become aware of thoughts, images, and feelings, but don't concen-trate on them. Just allow them to pass on.

Here's what you should do to elicit the relax-ation response:

- Sit quietly in a comfortable position.

- Close your eyes.

- Relax all your muscles, beginning at your feet and progressing up to your face. Keep them relaxed.

- Breathe in through your nose. Become aware of your breathing. As you breathe out through your mouth, say the word you chose silently to yourself. Try to empty all

Body-Scan Script

As you get into a comfortable position, allowing yourself to begin to sink comfortably into the surface below you, you may perhaps begin to allow your eyes gradually to close . . . From there, turn your attention to your breath . . . Breathing in, allowing the breath gradually to go all the way down to your belly. and then breathing out . . . And again, breathing in . . . and out . . . noticing the natural rhythm of your breathing . . .

Now allowing your attention to focus on your feet. Starting with your toes, notice whatever sensations are there—warmth, coolness, whatever's there . . . simply feel it. Using your mind's eye, imagine that as you breathe in, the breath goes all the way down into your toes, bringing with it new refreshing air . . . And now noticing the sensations elsewhere in your feet. not judging or thinking about what you're feeling, but simply becoming aware of the experience of your feet as you allow yourself to be fully supported by the surface below you . . .

Next focus on your lower legs and knees. These muscles and joints do a lot of work for us, but often we don't give them the attention they deserve. So now breathe down into the knees, calves, and ankles, noticing whatever sensations appear . . . See if you can simply stay with the sensations . . . breathing in new fresh air, and as you exhale, releasing tension and stress and allowing the muscles to relax and soften . . .

Now move your attention to the muscles, bones, and joints of the thighs, buttocks, and hips . . . breathing down into the upper legs, noticing whatever sensations you experience. It may be warmth, coolness, a heaviness or lightness. You may become aware of the contact with the surface beneath you, or perhaps the pulsing of your blood. Whatever's there . . . what matters is that you are taking time to learn to relax . . . deeper and deeper, as you breathe . . . in . . . and out.

Move your attention now to your back and chest. Feeling the breath fill the abdomen and chest . . . Noticing whatever sensations are there . . . not judging or thinking, but simply observing what is right here right now. allowing the fresh air to nourish the muscles, bones, and joints as you breathe in, and then exhaling any tension and stress.

Now focus on the neck, shoulders, arms, and hands. Inhaling down through the neck and shoulders, all the way down to the fingertips. Not trying too hard to relax, but simply becoming aware of your experience of these parts of your body in the present moment . . .

Turning now to your face and head, notice the sensations beginning at the back of your head, up along your scalp, and down into your forehead . . . Then become aware of the sensations in and around your eyes and down into your cheeks and jaw . . . Continue to allow your muscles to release and soften as you breathe in nourishing fresh air, and allow tension and stress to leave as you breathe out . . .

As you drink in fresh air, allow it to spread throughout your body, from the soles of your feet all the way up through the top of your head . . . And then exhale any remaining stress and tension . . . and now take a few moments to enjoy the stillness as you breathe in . . . and out . . . Awake, relaxed, and still . . .

Now as the body scan comes to a close, coming back into the room, bringing with you whatever sensations of relaxation . . . comfort . . . peace, whatever's there . . . knowing that you can repeat this exercise at any appropriate time and place of your choosing . . . And when you're ready open your eyes.

thoughts from your mind; concentrate on your word, sound, or symbol.

■ Continue this for 10 to 20 minutes. You may open your eyes to check the time, but do not use an alarm. When you finish, sit quietly for several minutes, at first with your eyes closed. Do not stand up for a few minutes.

■ Maintain a passive attitude, and let relaxation occur at its own pace. When distracting thoughts occur, ignore them by not dwelling on them, and return to repeating the word you chose. Do not worry about whether you are successful in achieving a deep level of relaxation.

■ Practice this once or twice daily.

Distraction

Our minds have trouble focusing on more than one thing at a time; therefore, we can lessen the intensity of symptoms by training our minds to focus attention on something other than our bodies and their sensations. This technique, called distraction or attention refocusing, is particularly helpful for those people who feel that their symptoms are painful or overwhelming or worry that every bodily sensation might indicate a new or worsening symptom or health problem. (It is important to mention that with distraction you are not ignoring the symptoms but choosing not to dwell on them.)

Sometimes it may be difficult to put anxious thoughts out of your mind. When you try to suppress any thought, you may end up thinking more about it. For example, try not thinking about a tiger charging at you. Whatever you do, don't let the thought of a tiger enter your mind. You'll probably find it nearly impossible not to think about the tiger.

Although you can't easily stop thinking about something, you can distract yourself and redirect your attention elsewhere. For example, think about the charging tiger again. Now stand up suddenly, slam your hand on the table,

and shout *"Stop!"* What happened to the tiger? Gone—at least for the moment.

Distraction works best for short activities or times in which symptoms may be anticipated. For example, if you know climbing stairs will be painful or cause discomfort or that falling asleep at night is difficult, you might try one of the following distraction techniques:

■ Make plans for exactly what you will do after the unpleasant activity passes. For example, if climbing stairs is uncomfortable or painful, think about what you need to do once you get to the top. If you have trouble falling asleep, try making plans for some future event, being as detailed as possible.

■ Think of a person's name, a bird, a flower, or whatever, for every letter of the alphabet. If you get stuck on one letter, go on to the next. (These are good distractions for pain as well as for sleep problems.)

■ Challenge yourself to count backward from 100 by threes (100, 97, 94, . . .).

■ To get through unpleasant daily chores (such as sweeping, mopping, or vacuuming), imagine your floor as a map of a country or continent. Try naming all the states, provinces, or countries, moving east to west or north to south. If geography does not appeal to you, imagine your favorite store and where each department is located.

■ Try to remember words to favorite songs or the events in an old story.

■ Try the *"Stop!"* technique. If you find yourself worrying or entrapped in endlessly repeating negative thoughts, stand up suddenly, slap your hand on the table or your thigh, and shout *"Stop!"* You can practice this technique whenever your mind endlessly repeats negative thoughts. With practice, you won't have to shout out loud. Just whispering *"Stop!"* or tightening your vocal cords and moving your tongue as if saying *"Stop!"* will often work. Some people imagine a large stop sign. Others put a rubber band on their wrist and snap it hard to break the chain of negative thought. Or just pinch yourself. Do anything that redirects your attention.

■ You might redirect your attention to a pleasurable experience:

• Look outside at something in nature.

• Try to identify all the sounds around you.

• Massage your hand.

• Smell a sweet or pungent odor.

There are, of course, many variations to these examples, all of which help you refocus attention away from your problem.

So far we have discussed short-term refocusing strategies that involve using only the mind for distraction. Distraction also works well for long-term projects or symptoms that tend to last longer, such as depression and some forms of chronic pain.

In these cases, the mind is focused not internally but externally on some type of activity. If you are somewhat depressed or have continuous unpleasant symptoms, find an activity that interests you, and distract yourself from the problem. The activity can be almost anything, from gardening to cooking to reading or going to a movie, even doing volunteer work. One of the marks of a successful self-manager is that he or she has a variety of interests and always seems to be doing something.

Positive Thinking and Self-Talk

All of us talk to ourselves all the time. For example, when waking up in the morning, we think, "I really don't want to get out of bed. I'm tired and don't want to go to work today." Or at the end of an enjoyable evening, we think, "Gee, that was fun. I should get out more often." What we think or say to ourselves is called our self-talk. The way we talk to ourselves tends to come from how and what

we think about ourselves. Our thoughts can be positive or negative, and so is our self-talk. Therefore, self-talk can be an important self-management tool when it's positive thinking or a weapon that hurts or defeats us when it's habitually negative thinking.

All of our self-talk is learned from others and becomes a part of us as we grow up. It comes in many forms, unfortunately mostly negative.

Negative self-statements are usually in the form of phrases that begin with something like "I just can't do . . . ," "If only I could . . . ," "If only I didn't . . . ," "I just don't have the energy . . . ," or "How could I be so stupid?" This type of negative thinking represents the doubts and fears we have about ourselves in general and about our abilities to deal with our condition and its symptoms. It damages our self-esteem, attitude, and mood. Negative self-talk makes us feel bad and makes our symptoms worse.

What we say to ourselves plays a major role in determining our success or failure in becoming good self-managers. Negative thinking tends to limit our abilities and actions. If we tell ourselves "I'm not very smart" or "I can't" all the time, we probably won't try to learn new skills because this just doesn't fit with what we think about ourselves. Soon we become prisoners of our own negative beliefs. Fortunately, self-talk is not something fixed in our biological makeup, and therefore it is not completely out of our control. We can learn new, healthier ways to think about ourselves so that our self-talk can work for us instead of against us. By changing the negative, self-defeating statements to positive ones, we can manage symptoms more effectively. This change, like any habit, requires practice and includes the following steps:

1. **Listen carefully to what you say to or about yourself, both out loud and silently.** If you find yourself feeling anxious, depressed, or angry, try to identify some of the thoughts you were having just before these feelings started. Then write down all the negative self-talk statements. Pay special attention to the things you say during times that are particularly difficult for you. For example, what do you say to yourself when getting up in the morning with pain, while doing those exercises you don't really like, or at those times when you are feeling blue? Challenge these negative thoughts by asking yourself questions to identify what about the statement is really true or not true. For example, are you exaggerating the situation, generalizing, worrying too much, or assuming the worst? Are you thinking in terms of black and white? Could there be gray? Maybe you are making an unrealistic or unfair comparison, assuming too much responsibility, taking something too personally, or expecting perfection. Are you making assumptions about what other people think about you? What do you know for a fact? Look at the evidence so that you are better able to change these negative thoughts and statements.

2. **Next, work on changing each negative statement to a more positive one, or find some positive statement to replace the negative one.** Write these down. For example, negative statements such as "I don't want to get up," "I'm too tired and I hurt," "I can't do the things I like anymore, so why bother?" or "I'm good for nothing" become positive messages such as "I'm feeling pretty good today, and I'm going to do something I enjoy," "I may not be able to do everything I used to, but there are still a lot of things I

can do," "People like me, and I feel good about myself," or "Other people need and depend on me; I'm worthwhile."

3. **Read and rehearse these positive statements, mentally or with another person.** It is this conscious repetition or memorization of the positive self-talk that will help you replace those old, habitual negative statements.

4. **Practice these new statements in real situations.** This practice, along with time and patience, will help the new patterns of thinking become automatic.

5. **Rehearse success.** When you aren't happy with the way you handled a particular situation, try this exercise:

   • Write down three ways that it could have gone better.

   • Write down three ways it could have gone worse.

   • If you can't think of alternatives to the way you handled it, imagine what someone whom you greatly respect would have done.

   • Or think what advice you would give to someone else facing a similar situation.

Remember that mistakes aren't failures. They're good opportunities to learn. Mistakes give you the chance to rehearse other ways of handling things. This is great practice for future crises.

As you first do this, you may find it hard to change negative statements into more positive ones. A shortcut is to use either a thought stopper or a positive affirmation. A thought stopper can be anything that is meaningful to you. For example, a puppy, a polar bear, or a redwood tree. When you have a negative thought, replace it with your thought stopper. We know it sounds silly, but try it.

A positive affirmation is a positive phrase that you can use over and over. For example, "I am getting better every day" or "I can do this" or "God loves me." Again, you use this to replace negative thoughts.

Imagery

You may think that "imagination" is all in your mind. But the thoughts, words, and images that flow from your imagination can have very real affects on your body. Your brain often cannot distinguish whether you are imagining something or if it is really happening. Perhaps you've had a racing heartbeat, rapid breathing, or tension in your neck muscles while watching a movie thriller. These sensations were all produced by images and sounds on a film. During a dream, maybe your body responded with fear, joy, anger, or sadness—all triggered by your imagination. If you close your eyes and vividly imagine yourself by a still, quiet pool or relaxing on a warm beach, your body responds to some degree as though you were actually there.

Guided imagery and visualization allow you to use your imagination to relieve symptoms. These techniques will help you focus your thoughts on healing images and suggestions.

Guided Imagery

This tool is like a guided daydream. It allows you to divert your attention, refocusing your mind away from your symptoms and transporting you to another time and place. It has the added benefit of helping you achieve deep relaxation by picturing yourself in a peaceful environment.

With guided imagery, you focus your mind on a particular image. Imagery usually involves your sense of sight, focusing on visual images. Adding other senses—smells, tastes, and sounds—makes the guided imagery even more vivid and powerful.

Some people are highly visual and easily see images with their "mind's eye." But if your images aren't as vivid as scenes from a great movie, don't worry; it's normal for the intensity of imagery to vary. The important thing is to focus on as much detail as possible and to strengthen the images by using all your senses. Adding real background music can also increase the impact of guided imagery.

With guided imagery, you are always completely in control. You're the movie director. You can project whatever thought or feeling you want onto your mental screen. If you don't like a particular image, thought, or feeling, you can redirect your mind to something more comfortable; you can use other images to get rid of unpleasant thoughts (for example, you might put them on a raft and watch them float away, sweep them away with a large broom, or erase them with a giant eraser); or you can open your eyes and stop the exercise.

The guided imagery scripts presented on pages 78 and 79 can help take you on this mental stroll. Here are some ways to use imagery:

- Read the script over several times until it is familiar. Then sit or lie down in a quiet place and try to reconstruct the scene in your mind. The script should take 15 to 20 minutes to complete.

- Have a family member or friend read you the script slowly, pausing for about 10 seconds wherever there is a series of periods (. . .).

- Make a recording of the script, and play it to yourself whenever convenient.

- Use a prerecorded tape, CD, or digital audio file that has a similar guided imagery script (see examples in the "Other Resources" section at end of this chapter).

Visualization

This technique is similar to guided imagery. Visualization allows you to create your own images, which is different from guided imagery, where the images are suggested to you. It is another way of using your imagination to create a picture of yourself in any way you want, doing the things you want to do. All of us use a form of visualization every day—when we dream, worry, read a book, or listen to a story. In all these activities the mind creates images for us to see. We also use visualization intentionally when making plans for the day, considering the possible outcomes of a decision we have to make, or rehearsing for an event or activity. Visualization can be done in different ways and can be used for longer periods of time or while you are engaged in other activities.

One way to use visualization to manage symptoms is to remember pleasant scenes from your past or create new scenes. To practice visualization, try to remember every detail of a special holiday or party that made you happy. Who was there? What happened? What did you do or talk about? You can also try this by remembering a vacation or some other memorable and pleasant event.

Visualization can be used to plan the details of some future event or to fill in the details of a fantasy. For example, how would you spend a million dollars? What would be your ideal romantic encounter? What would your ideal home or garden look like? Where would you go and what would you do on your dream vacation? Another form of visualization involves using your mind to think of symbols that represent the discomfort or pain felt in different parts of your body. For example, a painful joint might be red or a tight chest might have a constricting band around it. After forming these images, you then try to change them. The red color might fade until there is no more color, or the constricting band will stretch and stretch until it falls off; these new images then cause the way you think of the pain or discomfort to change.

Visualization helps build confidence and skill and therefore is a useful technique to help you set and accomplish your personal goals (see Chapter 2). After you write your weekly action plan, take a few minutes to imagine yourself taking a walk, doing your exercises, or taking your medications. You are mentally rehearsing the steps you need to take in order to achieve your goal successfully.

Imagery for Different Conditions

You have the ability to create special imagery to help (though not cure) specific symptoms or illnesses. Use any image that is strong and vivid for you—this often involves using all your senses to create the image—and one that is meaningful to you. The image does not have to be accurate for it to work. Just use your imagination and trust yourself. Here are examples of images that some people have found useful:

For Tension and Stress

A tight, twisted rope slowly untwists.

Wax softens and melts.

Tension swirls out of your body and down the drain.

For Healing of Cuts and Injuries

Plaster covers over a crack in a wall.

Cells and fibers stick together with very strong glue.

A shoe is laced up tight.

Jigsaw puzzle pieces come together.

For Arteries and Heart Disease

A miniature Roto-Rooter truck speeds through your arteries and cleans out the clogged pipes.

Water flows freely through a wide, open river.

A crew in a small boat rows in sync, easily and efficiently pulling the slender boat across the smooth water surface.

For Asthma and Lung Disease

The tiny elastic rubber bands that constrict your airways pop open.

A vacuum cleaner gently sucks the mucus from your airways.

Waves calmly rise and fall on the ocean surface.

For Diabetes

Small insulin keys unlock doors to hungry cells and allow nourishing blood sugar in.

An alarm goes off, and a sleeping pancreas gland awakens to the smell of freshly brewed coffee.

For Cancer

A shark gobbles up the cancer cells.

Tumors shrivel up like raisins in the hot sun and then evaporate completely into the air.

The faucet that controls the blood supply to the tumor is turned off, and the cancer cells starve.

Radiation or chemotherapy enters your body like healing rays of light and destroy cancer cells.

For Infections

White blood cells with flashing red sirens arrest and imprison harmful germs.

An army equipped with powerful antibiotic missiles attacks enemy germs.

A hot flame chases germs out of your entire body.

For a Weakened Immune System

Sluggish, sleepy white blood cells awaken, put on protective armor, and enter the fight against the virus.

White blood cells rapidly multiply like millions of seeds bursting from a single ripe seed pod.

For an Overactive Immune System (allergies, arthritis, psoriasis, etc.)

Overly alert immune cells in the fire station are reassured that the allergens have triggered a false alarm, and they go back to playing their game of poker.

The civil war ends with the warring sides agreeing not to attack their fellow citizens.

For Pain

All of the pain is placed in a large, strong metal box that is closed, sealed tightly and locked with a huge, strong padlock.

You grasp the TV remote control and slowly turn down the pain volume until you can barely hear it; then it disappears entirely.

The pain is washed away by a cool, calm river flowing through your entire body.

For Depression

Your troubles and feelings of sadness are attached to big colorful helium balloons and are floating off into a clear blue sky.

A strong, warm sun breaks through dark clouds.

You feel a sense of detachment and lightness, enabling you to float easily through your day.

Use any of these images, or make up your own. Remember, the best ones are vivid and have meaning to you. Use your imagination for health and healing.

Guided-Imagery Script: A Walk in the Country

You're giving yourself some time to quiet your mind and body. Allow yourself to settle comfortably, wherever you are right now. If you wish, you can close your eyes. Breathe in deeply, through your nose, expanding your abdomen and filling your lungs; and, pursing your lips, exhale through your mouth slowly and completely, allowing your body to sink heavily into the surface beneath you . . . And once again breathe in through your nose and all the way down to your abdomen, and then breathe out slowly through pursed lips—letting go of tension, letting go of anything that's on your mind right now and just allowing yourself to be present in this moment . . .

Imagine yourself walking along a peaceful old country road. The sun is gently warming your back . . . the birds are singing . . . the air is calm and fragrant . . .

With no need to hurry, you notice your walking is relaxed and easy. As you walk along in this way, taking in your surroundings, you come across an old gate. It looks inviting and you decide to take the path through the gate. The gate creaks as you open it and go through.

You find yourself in an old, overgrown garden—flowers growing where they've seeded themselves, vines climbing over a fallen tree, soft green wild grasses, shade trees.

You notice yourself breathing deeply . . . smelling the flowers . . . listening to the birds and insects . . . feeling a gentle breeze cool against your skin. All of your senses are alive and responding with pleasure to this peaceful time and place . . .

When you're ready to move on, you leisurely follow the path out behind the garden, eventually coming to a more wooded area. As you enter this area, your eyes find the trees and plant life restful. The sunlight is filtered through the leaves. The air feels mild and a little cooler… You savor the fragrance of trees and earth… and gradually become aware of the sound of a nearby stream. Pausing, you allow yourself to take in the sights and sounds, breathing in the cool and fragrant air several times . . . And with each breath, you notice how refreshed you are feeling…

Continuing along the path for a while, you come to the stream. It's clear and clean as it flows and tumbles over the rocks and some fallen logs. You follow the path easily along the creek for a way, and after awhile, you come out into a sunlit clearing, where you discover a small waterfall emptying into a quiet pool of water.

You find a comfortable place to sit for a while, a perfect niche where you can feel completely relaxed.

You feel good as you allow yourself to just enjoy the warmth and solitude of this peaceful place…

After awhile, you become aware that it is time to return. You arise and walk back down the path in a relaxed and comfortable way, through the cool and fragrant trees, out into the sun-drenched overgrown garden . . . One last smell of the flowers, and out the creaky gate.

You leave this country retreat for now and return down the road. You notice you feel calm and rested. You feel grateful and remind yourself that you can visit this special place whenever you wish to take some time to refresh yourself and renew your energy.

And now, preparing to bring this period of relaxation to a close, you may want to take a moment to picture yourself carrying this experience of calm and refreshment with you into the ordinary activities of your life . . . And when you're ready, take a nice deep breath and open your eyes.

Guided-Imagery Script: A Walk on the Beach

Begin by getting into a comfortable position, whether you are seated or lying down. Loosen any tight clothing to allow yourself to be as comfortable as possible. Uncross your legs and allow your hands to fall by your sides or rest in your lap, and if you are at all uncomfortable shift to a more comfortable position.

When you are ready, you may allow your eyes gradually to close and turn your attention to your breathing. Allow your belly to expand as you breathe in, bringing in fresh new air to nourish your body. And then breathing out. Notice the rhythm of your breathing—in . . . and out . . . without trying to control it in any way at all. Simply attend to the natural rhythm of your breath . . .

And now in your mind's eye, imagine yourself standing on a beautiful beach. The sky is a brilliant blue, and as some fluffy white clouds float slowly by, you drink in the beautiful colors . . . The temperature is not too hot and not too cold. The sun is shining, and you close your eyes, allowing the warmth of the sun to wash over you . . . You notice a gentle breeze caressing your face, the perfect complement to the sunshine.

Then you find yourself turn turning and looking out over the vastness of the ocean . . . you become aware of the sound of the waves gently washing up on shore . . . You notice the firmness of the wet sand beneath your feet, or If you decide to take off your shoes, you may enjoy the feeling of standing, in the cool, wet sand . . . perhaps you allow the surf roll up and gently wash across your feet, or perhaps you stay just out of its reach…

In the distance you hear some seagulls calling to one another and look out to see the birds gracefully gliding through the air. And as you stand there, notice how easy it is to be here, perhaps noticing some sensations of relaxation, comfort, or peace—whatever's there . . .

Now take a walk along the shore. Turn and begin to stroll casually along the beach, enjoying the sounds of the surf, the warmth of the sun, and the gentle massage of the breeze. As you move along, taking your time, your stride becomes lighter, easier . . . you notice the scent of the ocean . . . you pause to take in the freshness of the air . . . And then you continue on your way, enjoying the peacefulness of this place.

After a time, you decide to rest a while, and find a comfortable place to sit or lie down . . . and simply allow yourself to take some time to enjoy this, your special place . . .

And now, when you feel ready to return, you stand and begin walking back down the beach in a comfortable, leisurely way, taking with you any sensations of relaxation, comfort, peace, joy—Whatever's there . . . Noticing how easy it is to be here. Continuing back until you reach the place where you began your walk . . .

And now pausing to take one last long look around. Enjoying the vibrant colors of the sky and the sea . . . The gentle sound of the waves washing up on the shore. The warmth of the sun, the cool of the breeze . . .

And as you prepare to leave this special place, taking with you any sensations of joy, relaxation, comfort, peace, whatever's there. Knowing that you may return at any time appropriate time and place of your choosing.

And now bringing your awareness back into the room, focusing on your breathing . . . in and out . . . Taking a few more breaths . . . and when you're ready, opening your eyes.

Prayer and Spirituality

There is strong evidence in the medical literature of the relationship between spirituality and health. According to the American Academy of Family Physicians,* spirituality is the way we can find meaning, hope, comfort, and inner peace in our lives. Many people find spirituality through religion. Some find it through music, art, or a connection with nature. Others find it in their values and principles.

Many people are religious and share their religion with others. Others do not have a specific religion but do have spiritual beliefs. Our religion and beliefs can bring a sense of meaning and purpose to our life, help us put things into perspective, and set priorities. Our beliefs may help us find comfort during difficult times. They can help us with acceptance and motivate us to make difficult changes. Being part of a spiritual or religious community offers a source of support when needed and the opportunity to help others.

Recent studies find that people who belong to a religious or spiritual community or who regularly engage in religious activities, such as prayer or study, have improved health. There are many types of prayer--any of which may contribute to improved health: asking for help, direction, forgiveness, offering words of gratitude, praising, and blessing, among others. In addition, many religions have a tradition of contemplation or meditation. Prayer does not need a scientific explanation. It is probably the oldest of all self-management tools.

Although religion and spirituality cannot be "prescribed," we encourage you to explore your own beliefs. If you are religious, try practicing prayer more consistently. Also, if you are religious, consider telling your doctor and care team. Most won't ask. Help them understand the importance of your beliefs in managing your health and life. Most hospitals have chaplains or pastoral counselors. Even if you are not in the hospital, they will probably talk with you. Choose someone you feel comfortable with. Their advice and counsel can supplement your medical and psychological care.

---

*Adapted or reprinted with permission from "Spirituality and Medical Practice: Using the HOPE Questions as a Practical Tool for Spiritual Assessment," January 1, 2001, Vol 63, No 1, *American Family Physician* Copyright © 2001 American Academy of Family Physicians. All Rights Reserved.

Other Techniques That Use Your Mind

There additional valuable techniques you can consider which can clear your mind, positively shift your emotional state, as well as reduce tension and stress.

Mindfulness

Mindfulness involves simply keeping your attention in the present moment, without judging it as happy or sad, good or bad. It encourages living each moment—even painful ones—as fully and as mindfully as possible. Mindfulness is more than a relaxation technique; it is an attitude toward living. It is a way of calmly and consciously observing and accepting whatever is happening, moment to moment.

This may sound simple enough, but our restless, judging minds make it surprisingly difficult. As a restless monkey jumps from branch to branch, our mind jumps from thought to thought.

In mindfulness, you focus the mind on the present moment. The "goal" of mindfulness is simply to observe—with no intention of changing or improving anything. But people are positively changed by the practice. Observing and accepting life just as it is, with all its pleasures, pains, frustrations, disappointments, and insecurities, often enables you to become calmer, more confident, and better able to cope with whatever comes along.

To develop your capacity for mindfulness, sit comfortably on the floor or on a chair with your back, neck and head straight, but not stiff. Then:

- Concentrate on a single object, such as your breathing. Focus your attention on the feeling of the air as it passes in and out of your nostrils with each breath. Don't try to control your breathing by speeding it up or slowing it down. Just observe it as it is.

- Even when you resolve to keep your attention on your breathing, your mind will quickly wander off. When this occurs, observe where your mind went: perhaps to a memory, a worry about the future, a bodily ache, or a feeling of impatience. Then gently return your attention to your breathing.

- Use your breath as an anchor. Each time a thought or feeling arises, momentarily

acknowledge it. Don't analyze it or judge it. Just observe it, and return to your breathing.

- Let go of all thoughts of getting somewhere, or having anything special happen. Just keep stringing moments of mindfulness together, breath by breath.

- At first, practice this for just five minutes, or even one minute at a time. You may wish to gradually extend the time to ten, twenty or thirty minutes.

Because the practice of mindfulness is simply the practice of moment-to-moment awareness, you can apply it to anything: eating, showering, working, talking, running errands, or playing with your children. Mindfulness takes no extra time. Considerable research has demonstrated the benefits of mindfulness practice in relieving stress, easing pain, improving concentration, and relieving a variety of other symptoms.

Quieting Reflex

This technique was developed by a physician named Charles Stroebel. It will help you deal with short-term stress such as the urge to eat or smoke, road rage, or other annoyances. It relieves muscle tightening, jaw clenching, and holding your breath by activating the sympathetic nervous system.

It should be practiced frequently throughout the day, whenever you start to feel stressed. It can be done with your eyes opened or closed.

1. Become aware of what is annoying you: a ringing phone, an angry comment, the urge to smoke, a worrisome thought—whatever.

2. Repeat the phrase "Alert mind, calm body" to yourself.

3. Smile inwardly with your eyes and your mouth. This stops facial muscles from making a fearful or angry expression. The inward smile is a feeling. It cannot be seen by others.

4. Inhale slowly to the count of 3, imagining that the breath comes in through the bottom of your feet. Then exhale slowly. Feel your breath move back down your legs and out through your feet. Let your jaw, tongue, and shoulder muscles go limp.

With several months' practice the quieting reflex becomes an automatic skill.

Nature Therapy

Many of us suffer from what has been called "nature deficit disorder," but it can be readily cured with regular doses of the outdoors. For thousands of years exposure to natural environments has been recommended for healing. Taking a break from artificial lighting, excessive computer and TV screen time, and indoor environments can be restorative. A brief walk in a park or a longer planned visit to a beautiful outdoor environment can restore the mind and body. Or bring nature indoors with plants, pets, and nature photography. Even a few minutes of playing with or stroking a pet can lower blood pressure and calm a restless mind.

Worry Time

Worrisome negative thoughts feed anxiety. Ignored problems have a way of thrusting themselves back into our consciousness. You'll find it easier to set aside worries if you make time to deal with them.

Set aside 20 to 30 minutes a day as your "worry time." Whenever a worry pops into your mind, write it down and tell yourself that you'll deal with it during worry time. Jot down the little things (Did Linda take her lunch to school?) along with the big ones (Will our children be able to find jobs?). During your scheduled worry time, don't do anything except worry, brainstorm, and write down possible solutions. For each of your worries, ask yourself the following questions:

■ What is the problem?

■ How likely is it that the problem will occur?

■ What's the worst that could happen?

■ What's the best that could happen?

■ How would I cope with the problem?

■ What are possible solutions?

■ What is my plan of action?

Be specific. Instead of worrying about what might happen if you lose your job, ask yourself how likely it is that you will lose your job. And if you do, what will you do, with whom, and by when? Write a job search plan.

If you're anxious about getting seasick on the ocean and not making it to the bathroom in time, imagine how you would manage the situation. Ask yourself if any of this is really unbearable. Tell yourself you might feel uncomfortable or embarrassed, but you'll survive.

Remember, if a new worry pops up during the rest of the day, jot it down. Then distract yourself by refocusing intently on whatever you are doing.

Scheduling a definite worry time cuts the amount of time spent worrying by at least a third. If you look at your list of worries later, you'll find that the vast majority of them never materialized. Or they were not nearly as bad as you had anticipated.

A Healthy Perspective

Sometimes you can relieve stress and break the cycle of negative thoughts by shifting your perspective. If you find yourself upset, ask, "How important will this be in an hour, a day, a month, or a year?" This reframing often helps surface things that are really important and need action versus the more minor annoyances that capture our attention.

Practice Gratitude

One of the most effective ways to improve your mood and overall happiness is by focusing your attention on what's going well in your life. For what are you grateful? Psychologists have done research to demonstrate that people can increase their happiness by gratitude exercises. We encourage you to try these three:

- **Write a letter of thanks.** Write and then deliver a letter of gratitude to someone who had been especially kind to you but had never been properly thanked. Perhaps it's a teacher, a mentor, a friend, or a family member. Express your appreciation for the person's kindness. The letter will have more impact if you include some specific examples of what the recipient has done for you. Describe how the actions made you feel. Ideally, read your letter out loud to the person, if possible, face-to-face. Be aware of how you feel, and watch the other person's reaction.

- **Acknowledge at least three good things every day.** Each night before bed, write down at least three things that went well today. No event or feeling is too small to note. By putting your gratitude into words, you increase appreciation and memory of your blessings. Knowing that you will need to write each night changes your mental filters during the whole day. You will tend to seek out, look for, and specially note the good things that happen. If doing this daily is too much or begins to seem like a routine chore, do it once a week.

- **Make a list of the things you take for granted.** For example, if your chronic illness has affected your lungs, you can still be grateful that your kidneys are working. Perhaps you can celebrate a day in which you don't have a headache or backache. Counting your blessings can add up to a better mood and more happiness.

Compile a List of Strengths

Make a personal inventory of your talents, skills, achievements, and qualities, big and small. Celebrate your accomplishments. When something goes wrong, consult your list of positives, and put the problem in perspective. It then becomes just one specific experience, not something that defines your whole life.

Put Kindness into Practice

This world is plagued by acts of violence. When something bad happens, it's front-page news. As an antidote to this misery, despair, and cynicism, practice acts of kindness. Look for opportunities to give without expecting anything in return. Here are some examples:

- Hold the door open for the person behind you.

- Give an unexpected gift of movie or concert tickets.

- Send an anonymous gift to a friend who needs cheering up.

- Help someone with a heavy load.

- Tell positive stories you know of helping and kindness.

- Cultivate an attitude of gratefulness for the kindness you have received.

- Plant a tree.

- Smile and let people cut ahead of you in line or on the freeway.

- Pick up litter.

- Give another driver your parking space.

Be creative. Such kindness is contagious, and it has a ripple effect. In one study, the people who were given an unexpected treat (cookies) were later more likely to help others.

Write Away Stress

It's hard work to keep our deep negative feelings hidden. Over time, this cumulative stress undermines our body's defenses and seems to weaken our immunity. Confiding our feelings to others or writing them down puts them into words and helps us sort them out. Words help us understand and absorb a traumatic event and eventually put it behind us. It gives us a sense of release and control.

The psychologist Jamie Pennebaker described in his book *Opening Up* a series of studies looked at the healing effects of confiding or writing. One group was asked to express their deepest thoughts and feelings about something bad that had happened to them. Another group wrote about ordinary matters such as their plans for the day. Both groups wrote for 15 to 20 minutes a day for 3 to 5 consecutive days. No one read what either group had written.

The results were surprisingly powerful. When compared with the people who wrote about ordinary events, the ones who wrote about their bad experiences reported fewer symptoms, fewer visits to the doctor, fewer days off from work, improved mood, and a more positive outlook. Their immune function was enhanced for at least 6 weeks after writing. This was especially true for those who expressed previously undisclosed painful feelings.

Try the "write thing" when something is bothering you: when you find yourself thinking (or dreaming) too much about an experience; when you avoid thinking about something because it is too upsetting; when there's something you would like to tell others but don't for fear of embarrassment or punishment.

Here are some guidelines for writing as a way to help you deal with any traumatic experience:

- Set a specific schedule for writing. For example, you might write 15 minutes a day for 4 consecutive days, or 1 day a week for 4 weeks.

- Write in a place where you won't be interrupted or distracted.

- Don't plan to share your writing—that could stop your honest expression. Save what you write or destroy it, as you wish.

- Explore your very deepest thoughts and feelings and analyze why you feel the way you do. Write about your negative feelings such as sadness, hurt, hate, anger, fear, guilt, or resentment.

- Write continuously. Don't worry about grammar, spelling, or making sense. If clarity and coherence come as you continue to write, so much the better. If you run out of things to say, just repeat what you have already written.

- Even if you find the writing awkward at first, keep going. It gets easier. If you just cannot write, try talking into a tape recorder for 15 minutes about your deepest thoughts and feelings.

- Don't expect to feel better immediately. You may feel sad or depressed when your deepest feelings begin to surface. This usually fades within an hour or two or a day or two. The overwhelming majority of people report feelings of relief, happiness, and contentment soon after writing for a few consecutive days.

- Writing may help you clarify what actions you need to take. But don't use writing as

a substitute for taking action or as a way of avoiding things.

Once established, relaxation, imagery, and positive thinking can be some of the most powerful tools you can add to your self-management tool box. They will help you manage symptoms as well as master the other skills discussed in this book.

As with exercise and other acquired skills, using your mind to manage your health condition requires both practice and time before you begin to notice the benefits. So if you feel you are not accomplishing anything, don't give up. Be patient and keep on trying.

Suggested Further Reading

Ben-Shahar, Tal. *Happier: Learn the Secrets to Daily Joy and Lasting Fulfillment.* New York: McGraw-Hill, 2007.

Benson, Herbert, and Miriam Z. Klipper. *The Relaxation Response.* San Francisco: Quill, 2000.

Benson, Herbert, and Eileen M. Stuart. *The Wellness Book: The Comprehensive Guide to Maintaining Health and Treating Stress-Related Illness.* New York: Fireside, 1993.

Borysenko, Joan. *Inner Peace for Busy People: 52 Simple Strategies for Transforming Your Life.* Carlsbad, Calif.: Hay House, 2003.

Boroson, Martin. *One Moment Meditation.* New York: Winter Road Publishing, 2009.

Burns, David D. *The Feeling Good Handbook,* rev. ed. New York: Plume, 1999.

Caudill, Margaret. *Managing Pain Before It Manages You.* New York: Guilford Press, 2008.

Cousins, Norman. *Head First: The Biology of Hope and the Healing Power of the Human Spirit.* New York: Dutton, 1990.

Craze, Richard. *Teach Yourself Relaxation,* 3rd ed. New York: McGraw-Hill, 2009.

Davis, Martha, Elizabeth Eshelman, and Matthew McKay. *The Relaxation and Stress Reduction Workbook.* Oakland, Calif.: New Harbinger, 2008.

Diener, Ed, and Robert Biswas-Diener. *Happiness: Unlocking the Mysteries of Psychological Wealth.* Malden, Mass.: Blackwell, 2008.

Dossey, Larry. *Prayer Is Good Medicine.* San Francisco: HarperCollins, 1996.

Emmons, Robert A. *Thanks! How the New Science of Gratitude Can Make You Happier.* New York: Houghton Mifflin, 2007.

Funk, Mary Margaret. *Tools Matter for Practicing the Spiritual Life.* New York: Continuum, 2004.

Grenville-Cleave. *Introducing Positive Psychology: A Practical Guide.* London: Totem Books/Icon Books, 2012

Kabat-Zinn, Jon. *Coming to Our Senses: Healing Ourselves and the World Through Mindfulness.* New York: Hyperion, 2005.

Kabat-Zinn, Jon. *Full Catastrophe Living: Using the Wisdom of Your Body and Mind to Face Stress, Pain, and Illness.* New York: Delta, 2005.

Kabat-Zinn, Jon. *Wherever You Go, There You Are: Mindfulness Meditation in Everyday Life.* New York: Hyperion, 2005.

Keating, Thomas. *Open Mind, Open Heart: The Contemplative Dimension of the Gospel.* New York: Continuum, 2006.

Keating, Thomas, and Gustave Reininger, eds. *Centering Prayer in Daily Life and Ministry.* New York: Continuum, 1998.

Lyubomirsky, Sonia. *The How of Happiness: A New Approach to Getting the Life You Want.* New York: Penguin, 2008.

McKay, Matthew, Martha Davis, and Patrick Fanning. *Thoughts and Feelings: Taking Control of Your Moods and Your Life,* 4th ed. Oakland, Calif.: New Harbinger, 2007.

Ornstein, Robert, and David Sobel. *Healthy Pleasures.* Cambridge, Mass.: Perseus, 1989.

Peale, Norman V. *Positive Imaging: The Powerful Way to Change Your Life.* New York: Ballantine Books, 1996.Remen, Rachel Naomi. *Kitchen Table Wisdom: Stories That Heal.* New York: Riverhead Books, 2006.

Seligman, Martin. *Authentic Happiness.* New York: Free Press, 2004.

Seligman, Martin. *Flourish: A Visionary New Understanding of Happiness and Well-Being.* New York: Free Press, 2011.

Siegel, Bernie S. *Help Me to Heal: A Practical Guidebook for Patients, Visitors, and Caregivers.* Carlsbad, Calif.: Hay House, 2003.

Sobel, David, and Robert Ornstein. *The Healthy Mind, Healthy Body Handbook* (also published under the title *The Mind and Body Health Handbook*). Los Altos, Calif.: DRX, 1996.

Stahl, Bob, and Elisha Goldstein. *A Mindfulness-Based Stress Reduction Workbook.* Oakland, Calif.: New Harbinger, 2010.

Wiseman, Richard. *59 Seconds: Think a Little, Change a Lot.* New York: Borzoi Books, 2009.

Other Resources

- ☐ Association of Cancer Online Resources (ACOR): http://www.acor.org/
- ☐ Greater Good Science Center: http://greatergood.berkeley.edu/
- ☐ The Happiness Project: http://www.happiness-project.com/
- ☐ Mental Health America, Live Your Life Well: http://www.liveyourlifewell.org/
- ☐ Naparstek, Belleruth. *Health Journeys Guided Imagery* [audio CDs]: http://www.healthjourneys.com/
- ☐ National Institute of Mental Health: http://www.nimh.nih.gov/
- ☐ Regan, Catherine. and Rick Seidel. *Relaxation for Mind and Body: Pathways to Healing* [audio CD]. Boulder, Colo.: Bull, 2012.
- ☐ StressStop: http://www.stressstop.com/
- ☐ Weil, Andrew, and Martin Rossman. *Self-Healing with Guided Imagery* [audio CD]. Louisville, Colo.: Sounds True, 2006.

The weakest and oldest among us can become some sort of athlete, but only the strongest can survive as spectators. Only the hardiest can withstand the perils of inertia, inactivity, and immobility.

—J. H. Bland and S. M. Cooper,
Seminars in Arthritis and Rheumatism (1984)

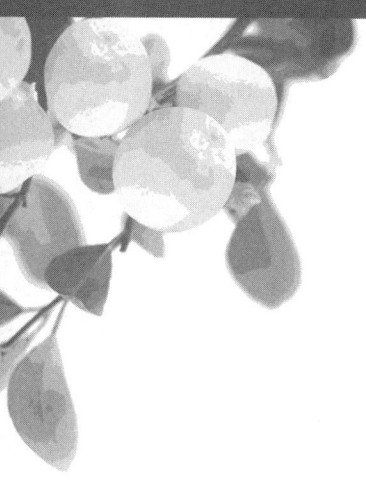

CHAPTER **6**

Exercise and Physical Activity for Every Body

ACTIVE PEOPLE ARE HEALTHIER AND HAPPIER than people who are not. This is true for all ages and conditions. Not moving enough can even cause or worsen illness.

You probably hear that regular physical activity is important, but if you have a chronic health problem, you may not know what to do or worry that you will do the wrong thing. Just 30 years ago, if you had arthritis, diabetes, or lung disease, it was hard to learn how to exercise. Now there is a lot of information. We will help you get started and be successful. Many countries have public health programs to help people understand the importance of physical activity and offer programs to get going. There are guidelines for children, young and older adults, people with chronic illness, and people with disabilities. These guidelines spell out what kinds of exercise or physical activities are best and how much you need. In this and the following three chapters, you will learn about these guidelines and learn about wise exercise choices. Of course, learning is not enough. It is up to you to make your life more enjoyable, comfortable, and healthier through physical activity. This advice is not intended to take the place of medical advice. If you have a prescribed exercise plan that differs from the suggestions here, take this book to your doctor or therapist and ask what she or he thinks about this program. We provide additional information and helpful exercise ideas for people with specific chronic illnesses in each of the chapters about those conditions.

Why Exercise?

Regular exercise can prevent or manage heart disease and diabetes. It improves blood pressure, blood sugar, and blood fat levels. Exercise can help maintain a good weight, which takes stress off weight-bearing joints. Exercise is also part of keeping bones strong and treating osteoporosis. There is evidence that regular exercise can help prevent blood clots, which is one of the reasons exercise can be of particular benefit to people with heart and vascular diseases. Regular exercise improves levels of strength, energy, and self-confidence and lessens feelings of stress, anxiety, and depression. Regular exercise can help you sleep better and feel more relaxed and happy.

In addition, strong muscles help people with arthritis protect their joints by improving stability and absorbing shock. Regular exercise also helps nourish joints and keeps cartilage and bone healthy. Regular exercise has been shown to help people with chronic lung disease improve endurance (and reduce trips to the emergency room). Many people with leg pain from poor circulation can walk farther and more comfortably with a regular exercise program. Studies of people with heart disease show that exercise improves heart health and quality of life.

The good news is that it doesn't take hours of painful, sweat-soaked exercise to achieve health benefits. Even short periods of moderate physical activity can improve health and fitness, reduce disease risks, and boost your mood. Being active also helps you feel more in control of your life and less at the mercy of your chronic illness. You don't have to kill yourself to save your life!

Developing an Exercise Program

For most people who are not already active, starting a regular exercise program means making a new habit or routine in your life. This usually involves setting aside a period of time on most days of the week to make exercise a part of your day. Exercise programs that are recommended in guidelines today talk about four types of fitness:

- **Flexibility.** Being flexible means you can move comfortably to do everything you need and want to do. Limited flexibility can cause pain, lead to injury, and make muscles work harder and tire more quickly. You lose flexibility when you are inactive and as a result of some diseases, but you can increase flexibility by doing gentle stretching exercises like those described in Chapter 7.

■ **Strength.** Muscles need to be exercised to maintain their strength. When inactive, muscles weaken and atrophy (shrink). When your muscles get weak, you feel weak and get tired quickly. Much of the disability and lack of mobility for people with chronic illness is due to muscle weakness. Exercise programs that ask muscles to do more work (such as lifting a weight) strengthen muscles.

■ **Endurance (aerobics).** Feeling energetic depends on the fitness of your heart, lungs, and muscles. The heart and lungs must work efficiently to send oxygen-rich blood to the muscles. The muscles must be fit enough to use the oxygen. Aerobic ("with oxygen") exercise uses the large muscles of your body in continuous activity such as walking, swimming, dancing, mowing the lawn, and riding a bike. Aerobic exercise improves cardiovascular fitness, lessens heart attack risk, and helps control weight. Aerobic exercise also promotes a sense of well-being, eases depression and anxiety, promotes restful sleep, and improves mood and energy levels.

■ **Balance.** Good balance helps keep you from falling. Strong and coordinated muscles in your trunk and legs are an important part of good balance. Flexibility, strength, and endurance also contribute to balance. Of course, there are other causes of falls (poor vision, poor lighting, tripping over rugs, getting dizzy), but being strong and coordinated are also very important. Certain exercises are especially good for improving balance.

Your Exercise Program

A complete program combines exercises to improve all four aspects of fitness: flexibility, strength, endurance, and balance. Chapter 7 shows you a number of flexibility and strengthening exercises and includes specific exercises for your posture and balance. Chapter 8 explains and gives examples of aerobic exercise for improving endurance. If you haven't exercised regularly in some time or have pain, stiffness, shortness of breath, or weakness that interferes with your daily activities, discuss exercise with your health care providers. Begin your exercise program by choosing some flexibility and strengthening exercises that you are willing to do every other day. Once you are able to exercise comfortably for at least 10 minutes at a time, you are ready to start adding some endurance or aerobic activities.

You may wonder how to choose the right exercises. The truth is that the best exercises for you are the ones that will help you do what you want to do. Often the most important decision to start a successful exercise program is to choose a goal (something you want to do) that exercise can help you reach. For example, climb 17 stairs so you can visit a special friend. Once you have a goal in mind, it is much easier to choose exercises that make sense to you. There is no doubt that we are all more successful exercisers if we know where we want exercise to take us. If you don't see how exercise can be helpful to you, it is hard to get excited about adding yet another task to your day.

Choose Your Goal and Make a Plan

1. **Choose something that you want to do but don't do now because of some physical reason.** For example, you might want to enjoy a shopping or fishing trip with your friends, mow the lawn, or take a family vacation.

2. **Think about why you don't do it or don't enjoy doing it now.** It might be that you get tired before everybody else, that it's too hard to get up from a low chair or bench, that climbing steps is painful or makes your legs tired, or that your shoulders are too weak or stiff to cast your fishing line or stow a carry-on bag.

3. **Decide what it is that makes it hard to do what you want.** For example, if getting up from a low seat is difficult, it may be that your hips or knees are stiff and your leg muscles are weak. In this case, look for flexibility and strengthening exercises for hips and knees. If you decide that a major problem is that your shoulders are stiff and your arms too weak to handle a carry-on bag for a plane trip, choose flexibility and strengthening exercises for your shoulders and arms.

4. **Design your exercise plan.** To start, read Chapter 7 and choose no more than 10 to 12 exercises. Begin by doing each exercise five times. As you get comfortable, you can do more. If you want to improve your endurance, read Chapter 8 about aerobic exercise. Start off with short times and build up gradually. Health and fitness take time to build, but every day you exercise you are healthier and being successful. That's why it's so important to make sure you keep it up.

Overcoming Your Exercise Barriers

Health and fitness make sense. Yet when faced with being more physically active, people often come up with many excuses, concerns, and worries. These barriers can prevent you from taking the first step. Here are some common barriers and possible solutions:

"I don't have enough time." We all have the same amount of time; we just use it differently. It's a matter of priorities. Some people find time for television but not for exercise. Exercise doesn't take a lot of time. Just 15 minutes a day is a good start, and it's much better than nothing. You may be able to work exercise into your day: watch television while pedaling a stationary bicycle or arrange a "walking meeting" to discuss business or family matters. If you add three 10-minute walks, you have 30 minutes of exercise for the day.

"I'm too tired." When you're out of shape or depressed, you may feel tired. You have to break out of the "too tired" cycle. Try an experiment: next time you are too tired, take a short walk (5 minutes or even 2). You may be surprised that this gives you energy. As you get into shape, you will recognize the difference between feeling listless and feeling physically tired.

"I'm too old." You're never too old for physical activity. No matter what your level of fitness or your age, you can always find ways to increase your activity, energy, and sense of well-being. Fitness is especially important as we age.

"I'm too sick." It may be true that you are too sick for a vigorous or strenuous exercise program, but you can usually find some ways to be more active. Remember, you can start with exercise 1 minute at a time, several times a day. Better fitness helps you cope with your illness and prevent further problems.

"I get enough exercise." This may be true, but for most people, their jobs and daily activities do not provide enough sustained exercise at a moderate level to keep them fit and energetic.

"Exercise is boring." You can make it more interesting and fun. Exercise with other people. Entertain yourself with a headset and musical tapes, or listen to the radio. Vary your activities and your walking routes. You might find exercise time good thinking time.

"Exercise is painful." The old saying "No pain, no gain" is simply wrong. Health benefits come from moderate-intensity physical activity. If you feel more pain when you finish than before you started, take a close look at what you are doing. You may be exercising improp-

erly or overdoing it. Talk with your instructor, therapist, or doctor. You may simply need to be less vigorous or change the type of exercise that you're doing. For some conditions, such as arthritis, exercise actually reduces pain.

"I'm too embarrassed." For some people the thought of donning a skin-tight designer exercise outfit and trotting around in public is delightful, but for others it is downright distressing. The options for physical activity range from exercise in the privacy of your own home to group social activities. You will be able to find something that suits you.

"I'm afraid I might fall." Check where you will exercise for fall safety (good lighting, well-maintained parking lots and walkways, handrails, and uncluttered floors). Choose exercises that feel safe—chair exercise, water exercise, or recumbent bicycling provide a lot of support as you get started. Remember, strong and flexible legs and ankles and staying active so that you stay coordinated reduce the risks of falls. Your doctor or therapist may recommend a cane, walking stick, or walker to enhance your balance, but it is important to have a therapist fit it to you and to learn how to use it safely. Using a cane or walker that doesn't fit or is used improperly can cause a fall.

"I'm afraid I'll have a heart attack." In most cases, the risk of a heart attack is greater for people who are not physically active than for those who exercise regularly. But if you are worried about this, check with your doctor. Especially if your illness is under control, it's probably safer to exercise than not to exercise.

"It's too cold (hot, dark, etc.)." If you are flexible and vary your type of exercise, you can generally work around the changes in weather that make certain types of exercise more difficult. Consider indoor activities such as stationary bicycling, swimming, or mall walking when weather is a barrier.

"I'm afraid I won't be able to do it right or won't be successful." Many people don't start a new project because they are afraid they will fail. If you feel this way, remember two things. First, whatever activities you are able to do—no matter how short or "easy"—will be much better than doing nothing. Be proud of what you have done, not guilty about what you haven't done. Second, new projects often seem overwhelming—until we get started and learn to enjoy each day's adventures and successes.

Perhaps you have some other barriers. Be honest with yourself about your worries. Talk to yourself and others to develop positive thoughts about exercise. If you get stuck, ask others for suggestions, or try some of the positive thinking suggestions in Chapter 5.

Better Balance

Sometimes people decide that the best way not to fall is to spend more time sitting. At first you might think that if you are not up walking around, you won't be at risk for falling. However, inactivity causes weakness, stiffness, slower reflexes, slower muscles, and even social isolation and depression. All of these harm your balance and increase your risk of falling. Even simple things such as getting up or sitting down in a chair, going to the bathroom, or going down a step can cause problems.

Other physical conditions such as weakness, dizziness, stiffness, poor eyesight, loss of feeling in feet, or inner ear problems can cause a fall, as can the side effects of medications. Falls can also be caused by the space around you: poor lighting, uneven ground, rugs, and cluttered floors. To avoid falls, reduce all these risks and keep yourself strong, flexible, and coordinated. Research shows that people who have strong legs and ankles, are flexible, and do things that require them to balance have less fear of falling and actually fall less.

If you have fallen or are afraid that you may fall, talk with your health care provider and get your balance checked to make sure there are no vision or inner ear problems or medication problems that need to be fixed. Make sure your home is safe. Exercising to keep yourself strong, flexible, and active also helps protect you from falling. Look in Chapter 7 for the balance exercises marked "BB" and exercises 27–32.

Preparing to Exercise

Committing to regular exercise is a big deal for everyone. If you have a chronic illness, you may also have many daily challenges and special exercise needs. People with arthritis, for example, must learn how to adapt exercise to changes in their arthritis and joint problems. People with heart or lung disease should not "exercise through" serious symptoms such as chest pain, palpitations (irregular heartbeat), shortness of breath, or excessive fatigue. They should notify their doctors if these happen or new symptoms appear. If your illness is not under good control, if you have been inactive for more than six months, or if you have questions about starting an exercise program, it is best to check with your doctor or therapist. Take this book with you and discuss your exercise ideas, or make a list of your questions.

We hope this chapter helps you learn to meet your needs and enjoy the benefits of physical activity. Start by knowing your own needs and limits and respect your body. Talk to other people like you who exercise. Talk with your doctor and other health professionals who understand your kind of chronic illness. Always pay attention to your own experience. That helps you know your body and make wise choices.

Physical Activity Guidelines

Many countries now have guidelines for what kinds of physical activity, and how much, people should do to be healthy. The guidelines are pretty much the same all over the world and include adults with and without chronic illness and disability. When you read the guidelines, it is important to remember that they are goals to work toward; they are not the starting point. On average, only about 25% of people in any country exercise enough to meet these guidelines. So don't worry that everyone else can do these but you. Your goal is to gradually and safely increase your physical activity to a level that is right for you. You may be able to get to exercise at that level, but maybe you won't. The important point is to use the information to get you started to be more active and healthier in a way that is right for you. Start doing what you can. Even a few minutes of activity several times a day is a good beginning. The important thing is to do something that works for you, make it a habit, and gradually increase your time or number of days a week as you can. The guidelines presented here are from the U.S. Department of Health and Human Services and came out in

2008. Remember, they are a guide to where you could go, not where you should be now. Chapters 7 and 8 will give you more information to help you get started on your exercise plan.

Physical Activity Guidelines

Moderate aerobic (endurance) exercise for at least 150 minutes (2.5 hours) a week or vigorous intensity activity for at least 75 minutes a week.

Aerobic activity should be performed at least 10 minutes at a time spread out through the week.

Moderate-intensity muscle-strengthening exercise of all major muscle groups should be done at least 2 days a week.

If people cannot meet the guidelines, they should be as active as they can and avoid inactivity.

Examples of 150 Minutes a Week of Moderate Aerobic Activity

A 10-minute walk at moderate intensity three times a day, 5 days a week

A 20-minute bike ride at moderate intensity 3 days a week and a 30-minute walk 3 days a week

A 30-minute aerobic dance class at moderate intensity twice a week and three 10-minute walks 3 days a week

Gardening and yard work (digging, raking, lifting) 30 minutes a day, 5 days a week.

Examples of Muscle-Strengthening Exercise

Twice a week do ten exercises 8 to 12 times each with enough weight or resistance that you feel tired when you finish each exercise.

Do yoga twice a week.

You can lift weights, use bands, or just work against your own body weight to do exercises for your arms, trunk, and legs.

Opportunities in Your Community

Many people who exercise regularly do so with at least one other person. Two or more people can keep each other motivated, and a whole class can become a circle of friends. On the other hand, exercising alone gives you the most freedom. You may feel that there are no classes that would work for you or there is no buddy with whom to exercise. If so, start your own program; as you progress, you may find that these feelings change.

Most communities offer a variety of exercise classes, including special programs for people over 50, adaptive exercises, mall walking, fitness trails, tai chi, and yoga. Check with the local Y, community and senior centers, parks and recreation programs, adult education classes, organizations for specific diseases (arthritis, diabetes, cancer, heart disease), and community colleges. There is a great deal of variation in these programs, as well as in the training of the exercise staff. By and large, the classes are inexpensive, and the staff in charge of planning respond to people's needs. Public health offices often sponsor classes that are appropriate for a wide range of ages and needs.

Hospitals often have medically supervised classes for people with heart or lung disease (cardiac or pulmonary rehabilitation classes). Occasionally, people with other chronic illnesses can be included as well. These programs tend to be more expensive than other community classes, but there is the advantage of medical supervision, if that's important to you.

Health and fitness clubs usually offer aerobic classes, weight training, cardiovascular equipment, and sometimes a heated pool. They charge membership fees. The following list describes some things to ask about when you search for community programs.

■ **Classes designed for moderate- and low-intensity exercise and for beginners.** You should be able to observe classes and participate in at least one class before signing up and paying.

■ **Safe and effective endurance, strength, balance, and flexibility components that are tailored to meet your needs.**

■ **Qualified instructors with experience working with people like you.** Knowledgeable instructors are more likely to understand special needs and be willing and able to work with you.

■ **Membership policies that allow you to pay by the class or for a short series of classes or let you freeze your membership at times when you can't participate.** Some fitness facilities offer different rates depending on how many services you use.

■ **Facilities that are easy to get to, park near, and enter.** Parking lots, dressing rooms, and exercise sites should be accessible and safe, with professional staff on site.

■ **A pool that allows "free swim" times when the water isn't crowded.** Also find out the policy about children in the pool; small children playing and making noise may not be good for your needs.

■ **Staff and other members who are friendly and easy to talk to.**

■ **An emergency management protocol and instructors certified in CPR and first aid.**

Note that there are many excellent exercise videotapes and DVDs for use at home. These vary in intensity, from very gentle chair exercises to more strenuous aerobic exercise. Ask your doctor, therapist, or voluntary agency for suggestions, or review the tapes yourself.

Putting Your Program Together

The best way to enjoy and stick with your exercise program is to suit yourself! Choose what you want to do, a place where you feel comfortable, and an exercise time that fits your schedule. If you want to have dinner on the table at 6:00, don't choose an exercise program that requires you to attend a 5:00 class. If you are retired and enjoy lunch with friends and an afternoon nap, it is wise to choose an early or midmorning exercise time.

Pick two or three activities that you think you would enjoy and that would be comfortable. Choose activities that can be easily worked into your daily routine. If an activity is new, try it out before going to the expense of buying equipment or joining a health club. By having more than one exercise, you can keep active and work around vacations, seasons, and changing problems with your condition. Variety also helps prevent overuse injuries and keep you from getting bored.

Having fun and enjoying yourself are benefits of exercise that often go unmentioned. Too often we think of exercise as serious business. However, most people who stick with a program do so because they enjoy it or how they feel because of exercise. They think of their exercise as recreation or a positive part of life rather than a chore. Start off with success in mind. Allow yourself time to get used to something new and meeting new people. You'll probably find that you look forward to exercise.

Experience, practice, and success help build a habit. Follow the self-management steps in Chapter 2 to make starting your program easier.

- **Keep your exercise goal in mind.** Review "Choose Your Goal and Make a Plan" earlier in this chapter.

- **Choose exercises you want to do.** Combine activities that move you toward your goal and those recommended by your health professionals. Select exercise and activities from the next two chapters to get started.

- **Choose the time and place to exercise.** Tell your family and friends about your plan.

- **Make an action plan with yourself.** Decide how long you'll stick with these particular exercises; 6 to 8 weeks is a reasonable time for any new program.

- **Start your program.** Remember to begin doing what you can and proceed slowly, especially if you haven't exercised in a while.

- **Keep an exercise diary or calendar.** A diary or journal lets you write more. Some people enjoy having a record of what they did and how they felt. Others like a simple calendar on which they note each exercise session.

- **Use self-tests to keep track of your progress.** You will find these at the end of the next two chapters. Record the date and results of the ones you choose.

- **Repeat the self-tests at regular intervals, record the results, and check the changes.**

- **Revise your program.** At the end of 6 to 8 weeks, decide what you liked, what worked, and what made exercising difficult. Make changes and draw up an action plan for another few weeks. You may decide to change some exercises, the place or time you exercise, or your exercise partner or group.

- **Reward yourself for a job well done.** Rewards come with improved health and endurance: enjoyable family outings, refreshing walks, trips to a concert or museum, or a day out fishing are great rewards. Pats on the back and a new exercise shirt can be fun too.

Keeping It Up

If you haven't exercised recently, you'll probably experience some new feelings and even discomfort. It's normal to feel sore muscles and tender joints and to be more tired in the evenings. Muscle or joint pain that lasts more than 2 hours after the exercise or feeling tired into the next day means that you probably did too much too fast. Don't stop; just don't work so hard the next day or work for a shorter time.

When you do aerobic exercise, it's natural to feel your heart beat faster, your breathing speed up, and your body get warmer. However, chest pain, feeling sick to your stomach, feeling dizzy, or being severely short of breath is a sign to contact your doctor. If this happens to you, stop exercising until you check with your doctor. (See Table 6.1.)

People who have a chronic illness often have additional sensations to sort out. It can be difficult to separate whether it is the illness, the exercise, or anxiety that is causing concern. You can find out a lot if you talk to someone else like you who has started an exercise program. Once you've sorted out the new feelings, you'll be able to exercise with more confidence.

Expect setbacks. During the first year, people often have two to three interruptions in their exercise schedule, often because of family needs, minor injuries, or illnesses not related to exercise. You may get off track for a while. Don't be discouraged. You may need a rest, a different schedule, or different activities. When you are feeling better and start again, begin at a lower, more gentle level. It can take you the same amount of time to get back into shape as you were out. For instance, if you missed 3 weeks, it may take at least that long to get back to your previous level. Go slowly. Be kind to yourself. You're in this for the long haul.

Think of your head as the coach and your body as your team. For success, all parts of the team need attention. Be a good coach. Encourage and praise yourself. Design "plays" you feel your team will like. Choose places that you like and are safe. A good coach knows his or her team, sets good goals, and helps the team succeed and get more confident. A good coach is loyal. A good coach does not belittle, nag, or make anyone feel guilty. Be a good coach to your team.

Besides a good coach, everyone needs a good cheerleader or two. Of course, you can be your own cheerleader, but being both coach and cheerleader is a lot to do. Successful exercisers usually have at least one family member or close friend who encourages them. Your cheerleader can exercise with you, help you get other chores done so you can exercise, praise you, or just consider your exercise time when making plans.

Table 6.1 **If Exercise Problems Occur**

Problem	Advice
Irregular or rapid heartbeat. Pain, tightness or pressure in the chest, jaw arms, or neck. Shortness of breath lasting past the exercise period.	Stop exercising. Talk with your doctor right away. Don't exercise until you have been cleared by your doctor.
Light-headedness, dizziness, fainting, cold sweat, or confusion.	Lie down with feet up or sit down with head between knees. Seek medical advice immediately.
Shortness of breath or calf pain from circulation or breathing problems.	Warm up by going slowly at first. Take short rests to recover and keep going.
Excessive tiredness after exercise, especially if you are still tired the next day.	Exercise less hard next time. If tiredness lasts, check with your doctor.

Sometimes cheerleaders pop up by themselves, but don't be bashful about asking for a hand.

With exercise experience you develop a sense of control over yourself and your illness. You learn how to choose your activity to fit your needs. You know when to do less and when to do more. You know that a change in symptoms or a period of inactivity is usually only temporary and doesn't have to feel like a disaster. You know you have the tools to get back on track. Give yourself a chance to succeed. Sticking with it and doing it your way makes you a sure winner.

Suggested Further Reading

Dahm, Diane, and Jay Smith, eds. *Mayo Clinic Fitness for Everybody*. Rochester, Minn.: Mayo Clinic Health Information, 2005.

Moffat, Marilyn, and Steve Vickery. *Book of Body Maintenance and Repair*. New York: Henry Holt, 1999.

Nelson, Miriam E., and Sarah Wernick. *Strong Women Stay Young*, rev. ed. New York: Bantam Books, 2005.

White, Martha. *Water Exercise: 78 Safe and Effective Exercises for Fitness and Therapy*. Champaign, Ill.: Human Kinetics, 1995.

Other Resources

Physical activity guidelines:

- ☐ Australia: http://www.health.gov.au/internet/main/publishing.nsf/content/health-pubhlth -strateg-active-recommend.htm

- ☐ Canada: http://www.phac-aspc.gc.ca/hp-ps/hl-mvs/pa-ap/

- ☐ Centers for Disease Control and Prevention, http://www.cdc.gov/physicalactivity/

- ☐ National Center for Physical Activity for people with disabilities, http://www.ncpad.org/

- ☐ National Institute on Aging, *Exercise and Physical Activity: Your Everyday Guide from the National Institute on Aging:* http://www.nia.nih.gov/HealthInformation/Publications/ ExerciseGuide/

- ☐ National Center for Injury Prevention and Control, *Check for Safety: A Home Fall Prevention Checklist for Older Adults* and *What YOU Can Do to Prevent Falls:* http://www.cdc.gov/ HomeandRecreationalSafety/Falls/fallsmaterial.htm

- ☐ U.S. Department of Health and Human Services: http://www.health.gov/paguidelines/

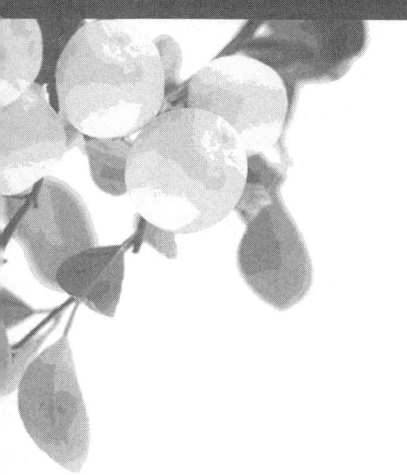

CHAPTER 7

Exercising for Flexibility, Strength, and Balance: Making Life Easier

YOU CAN USE THE EXERCISES IN THIS CHAPTER in several ways: to get ready for aerobic exercise; to improve flexibility, strength, and balance; to stretch and strengthen your back and chest for better posture and breathing; and to warm up and cool down for your aerobic exercise routines.

The exercises are arranged in order from the head and neck down to the toes. Most of the upper-body exercises may be done either sitting or standing. Exercises done lying down can be performed on the floor or on a firm mattress. We have labeled the exercises that are particularly important for breathing and good posture "VIP" (Very Important for Posture). Exercises to improve balance by strengthening and loosening legs and ankles are marked "BB" (Better Balance). There is also a section of balance exercises that are designed to help you practice balance skills.

If you see this symbol next to an exercise, this means that you can add weights (hand or ankle weights) to that exercise. This will make it a harder strengthening exercise. If you can do an exercise easily at least ten times, you can add weights. Start with 1 to 2 pounds (0.5 to 1.0 kg), and add weight gradually as you get stronger and the exercise gets easier. You can use homemade weights (cans, bags of beans, plastic bottles filled with water or sand) or buy weights in different sizes.

You can make a routine of exercises that flow together. Arrange them so you don't have to get up and down too often. Exercise to music if you wish. An exercise CD has been designed to go with this book; see details under "Other Resources" at the end of this chapter.

The following tips apply to all the exercises in this chapter:

- Move at a comfortable speed. Do not bounce or jerk.

- To loosen tight muscles and joints, stretch just until you feel tension, hold for 10 to 30 seconds, and then relax. Remember to breathe in and out.

- Stop if your body starts to hurt. Stretching should feel good, not painful.

- Start with no more than five repetitions of any exercise. Increase gradually as you make progress.

- Always do the same number of exercises for your left and right sides.

- Breathe naturally. Do not hold your breath. Count out loud to make sure you are breathing.

- If you have more symptoms (such as pain) that last more than 2 hours after exercising, do less next time. If an exercise gives you problems, stop and try another exercise. Don't quit exercising.

The following exercises are for both sides of the body and a full range of motion. If you are limited by muscle weakness or joint tightness, go ahead and do the exercise as completely as you can. *The benefit of doing an exercise comes from moving toward a certain position, not from being able to complete the movement perfectly.* In some cases you may find that after a while you can complete the movement and increase your available range of motion. At other times you will keep doing it your own way.

Neck Exercises

1. Heads Up (VIP)

This exercise relieves jaw, neck, and upper back tension or pain and is the start of good posture. You can do it while driving, sitting at a desk, sewing, reading, or exercising. Just sit or stand straight and gently slide your chin back. Keep looking forward as your chin moves backward.

You'll feel the back of your neck lengthen and straighten. To help, put your finger on your nose and then draw straight back from your finger. (Don't worry about a little double chin— you really look much better with your neck straight!)

Clues for Finding the Correct Position

- Ear over shoulder, not out in front
- Head balanced over neck and trunk, not in the lead
- Back of neck more vertical, not leaning forward
- Bit of double chin

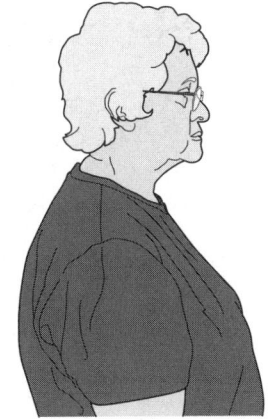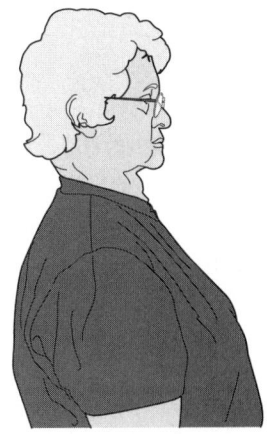

2. Neck Stretch

In heads-up position (Exercise 1) and with your shoulders relaxed, turn slowly to look over your right shoulder. Then turn slowly to look over your left shoulder. Next, tilt your head to the right and then to the left. Move your ear toward your shoulder. Do not move your shoulder up to your ear.

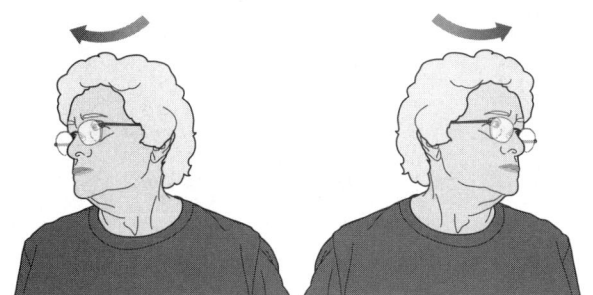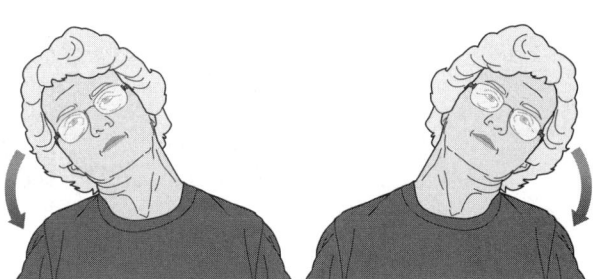

Hand and Wrist Exercises

A good place to do hand exercises is at a table that supports your forearms. Do them after washing dishes, after bathing or showering, or when taking a break from handwork. Your hands are warmer and more limber at these times.

3. Thumb Walk

Holding your wrist straight, form the letter O by lightly touching your thumb to each fingertip. After each O, straighten and spread your fingers. Use the other hand to help if needed.

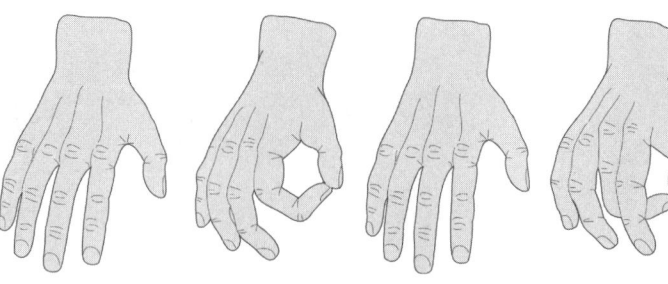

Shoulder Exercises

4. Shoulder Shape Up

In heads-up position (Exercise 1), slowly raise the shoulders to the ears; hold the position and then drop them. Next, raise the shoulders again to the ears and then begin to slowly rotate them backward by pinching the shoulder blades together; bring the shoulders down and forward to complete a circle. Return to the heads-up position. Finally, reverse the direction of the shoulder circles.

This is a good exercise if the neck stretch (Exercise 2) is difficult for you.

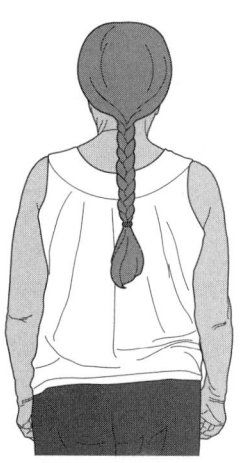 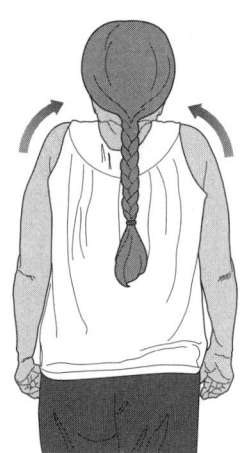 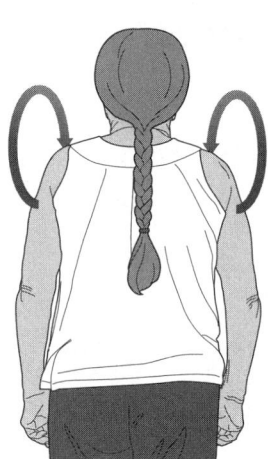

5. Good Morning (VIP)

Start with hands in gentle fists, palms down, and wrists crossed. Breathe in and stretch out your fingers while you uncross your arms and reach up for the sky. Breathe out as you stretch your arms and relax.

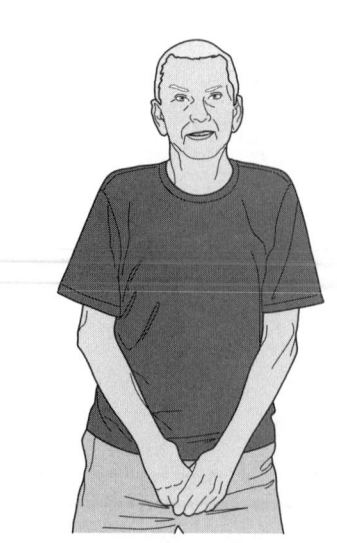 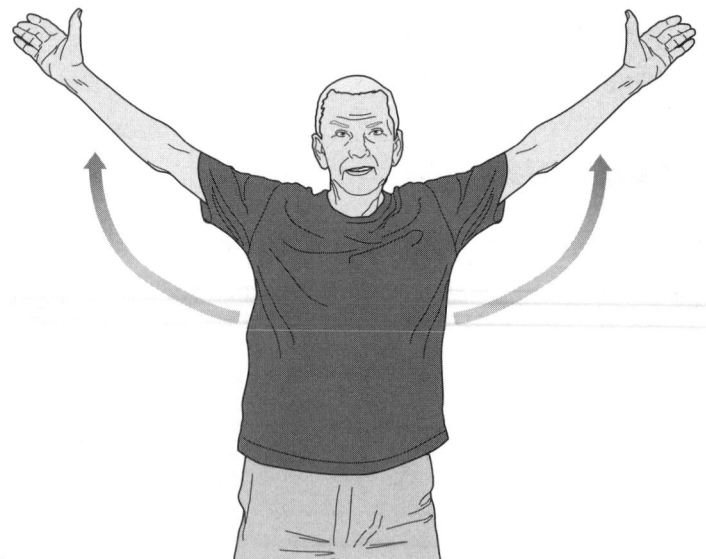

6. Wand Exercise

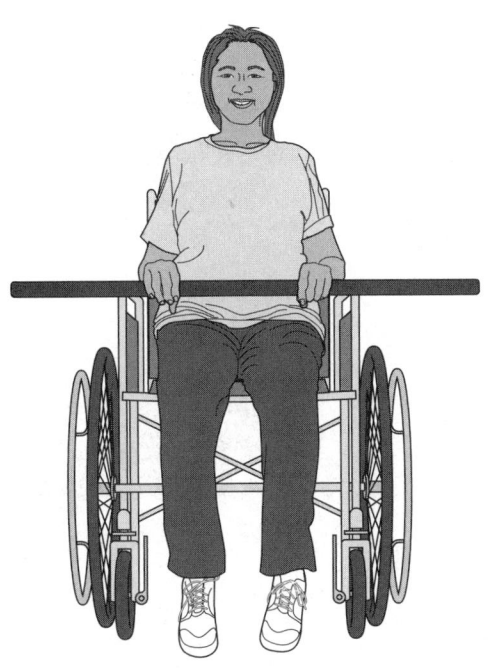 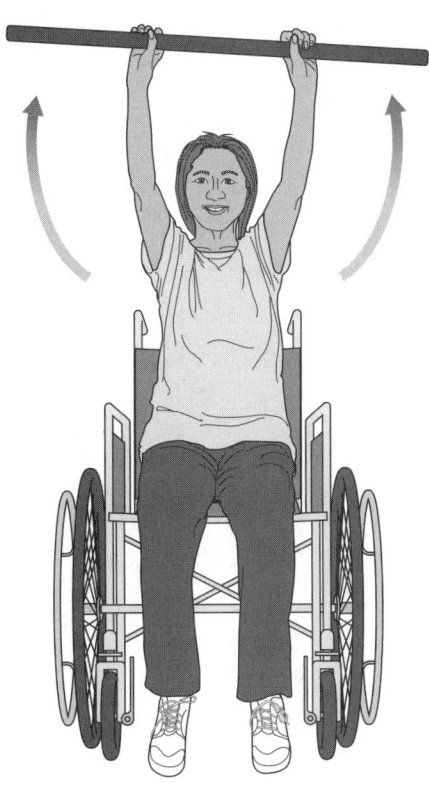

If one or both of your shoulders are tight or weak, you may want to give yourself a "helping hand." This shoulder exercise and the next allow the arms to help each other.

Use a yardstick, mop handle, or cane as your wand. Place one hand on each end, and raise the wand as high overhead as possible. You might try this in front of a mirror. This exercise can be done standing, sitting, or lying down.

7. Pat and Reach

This double-duty exercise helps increase flexibility and strength for both shoulders. Raise one arm up over your head, and bend your elbow to pat yourself on the back. Move your other arm to your back, bend your elbow, and reach up toward the other hand. Can your fingertips touch? Relax and switch arm positions. Can you touch on that side? For most people, one position will work better than the other. Do not worry if you cannot touch. Many people cannot touch, but you will improve as you practice. If you wish, you may use a towel as if you were drying your back; this can provide you with feedback and assist in the motion.

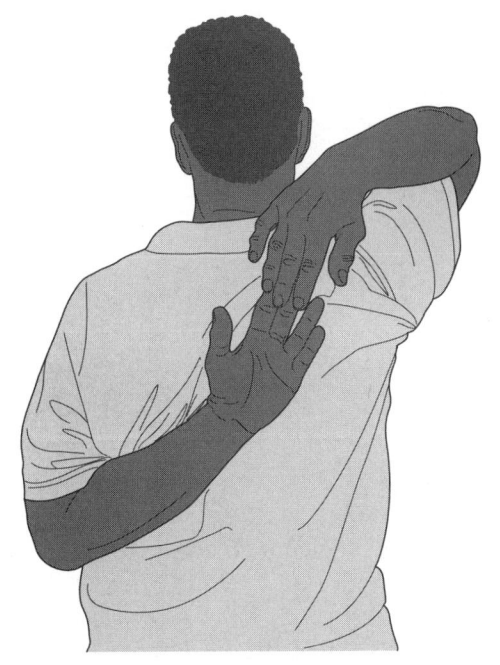

8. Shoulder Blade Pinch (VIP)

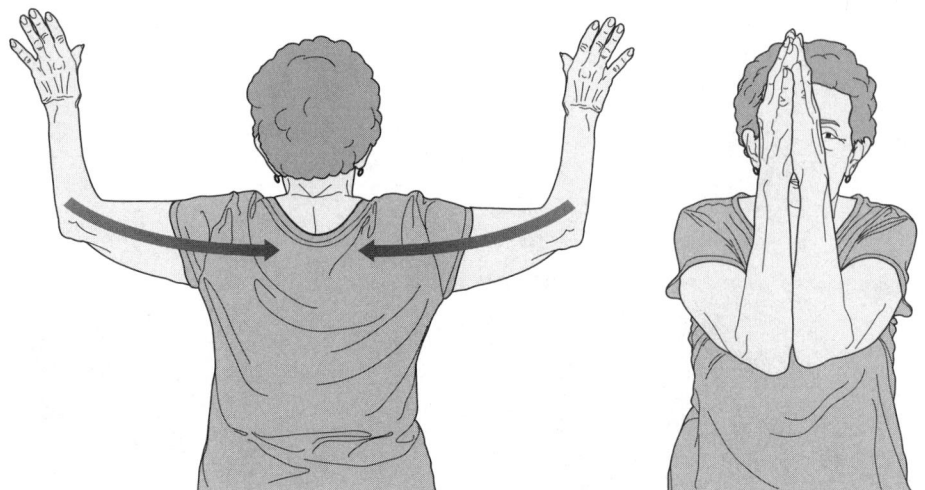

This is a good exercise to strengthen the middle and upper back and to stretch the chest, and it can be especially good for individuals with breathing problems. Sit or stand with your head in heads-up position (Exercise 1) and your shoulders relaxed. Raise your arms out to the sides with elbows bent. Pinch your shoulder blades together by moving your elbows as far back as you can. Hold briefly, and then slowly move your arms forward to touch elbows. If this position is uncomfortable, lower your arms or rest your hands on your shoulders.

Back and Abdominal Exercises

9. Knee to Chest Stretch

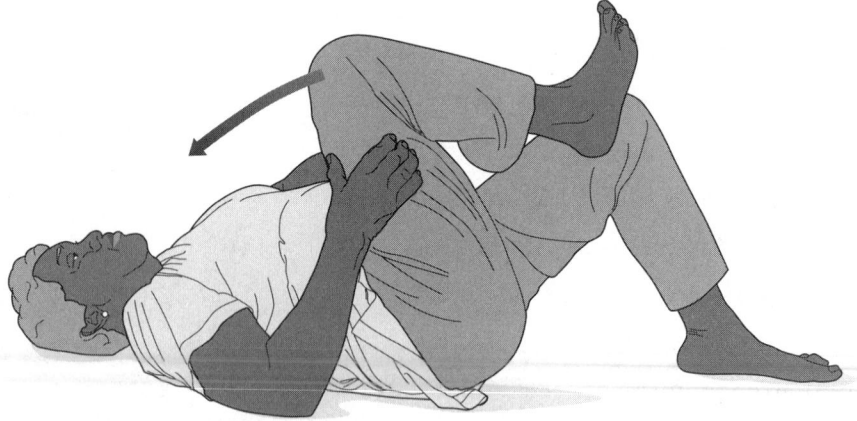

For a low back stretch, lie on the floor with knees bent and feet flat. Bring one knee toward your chest, using your hands to help. Hold your knee near your chest for 10 seconds, and lower the leg slowly. Repeat with the other knee. You can also tuck both legs at the same time if you wish. Relax and enjoy the stretch.

10. Pelvic Tilt (VIP)

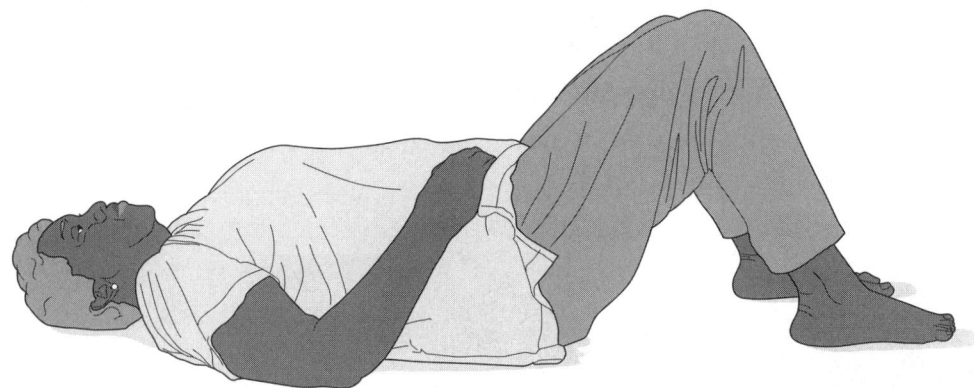

This is an excellent exercise for the low back and can help relieve low back pain. Lie on your back with knees bent, feet flat. Place your hands on your abdomen. Flatten the small of your back against the floor by tightening your stomach muscles and your buttocks. When you do this exercise, you will be tilting your tailbone forward and pulling your stomach back. Think about trying to pull your stomach in enough to zip a tight pair of trousers. Hold the tilt for 5 to 10 seconds. Relax. Arch your back slightly. Relax and repeat the pelvic tilt. Keep breathing. Count the seconds out loud. Once you've mastered the pelvic tilt lying down, practice it sitting, standing, and walking.

11. Back Lift (VIP)

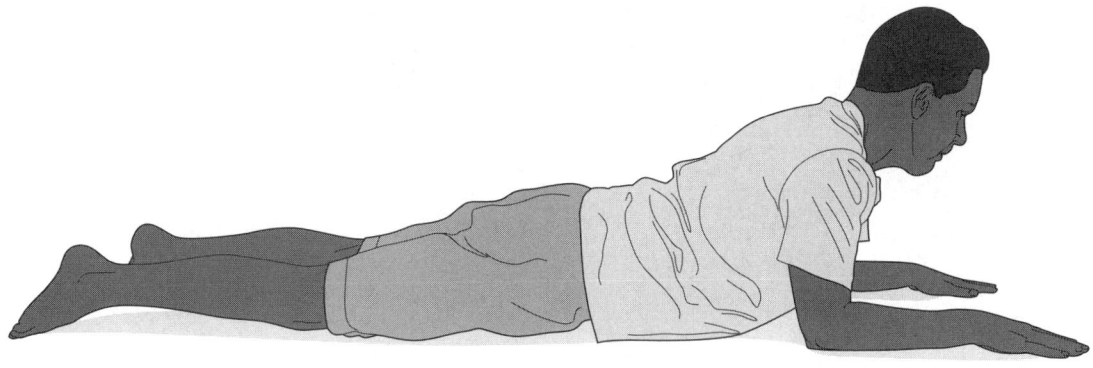

This exercise improves flexibility along your spine and helps you lift your chest for easier breathing. Lie on your stomach, and rise up onto your forearms. Keep your back relaxed, and keep your stomach and hips down. If this is comfortable, straighten your elbows. Breathe naturally and relax for at least 10 seconds. If you have moderate to severe low back pain, do not do this exercise unless it has been specifically prescribed for you.

To strengthen back muscles, lie on your stomach with your arms at your side or overhead. Lift your head, shoulders, and arms. Do not look up. Keep looking down with your chin tucked into that double-chin position. Count out loud as you hold for a count of 10. Relax.

You can also lift your legs, instead of your head and shoulders, off the floor.

Note that lifting both ends of your body at once is a fairly strenuous exercise. It may not be helpful for a person with back pain.

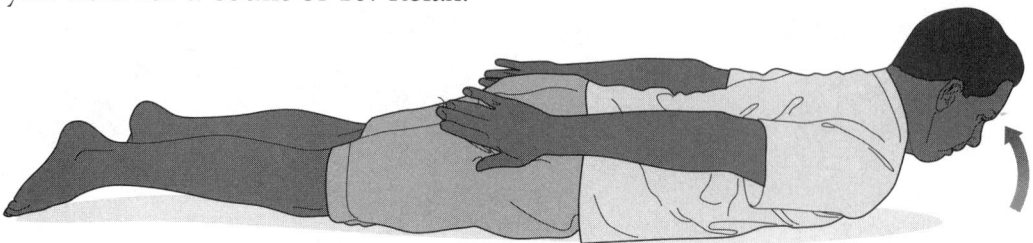

12. Low Back Rock and Roll

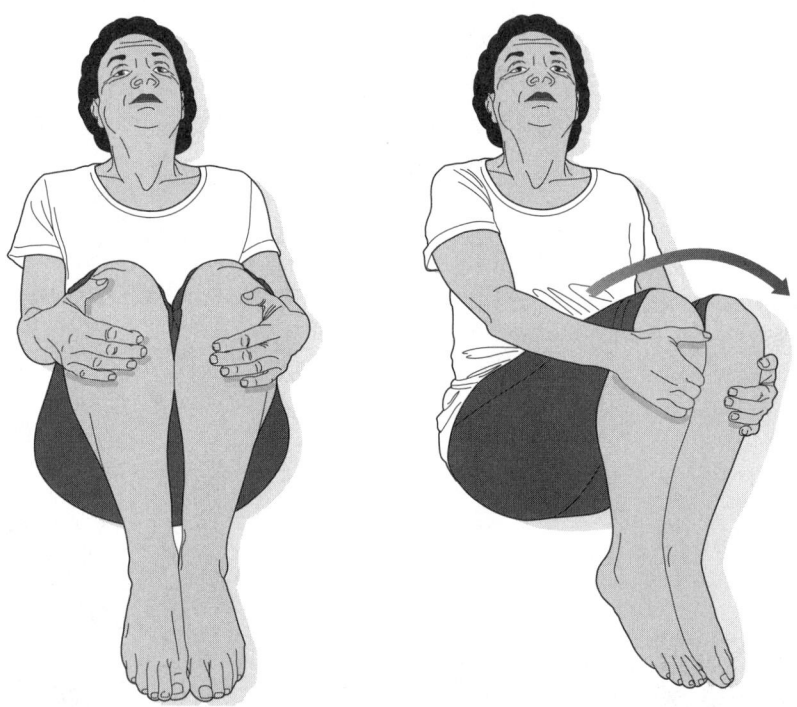

Lie on your back, and pull your knees up to your chest. You can keep holding on to your legs with your hands behind the thighs or stretch your arms out to your sides to lie on the floor at shoulder level. Rest in this position for 10 seconds, and then gently roll your hips and knees to one side and then the other. Rest and relax as you roll to each side. Keep your upper back and shoulders flat on the ground.

13. Curl-Up (BB)

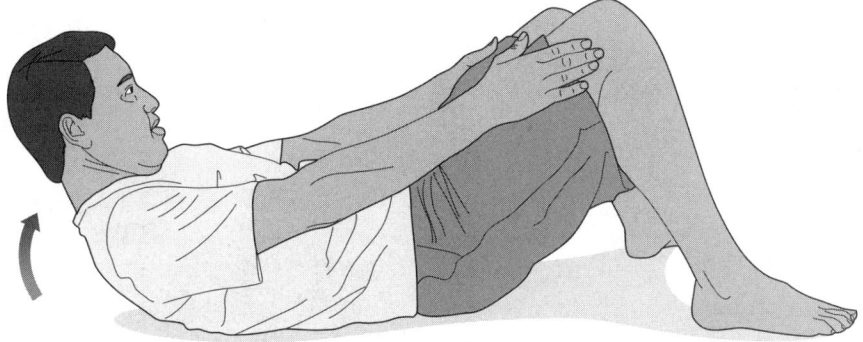

A curl-up, as shown here, is a good way to strengthen stomach muscles. Lie on your back, knees bent, feet flat. Do the pelvic tilt (Exercise 10). Slowly curl up in segments. Tuck your chin as you roll your head up and begin to lift the shoulders off the floor. Slowly uncurl back down, or hold for 10 seconds and slowly lower.

Breathe out as you curl up, and breathe in as you go back down. Do not hold your breath. If you have neck problems or if your neck hurts when you do this exercise, try the next one instead. Never tuck your feet under a chair or have someone hold your feet!

14. Roll-Out

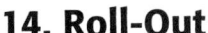

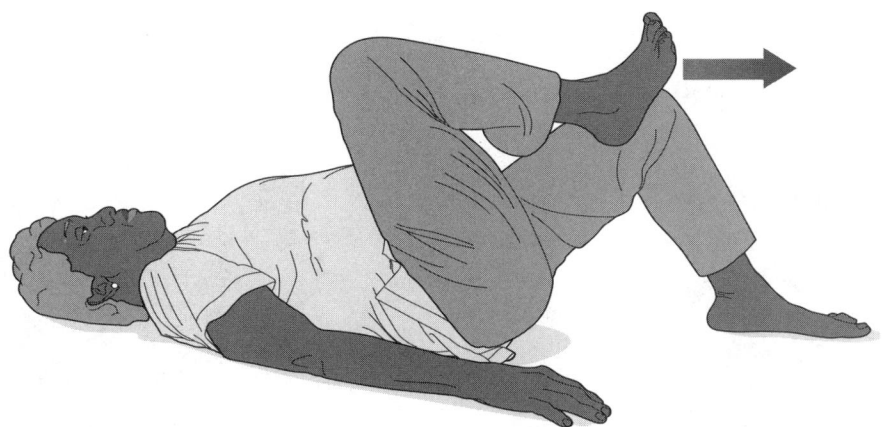

This is another good stomach strengthener, and it is easy on the neck. Use it instead of the curl-up (Exercise 13), or if neck pain is not a problem, do them both.

Lie on your back with knees bent and feet flat. Do the pelvic tilt (Exercise 10), and hold your lower back firmly against the floor.

Slowly and carefully, move one leg away from your chest as you straighten your knee. Move your leg out until you feel your lower

back start to arch. When this happens, tuck your knee back to your chest. Reset your pelvic tilt and roll your leg out again. Breathe out as your leg rolls out. Do not hold your breath. Repeat with the other leg.

You are strengthening your abdominal muscles by holding your pelvic tilt against the weight of your leg. As you get stronger, you'll be able to straighten your legs out farther and move both legs together.

Hip and Leg Exercises

15. Straight Leg Raises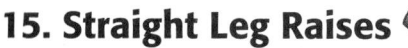

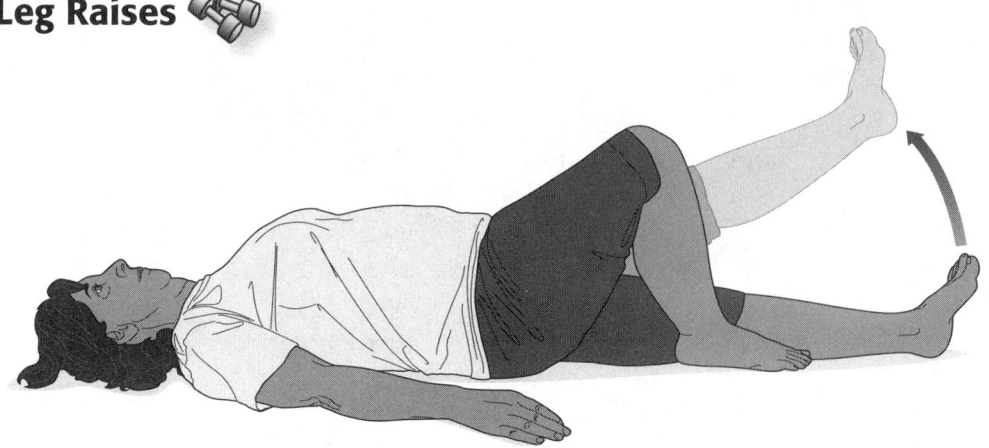

This exercise strengthens the muscles that bend the hip and straighten the knee. Lie on your back, knees bent, feet flat. Straighten one leg. Tighten the muscle on the upper surface of that thigh, and straighten the knee as much as possible. Keeping the knee straight, raise your leg a foot or two (up to 50 cm) off the ground. Do not arch your back. Hold your leg up, and count out loud for 10 seconds. Relax. Repeat with the other leg.

16. Hip Hooray (standing only)

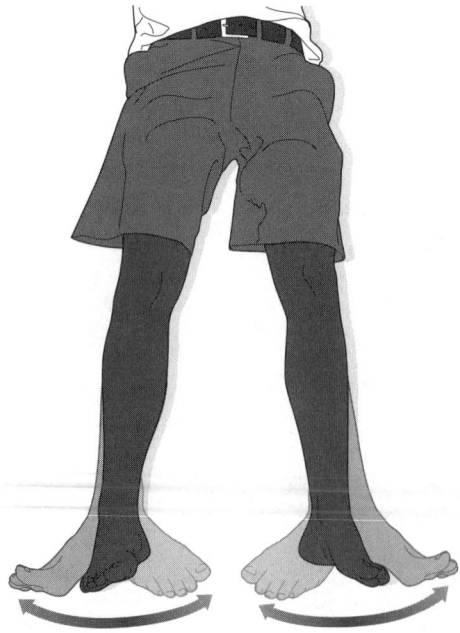

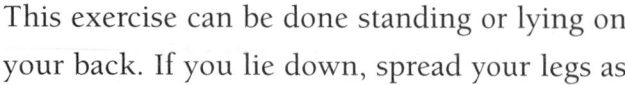

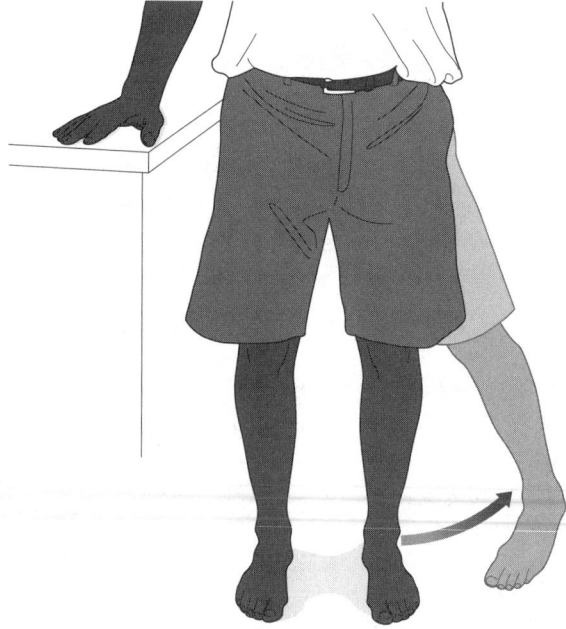

This exercise can be done standing or lying on your back. If you lie down, spread your legs as far apart as possible. Roll your legs and feet out like a duck, then in to be pigeon-toed, and then move your legs back together. If you are standing, move one leg out to your side as far as you can. Lead out with the heel and in with the toes.

Hold on to a counter for support. You can make the muscles work harder while you are standing by adding a weight to your ankle.

17. Back Kick (VIP) (BB)

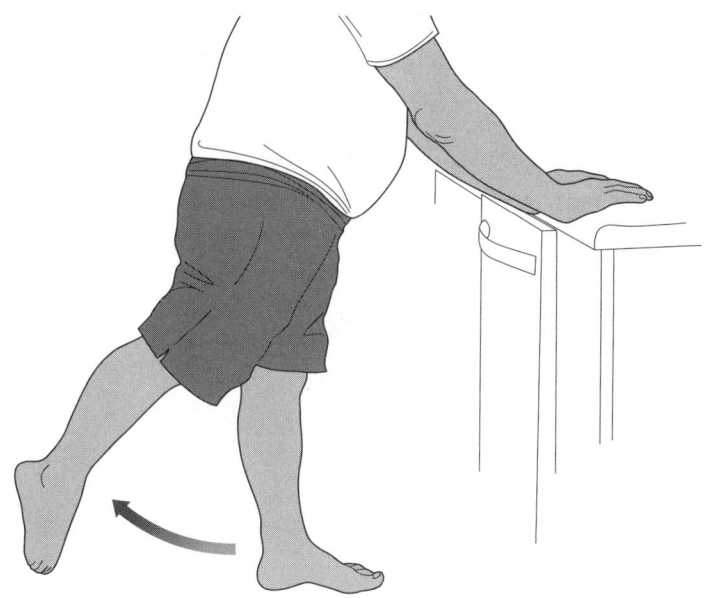

This exercise increases the backward mobility and strength of your hip. Hold on to a counter for support. Move the leg up and back, knee straight. Stand tall, and do not lean forward.

18. Knee Strengthener (BB)

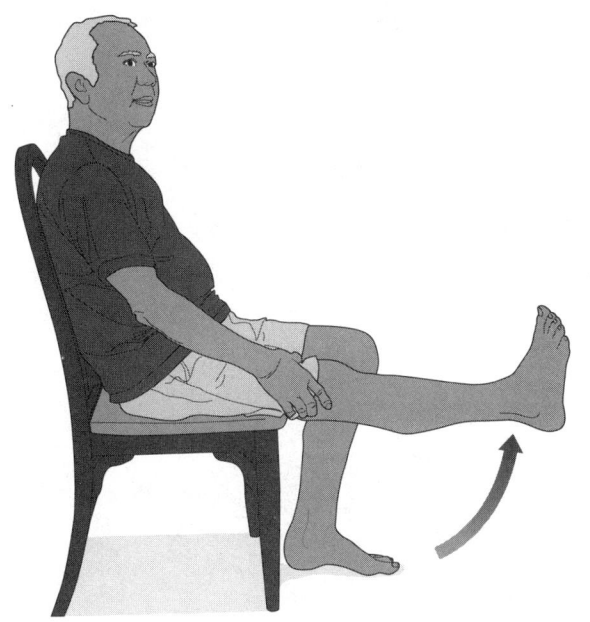

Strong knees are important for walking and standing comfortably. This exercise strengthens the knee. Sitting in a chair, straighten the knee by tightening up the muscle on the upper surface of your thigh. Place your hand on your thigh and feel the muscle work. If you wish, make circles with your toes. As your knee strengthens, see if you can build up to holding your leg out for 30 seconds. Count out loud. Do not hold your breath.

19. Power Knees

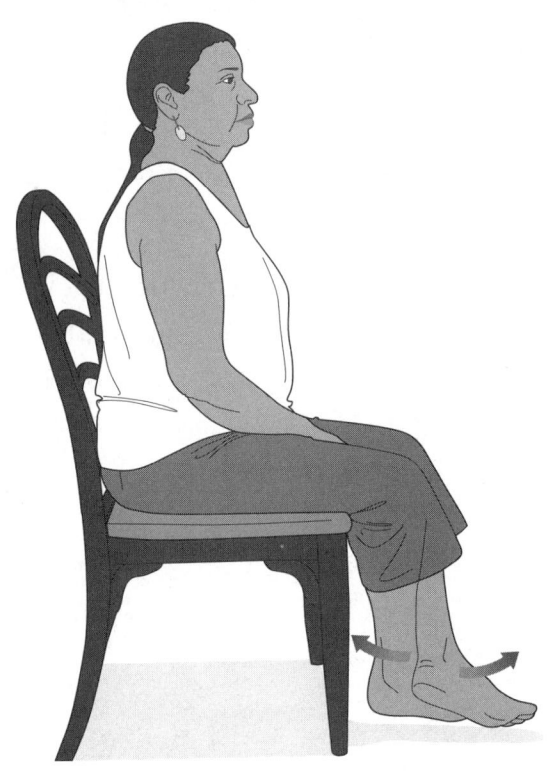

This exercise strengthens the muscles that bend and straighten your knee. Sit in a chair and cross your legs at the ankles. Your legs can be almost straight, or you can bend your knees as much as you like. Try several positions. Push forward with your back leg, and press backward with your front leg. Exert pressure evenly so that your legs do not move. Hold and count out loud for 10 seconds. Relax. Switch leg positions. Be sure to keep breathing. Repeat.

20. Ready-Go (BB)

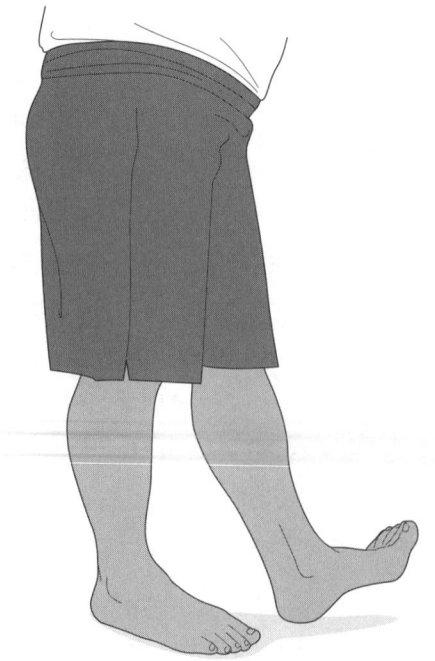

Stand with one leg slightly in front of the other with your heel on the floor as if ready to take a step with the front foot. Now tighten the muscles on the front of your thigh, making your knee firm and straight. Hold to a count of 10. Relax. Repeat with the other leg.

21. Hamstring Stretch

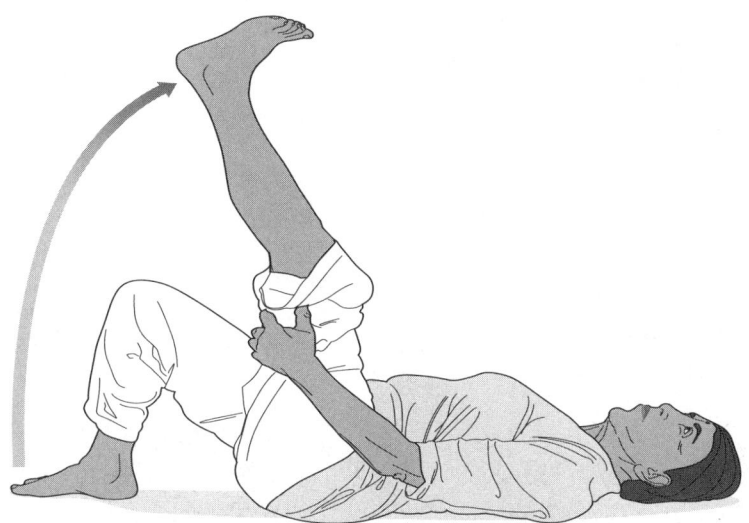

Do the self-test for hamstring tightness (page 122) to see if you need to do this exercise. If you have unstable knees or "back knee" (a knee that curves backward when you stand up), do not do this exercise.

If you do have tight hamstrings, lie on your back, knees bent, feet flat. Grasp one leg at a time behind the thigh. Holding the leg out at arm's length, slowly straighten the knee. Hold the leg as straight as you can as you count to 10. You should feel a slight stretch at the back of your knee and thigh.

Be careful with this exercise. It's easy to over-stretch and end up sore.

22. Achilles Stretch (BB)

This exercise helps maintain flexibility in the Achilles tendon, the large tendon at the back of your ankle. Good flexibility helps reduce the risk of injury, calf discomfort, and heel pain. The Achilles stretch is especially helpful for cooling down after walking or cycling and for people who get cramps in the calf muscles. If you have trouble with standing balance or spasticity (muscle jerks), you can do a seated version of this exercise. Sit in a chair with feet flat on the floor. Keep your heel on the floor and slowly slide your foot (one foot at a time) back to bend your ankle and feel some tension on the back of your calf (lower leg).

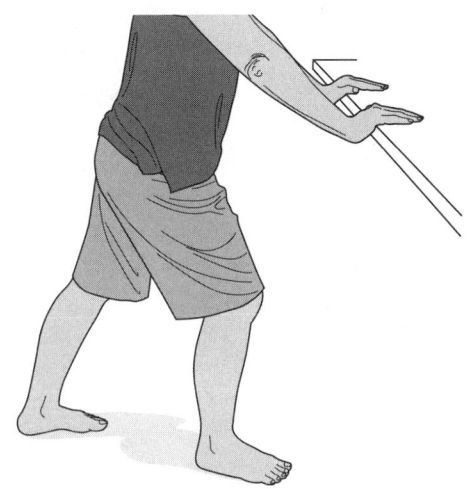

Stand at a counter or against a wall. Place one foot in front of the other, toes pointing forward and heels on the ground. Lean forward, bend the knee of the forward leg, and keep the back knee straight, heel down. You will feel a good stretch in the calf. Hold the stretch for 10 seconds. Do not bounce. Move gently. You can adjust this exercise to reach the other large calf muscle by slightly bending your back knee while you stretch the calf. Can you feel the difference? It's easy to get sore doing this exercise. If you've worn shoes with high heels for a long time, be particularly careful.

23. Tiptoes (BB)

This exercise will help strengthen your calf (lower leg) muscles and make walking, climbing stairs, and standing less tiring. It may also improve your balance. Hold on to a counter or table for support and rise up on your tiptoes. Hold for 10 seconds. Lower slowly. How high you go is not as important as keeping your balance and controlling your ankles. It is easier to do both legs at the same time. If your feet are too sore to do this standing, start doing it while sitting down. If this exercise makes your ankle jerk, stop doing it and talk to your therapist about other ways to strengthen these calf muscles if needed.

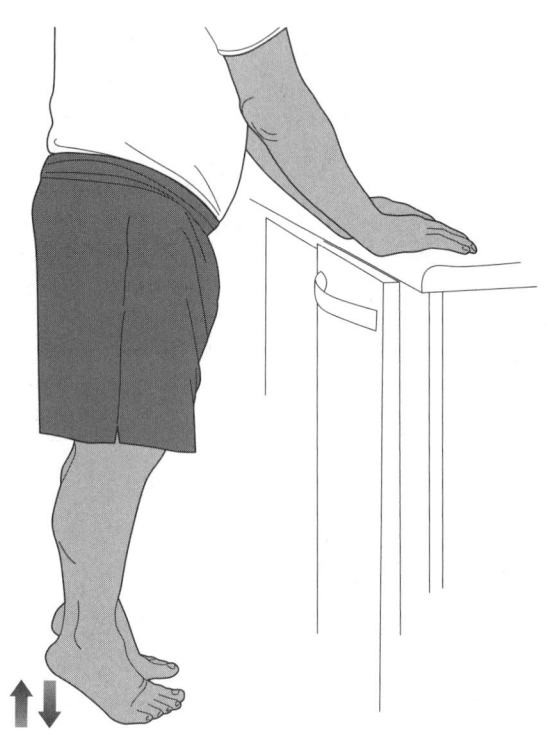

Ankle and Foot Exercises

Do these exercises sitting in a straight-backed chair with your feet bare. Have a bath towel and ten marbles next to you. These exercises are for flexibility, strength, and comfort. This is a good time to examine your feet and toes for any signs of circulation or skin problems and to check your nails to see if they need trimming.

24. Towel Grabber

Spread a towel out in front of your chair. Place your feet on the towel, with your heels near the edge closest to you. Keep your heels down and your foot slightly raised. Scoot the towel back underneath your feet by pulling it with your toes. When you have done as much as you can, reverse the toe motion and scoot the towel out again.

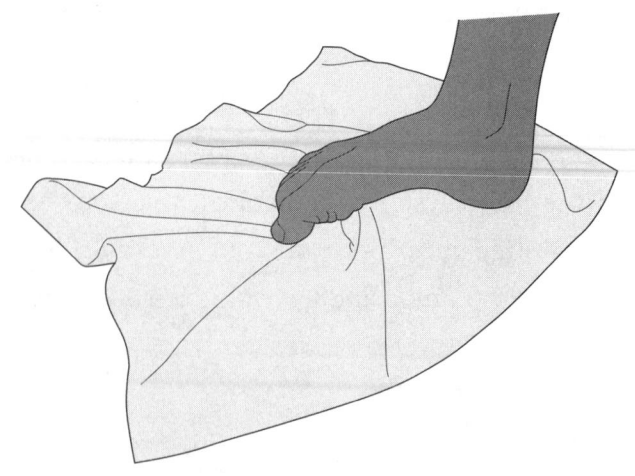

25. Marble Pickup

Do this exercise one foot at a time. Place several marbles on the floor between your feet. Keep your heel down, and pivot your toes toward the marbles. Pick up a marble with your toes, and pivot your foot to drop the marble as far as possible from where you picked it up. Repeat until all the marbles have been moved. Reverse the process and return all the marbles to the starting position. If marbles are difficult, try other objects, such as jacks, dice, or wads of paper.

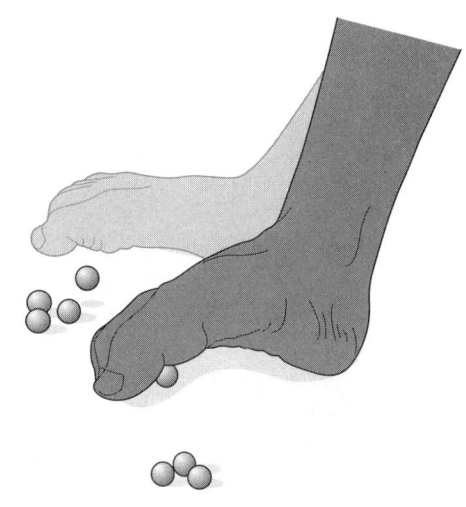

26. Foot Roll

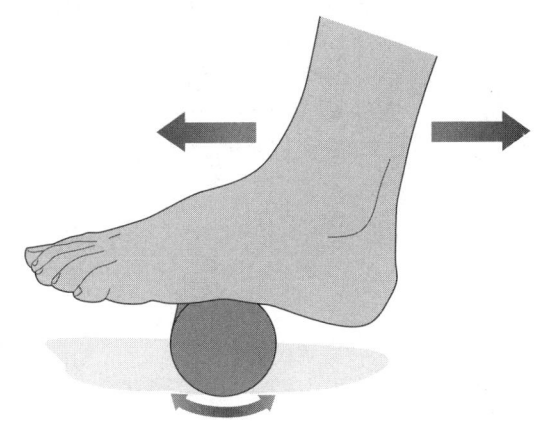

Place a rolling pin (or a large dowel or closet rod) under the arch of your foot, and roll it back and forth. It feels great and stretches the ligaments in the arch of the foot.

Balance Exercises

The exercises in this section are designed to let you practice balance activities in a safe and progressive way. The exercises are given in order of difficulty, so start with the first exercises and work up to the more difficult ones as your strength and balance improve. If you feel that your balance is particularly poor, exercise with someone else close by who can give you a supporting hand if needed. Always practice by a counter or stable chair that you can hold on to if necessary. Signs of improving balance are being able to hold a position longer or without extra support or being able to do the exercise or hold the position with your eyes closed. There may also be some balance exercise classes in your community to help continue your progress. Tai chi is a wonderful program to help you work on balance and strength. It is low-impact and gentle on your joints. The National Institute on Aging offers an exercise guide and video that includes other balance exercises, but you can use these to get started.

27. Beginning Balance

Stand quietly with your feet comfortably apart. Place your hands on your hips, and turn your head and trunk as far to the left as possible and then to the right. Repeat five to ten times. To increase the difficulty, do the same thing with your eyes closed.

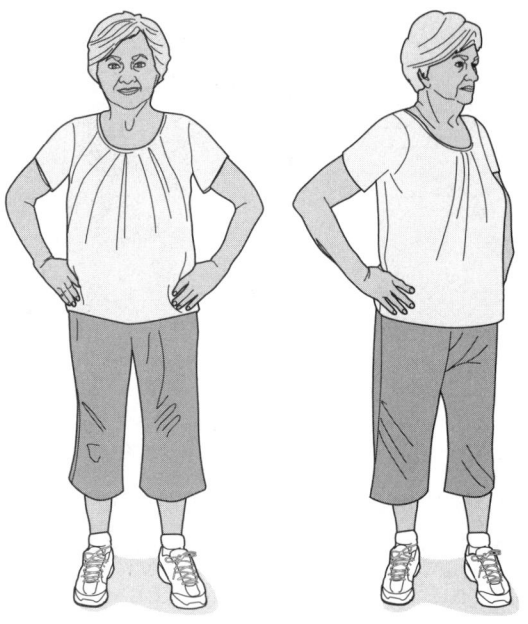 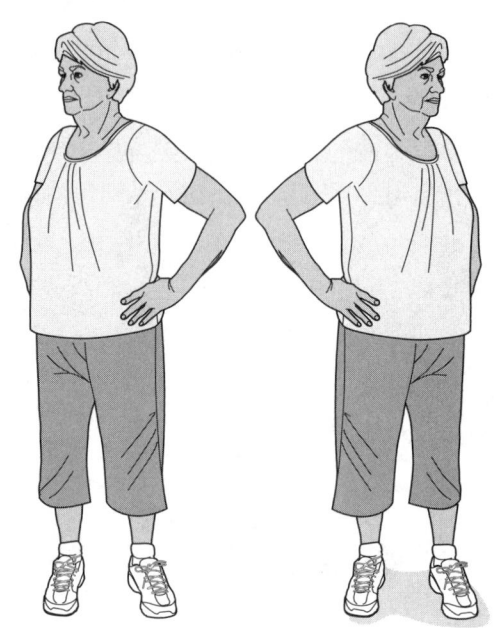

28. Swing and Sway

Using a counter or the back of a stable chair for support, do each of the following five to ten times:

1. Rock back on your heels and then go up on your toes.

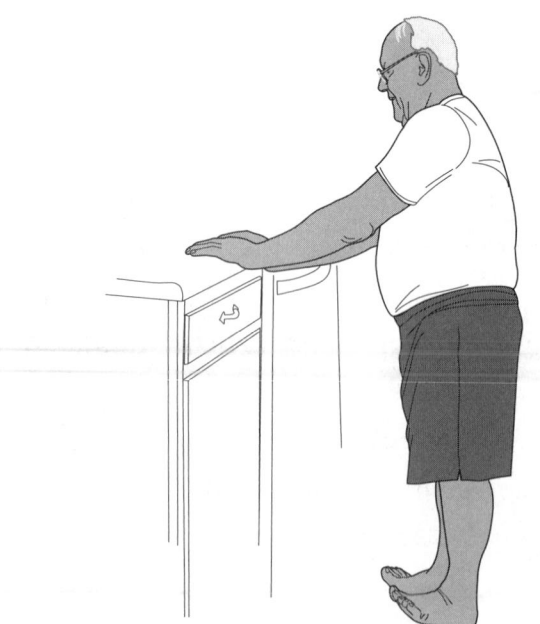 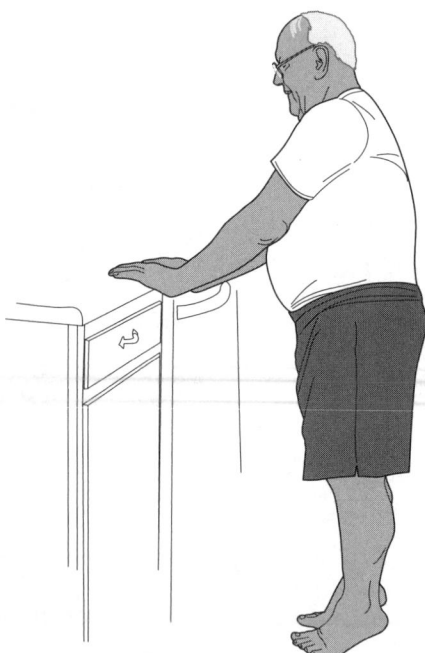

2. Do the box step (like dancing the waltz).

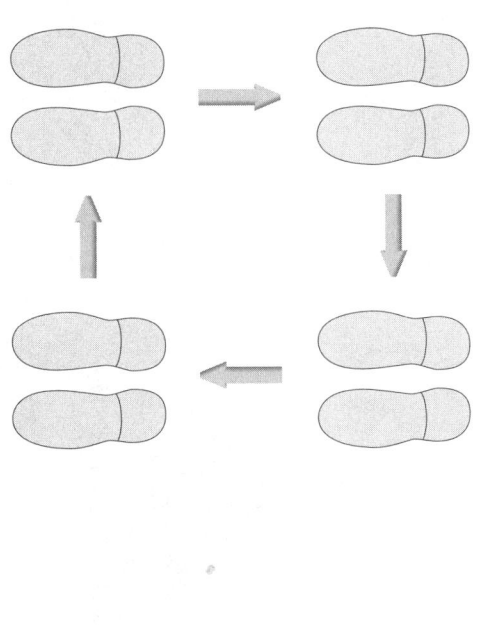

3. March in place, first with eyes open and then with eyes closed.

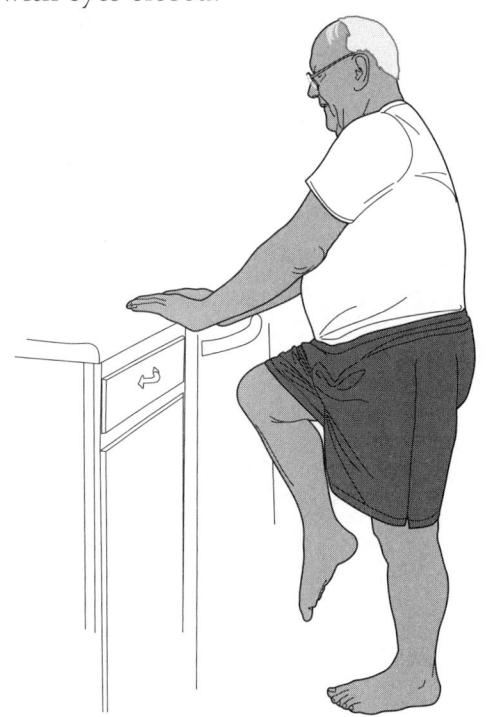

29. Base of Support

Do these exercises with standby assistance or standing close to a counter for support. The purpose of these exercises is to help you improve your balance by going from a larger to a smaller base of support. Work on being able to hold each position for 10 seconds. When you can do it with your eyes open, practice with your eyes closed.

1. Stand with feet together.

2. Stand with one foot out in front and the other back.

3. Stand heel to toe.

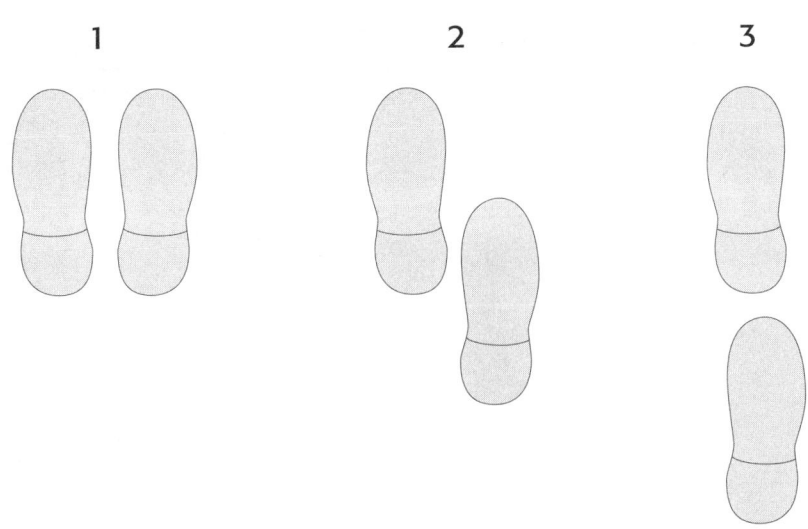

30. Toe Walk

The purpose of this exercise is to increase ankle strength and to give you practice balancing on a small base of support while moving. Stay close to a counter or support. Rise up on your toes and walk up and back along the counter. Once you are comfortable walking on your toes without support and with your eyes open, try it with your eyes closed.

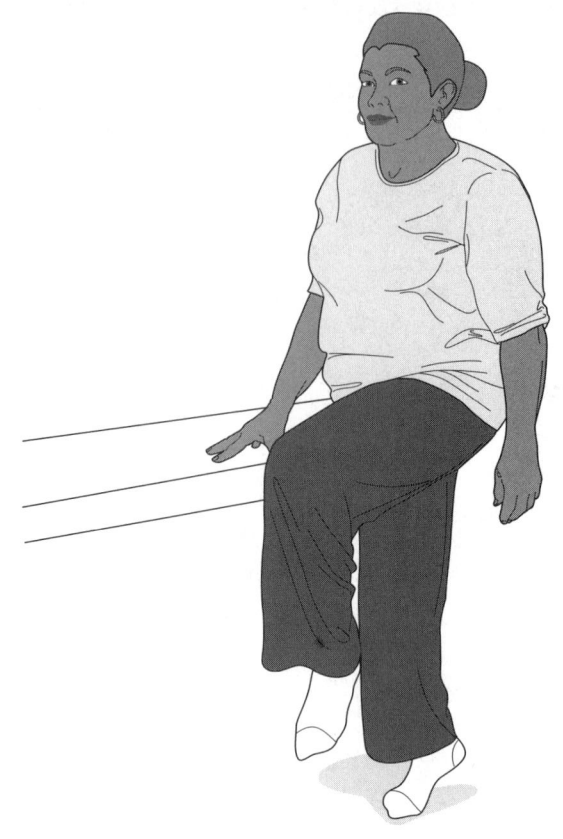

31. Heel Walk

The purpose of this exercise is to increase your lower leg strength and give you practice moving on a small base of support. Stay close to a counter for support. Raise your toes and forefoot and walk up and back along the counter on your heels. Once you are comfortable walking on your heels without support and with your eyes open, try it with your eyes closed.

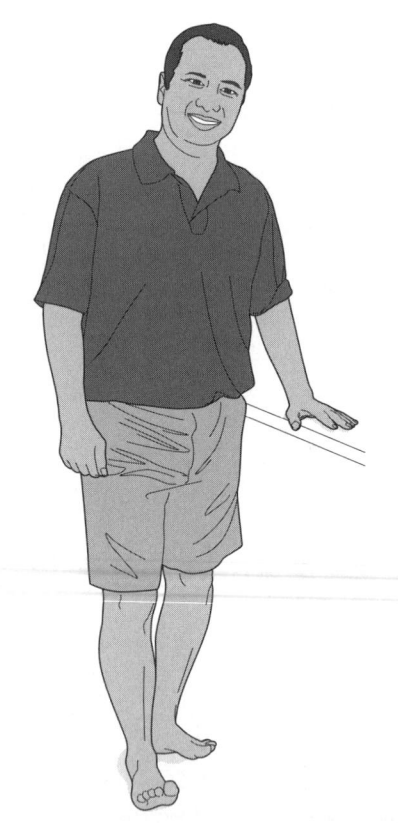

32. One-Legged Stand

Holding on to a counter or chair, lift one foot completely off the ground. Once you are balanced, lift your hand. The goal is to hold the position for 10 seconds. Once you can do this for 10 seconds without holding on, practice it with your eyes closed. Repeat for the other leg.

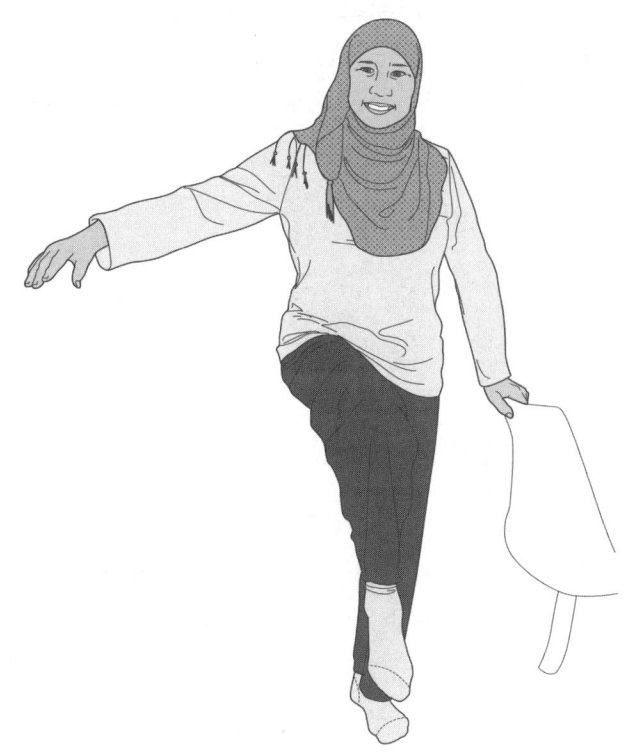

The Whole Body

33. The Stretcher

This exercise is a whole-body stretch to be done lying on your back. Start the motion at your ankles as explained here, or reverse the process if you want to start with your arms first.

1. Point your toes, and then pull your toes toward your nose. Relax.

2. Bend your knees. Then flatten your knees and let them relax.

3. Arch your back. Do the pelvic tilt (Exercise 10). Relax.

4. Breathe in and stretch your arms above your head. Breathe out and lower your arms. Relax.

5. Stretch your right arm above your head, and stretch your left leg by pushing away with your heel. Hold for a count of 10. Switch to the other side and repeat.

Self-Tests

Whatever our goals, we all need to see that our efforts make a difference. Because an exercise program produces gradual change, it's often hard to tell if the program is working and to recognize improvement. Choose several of these flexibility and strength tests to measure your progress. Not everyone will be able to do all the tests. Choose those that work best for you. Perform each test before you start your exercise program, and record the results. After every 4 weeks, do the tests again and check your improvement.

1. Arm Flexibility

Do Exercise 7 (pat and reach) for both sides of the body. Ask someone to measure the distance between your fingertips. *Goal:* Less distance between your fingertips.

2. Shoulder Flexibility

Stand facing a wall with your toes touching the wall. One arm at a time, reach up the wall in front of you. Hold a pencil, or have someone mark how far you reached. Also do this sideways, standing about 3 inches (8 cm) away from the wall. *Goal:* To reach higher.

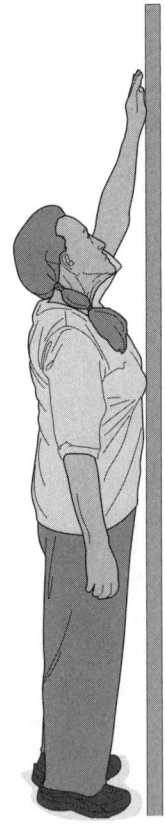 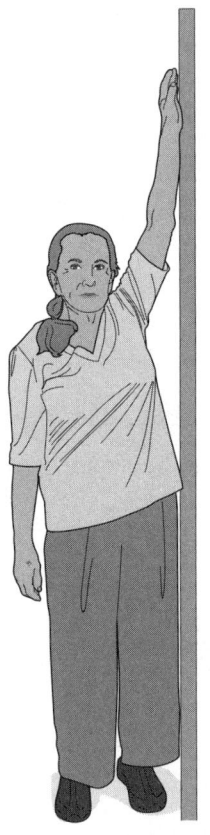

3. Hamstring Flexibility

Do the hamstring stretch (Exercise 21), one leg at a time. Keep your thigh (upper leg) perpendicular to your body. How much does your knee bend? How tight does the back of your leg feel? *Goal:* Straighter knee and less tension in the back of the leg.

4. Ankle Flexibility

Sit in a chair with your bare feet flat on the floor and your knees bent at a 90-degree angle. Keep your heels on the floor. Raise your toes and the front of your foot. Ask someone to measure the distance between the ball of your foot and the floor.

Goal: A distance of 1 to 2 inches (3 to 5 cm) between your foot and the floor.

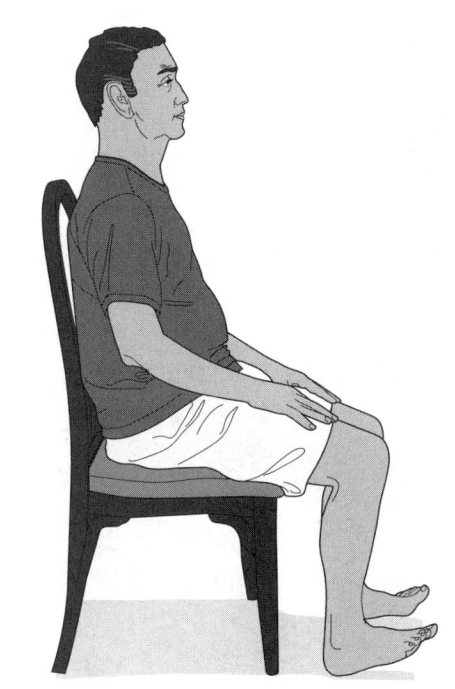

5. Abdominal Strength

Do the curl-up (Exercise 13). Count how many repetitions you can do before you get too tired to do more, or count how many you can do in 1 minute. *Goal:* More repetitions.

6. Ankle Strength

This test has two parts. Stand at a table or counter for support.

Do Exercise 23 (tiptoes) as quickly and as often as you can. How many can you do before you tire?

Stand with your feet flat. Put most of your weight on one foot, and quickly tap the floor with the front part of your other foot. How many taps can you do before you tire? *Goal:* A total of 10 to 15 repetitions of each movement.

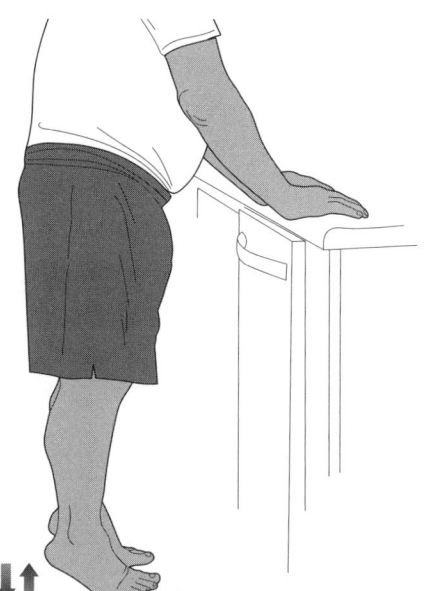

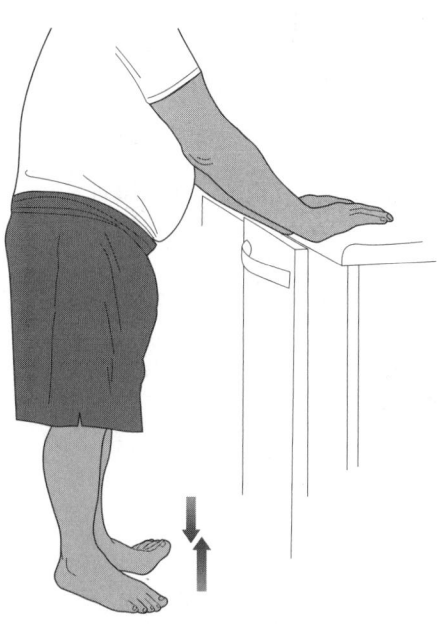

7. Balance

Do Exercise 31 (heel walk), and record how long you can stand on each foot without needing to reach for support. Record times with eyes open and closed. When you are ready to test your balance again, see if you can stand without support longer or if you can balance with eyes closed. The goal is to be able to balance on one foot with your eyes open and closed for 30 seconds each way.

Suggested Further Reading

Blahnik, Jay. *Full Body Flexibility*. Champaign, Ill.: Human Kinetics, 2007.

Knopf, Karl. *Stretching for 50+*. Berkeley, Calif.: Ulysses Press, 2005.

Knopf, Karl. *Weights for 50+*. Berkeley, Calif.: Ulysses Press, 2005.

Moccandanza, Roberto. *Stretching Basics*. New York: Sterling, 2007.

Torkelson, Charlene. *Get Fit While You Sit: Easy Workouts from Your Chair*. Alameda, Calif.: Hunter House, 1999.

Other Resources

☐ Asthma: *Don't Let Exercise-Induced Asthma Keep You Sidelined*, American Lung Association, http://www.lungusa.org/about-us/our-impact/top-stories/active-exercise-asthma.html

☐ *Exercise: Arthritis Self-Management*. [2-CD Audio] Bull Publishing Company, 2006

☐ Exercises for midlife adults and seniors: *Pep Up Your Life*, President's Council on Physical Fitness and Sport, http://www.nia.nih.gov/HealthInformation/Publications

☐ Flexibility, strength, and balance: *Sit and Be Fit* [DVDs], http://www.sitandbefit.org

☐ Physical activity: National Council on Aging, http://www.ncoa.org/improving-health/physical-activity

☐ Physical activity publications: National Institute on Aging, http://www.nia.nih.gov/HealthInformation/Publications [DVD also available]

☐ Preventing falls: National Council on Aging, http://www.ncoa.org/improving-health/falls-prevention

☐ Strength training: Centers for Disease Control and Prevention, *Growing Stronger for Older Adults*, http://www.cdc.gov/physicalactivity/growingstronger/index.htm

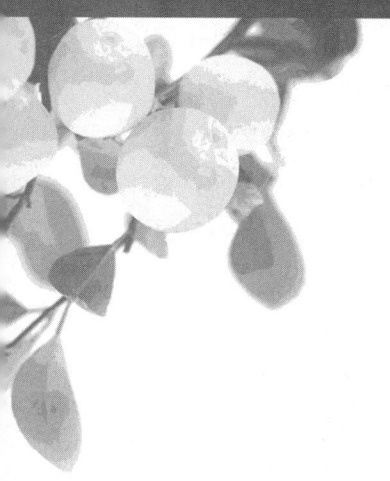

CHAPTER 8

Exercising for Endurance: Aerobic Activities

WHEN THINKING ABOUT AEROBIC (ENDURANCE) EXERCISE, many people are confused about what to do and how much to do. We describe the guidelines for aerobic, flexibility, and strengthening exercise in Chapter 6. Figuring out your very own program may be a challenge. The guidelines recommend that adults exercise at a moderate intensity for at least 150 minutes spread out through the week. There are many ways to work aerobic activities into your day. In this chapter you will learn about exercise effort, various aerobic activities, and how to put together a program that works for you. The most important thing is that some activity is better than none. If you start off doing what is comfortable and increase your efforts gradually, it is likely that you will build a healthy, lifelong habit. You will learn how to stay active and how to get back to activity even when changes in your condition may slow you down for a while. Generally, it is better to begin your program by underdoing rather than overdoing.

You can adjust your exercise effort and work toward your goal by using the three basic building blocks: frequency, time, and intensity.

- **Frequency** is how often you exercise. Most guidelines suggest doing at least some exercise most days of the week. Three to five times a week is a good choice for moderate-intensity aerobic exercise. Taking every other day off gives your body a chance to rest and recover.

- **Time** is the length of each exercise period. According to the guidelines, it is best if you can exercise at least 10 minutes at a time. You can add up 10-minute exercise periods all week to work toward 150 minutes. For example, three 10-minute walks a day for 5 days gets you to 150 minutes for the week. If 10 minutes is too much at first, start with what you can do and work toward 10 minutes.

- **Intensity** is your exercise effort—how hard you are working. Aerobic exercise is safe and effective at a moderate intensity. When you exercise at moderate intensity, you'll feel warmer, you'll breathe more deeply and faster than usual, and your heart will beat faster than normal. At the same time, you will feel that you can continue for a while longer. Exercise intensity is relative to your fitness. For an athlete, running a mile in 10 minutes is probably low-intensity exercise. For a person who hasn't exercised in a long time, a brisk 10-minute walk may be moderate to high intensity. For someone with severe physical limitations, a slow walk may be high intensity. The trick, of course, is to figure out what is moderate intensity for you. There are several easy ways to do this.

Talk Test

When exercising, talk to another person or yourself, or recite poems out loud. Moderate-intensity exercise allows you to speak comfortably. If you can't carry on a conversation because you are breathing too hard or are short of breath, you're working at a high intensity. Slow down to a more moderate level. The talk test is an easy and quick way to recognize your effort and regulate intensity. If you have lung disease, the talk test might not work for you. If that is the case, try using the perceived-exertion scale.

Perceived Exertion

Another way to monitor intensity is to rate how hard you're working on a scale of perceived exertion. There are two scales: 0 to 10 and 6 to 20. On the 0-to-10 scale, 0, at the low end of the scale, is lying down, doing no work at all, and 10 is equivalent to working as hard as possible, very hard work that you couldn't do for more than a few seconds. A good level for moderate aerobic exercise on the 0-to-10 scale is between 4 and 5.

On the 6-to-20 scale, 6 is considered the same as sitting quietly and 20 as working as hard as possible. On the 6-to-20 scale, moderate intensity is between 11 and 14.

Use whichever scale that you like better.

Heart Rate

Unless you're taking heart-regulating medicine (such as the beta-blocker propranolol), checking your heart rate is another way to measure exercise intensity. The faster the heart beats, the harder you're working. (Your heart also beats fast when you are frightened or nervous, but here we're talking about how your heart responds to physical activity.) Endurance exercise at moderate intensity raises your heart rate to a range between 55% and 70% of your safe maximum heart rate. The safe maximum heart rate declines with age, so your safe exercise heart rate gets lower as you get older. You can follow the general guidelines of Table 8.1 or calculate your own exercise heart rate using the formula we're about to give you. Either way, you need to know how to take your pulse.

Take your pulse by placing the tips of your index and middle fingers at your wrist below the base of your thumb. Move your fingers around, but don't push down, until you feel the pulsations of blood pumping with each heartbeat. Count how many beats you feel in 15 seconds. Multiply this number by 4. Start by taking your pulse whenever you think of it, and you'll soon learn the difference between your resting and exercise heart rates. Most people

have a resting heart rate between 60 and 100 beats per minute.

Here's how to calculate your own exercise heart rate range:

1. Subtract your age from 220:

   Example: $220 - 60 = 160$

   You: $220 - \rule{2cm}{0.15mm} = \rule{2cm}{0.15mm}$

2. To find the low end of your exercise heart rate range, multiply your answer in step 1 by 0.55:

   Example: $160 \times 0.55 = 88$

   You: $\rule{2cm}{0.15mm} \times 0.55 = \rule{2cm}{0.15mm}$

3. To find the upper end of your moderate intensity range, multiply your answer in step 1 by 0.7:

   Example: $160 \times 0.7 = 112$

   You: $\rule{2cm}{0.15mm} \times 0.7 = \rule{2cm}{0.15mm}$

The exercise heart rate range for moderate intensity in our example is from 88 to 112 beats per minute. What is yours?

You only need to count your pulse for 15 seconds, not a whole minute. To find your

Table 8.1 Moderate-Intensity Exercise Heart Rate, by Age

Age	Exercise Pulse (beats per minute)	Exercise Pulse (15-second count)
30s	105–133	26–33
40s	99–126	25–32
50s	94–119	24–30
60s	88–112	23–28
70s	83–105	21–26
80s	77–98	19–25
90 and above	72–91	18–23

15-second pulse for exercise, divide both the lower-end and upper-end numbers by 4. The person in our example should be able to count between 22 (88 ÷ 4) and 28 (112 ÷ 4) beats in 15 seconds while exercising.

The most important reason for knowing your exercise heart rate range is so that you can learn not to exercise too vigorously. After you've done your warm-up and 5 minutes of endurance exercise, take your pulse. If it's higher than the upper rate, don't panic. Just slow down a bit. You don't need to work so hard.

If you are taking medicine that regulates your heart rate, have trouble feeling your pulse, or think that keeping track of your heart rate is a bother, use the talk test or a perceived-exertion scale to monitor your exercise intensity.

Be FIT

You can design your own program by using the FIT approach. FIT stands for how often you exercise (F = Frequency), how hard you work (I = Intensity), and how long you exercise each day (T = Time). The guidelines recommend that you exercise at moderate intensity for a minimum of 150 minutes a week. You can build your exercise program by varying frequency, time, and activities. We are recommending moderate-intensity exercise, so you will start slowly and increase frequency and time as you work toward or even beyond 150 minutes each week. You can use different kinds or combinations of exercises. The following are programs of moderate intensity that reach 150 minutes each week:

A 10-minute walk at moderate intensity three times a day, 5 days a week

A 20-minute bike ride at moderate intensity (most on level ground) 3 days a week and a 30-minute walk 3 days a week

A 30-minute aerobic dance class at moderate intensity twice a week and three 10-minute walks 3 days a week

If you are just starting, you could begin like this:

- Take a 5-minute walk around the house three times a day, 6 days a week (total = 90 minutes).

- Take a water aerobics class for 40 minutes twice a week and two 10-minute walks on 2 other days a week (total = 120 minutes).

- Take a low-impact aerobic class once a week (50 minutes), mow the lawn for 30 minutes, and take two 20-minute walks (total = 120 minutes).

An easy way to remember the guideline goal for minimum physical activity is that you should accumulate 30 minutes of moderate physical activity on most days of the week. This could be a combination of walking, stationary bicycling, dancing, swimming, or chores that require moderate-intensity activity. It is important to remember that 150 minutes is a goal, not necessarily your starting point. If you begin exercising just 2 minutes at a time, you are likely to be able to reach the recommended 10 minutes three times a day. Almost everyone can reach the guideline goals and achieve important health benefits. If you have a setback and stop exercising for a while, start back exercising for less time and less vigorously than when you stopped. It takes some time to work back up again; be patient with yourself.

> **Be FIT**
>
> Here's a quick way to remember the three building blocks of your exercise program:
>
> F = Frequency (how often)
> I = Intensity (how hard)
> T = Time (how long)

Warming Up and Cooling Down

If you are going to exercise at moderate intensity, it is important to warm up first and cool down afterward.

Warming Up

Don't exercise cold. Before building to moderate intensity, you must prepare your body to do more strenuous work. This means doing at least 5 minutes of a low-intensity activity to allow your muscles, heart, lungs, and circulation to gradually increase their work. If you are going for a brisk walk, warm up with 5 minutes of slow walking. If you are riding a stationary bike, warm up on the bike with 5 minutes of easy pedaling. In an aerobic exercise class, you will warm up with a gentle routine before getting more vigorous. Warming up reduces the risk of injuries, soreness, and irregular heartbeat.

Cooling Down

A cool-down period after moderate-intensity exercise helps your body return to its normal resting state. Repeating the 5-minute warm-up activity or taking a slow walk helps your muscles gradually relax and your heart and breathing slow down. Gentle flexibility exercises during the cool-down can be relaxing, and gentle stretching after exercise helps reduce muscle soreness and stiffness.

Aerobic (Endurance) Exercises

We will examine a few common low-impact aerobic exercises. All of these exercises can condition your heart and lungs, strengthen your muscles, relieve tension, and help you manage your weight. Most of these exercises can also strengthen your bones (swimming and aqua aerobics are the exceptions).

Walking

Walking is easy, inexpensive, and safe, and it can be done almost anywhere. You can walk by yourself or with company. Walking is safer than jogging or running and puts less stress on the body. It's an especially good choice if you have been sedentary or have joint or balance problems.

If you walk to shop, visit friends, and do household chores, then you can probably walk for exercise. Using a cane or walker need not stop you from getting into a walking routine. If you are in a wheelchair, use crutches, or experience more than mild discomfort when you walk a short distance, you should consider some other type of aerobic exercise or consult a physician or therapist for help.

Be cautious the first two weeks of walking. If you haven't been doing much for a while, 5 or 10 minutes may be enough. Alternate brisk walks and slow walks to build up your time. Each week increase the brisk walking interval by no more than 5 minutes until you are up to 20 or 30 minutes. Remember that your goal is to walk most days of the week, at moderate intensity, to get up to at least 10 minutes at a time. Before starting, read these walking tips.

Walking tips

- **Choose your ground.** Walk on a flat, level surface. Walking on hills, uneven ground, soft earth, sand, or gravel is hard work and often leads to hip, knee, or foot pain. Fitness trails, shopping malls, school tracks, streets with sidewalks, and quiet neighborhoods are good places.

- **Always warm up and cool down with a stroll.** Walk slowly for 5 minutes to prepare your circulation and muscles for a brisker walk. Finish up with the same slow walk to let your body calm down gradually. Experienced walkers know they can avoid shin and foot discomfort if they begin and end with a stroll.

- **Set your own pace.** It takes practice to find the right walking speed. To find your speed, start walking slowly for a few minutes, then increase your speed to a pace that is slightly faster than normal for you. After 5 minutes, check your exercise intensity by using a perceived-exertion or talk test. If you are working too hard or feel out of breath, slow down. If you are below your desired intensity, try walking a little faster. Walk another 5 minutes and check your intensity again. If you are still below your target intensity, keep walking at a comfortable speed and simply check your intensity in the middle and at the end of each walk.

- **Increase your arm work.** You can use your arms to raise your heart rate into the target exercise range. (Note that many people with lung disease may want to avoid arm exercises, as they can cause more shortness of breath than other exercises.) Bend your elbows a bit, and swing your arms more vigorously. You might carry a 1- or 2-pound (0.5 or 1.0 kg) weight in each hand. You can purchase hand weights for walking; hold a can of food in each hand, or put sand, dried beans, or pennies in two small plastic beverage bottles or socks. The extra work you do with your arms increases your intensity of exercise without forcing you to walk faster than you find comfortable.

Shoes

Wear shoes of the correct length and width with shock-absorbing soles and insoles. Make sure they're big enough in the toe area. The rule of thumb is a thumb width between the end of your longest toe and the end of the shoe. You shouldn't feel pressure on the sides or tops of your toes. The heel counter should hold your heel firmly in the shoe when you walk.

Wear shoes with a continuous composite sole. Be sure your shoes are in good repair. Shoes with laces or Velcro let you adjust width as needed and give more support than slip-ons. If you have problems tying laces, consider Velcro closures or elastic shoelaces. Shoes with leather soles and a separate heel don't absorb shock as well as athletic and casual shoes. Good shoes do not need to be expensive; any shoes that meet the criteria we have just described will serve your purposes. Many people like shoes with removable insoles that can be exchanged for more shock-absorbing ones. You can find insoles in sporting goods stores and shoe stores. When you shop

for insoles, take your walking shoes with you. Try on the shoe with the insole inserted to make sure there's still enough room for your foot to be comfortable. Insoles come in different sizes and can be trimmed with scissors for a custom fit. If your toes take up extra room, try the three-quarter insoles that stop just short of your toes. If you have prescribed inserts in your shoes already, ask your doctor about insoles.

Avoid purchasing shoes that are too heavy or that have very thick, rubbery, or sticky soles that may create a tripping hazard.

Possible problems

If you have pain around your shins when you walk, you may not be spending enough time warming up. Try some ankle exercises (Chapter 7, Exercises 24–26) before you start walking. Start your walk at a slow pace for at least 5 minutes. Keep your feet and toes relaxed.

Sore knees are another common problem. Fast walking puts more stress on knee joints. To slow your speed and keep your heart rate up, try doing more work with your arms, as described earlier. Do the knee strengthener and ready-go exercises (Chapter 7, Exercises 18 and 20) in your warm-up.

Cramps in the calf and pain in the heel can be reduced by starting with the Achilles stretch (Chapter 7, Exercise 22). A slow walk to warm up is also helpful. If you have circulation problems in your legs and get cramps or pain in your calves while walking, alternate between comfortably brisk and slow walking. Slow down and give your circulation a chance to catch up before the pain is so intense that you have to stop. As you will see, such exercises may even help you gradually walk farther with less cramping or pain. If this doesn't help, check with your physician or therapist for suggestions.

Maintain good posture. Remember the heads-up position described in Chapter 7, and keep your shoulders relaxed to help reduce neck and upper back discomfort.

Swimming

Swimming is another good aerobic exercise. The buoyancy of the water lets you move your joints through their full range of motion and strengthen your muscles and cardiovascular system with less stress than on land. Because swimming involves the arms, it can lead to excessive shortness of breath. This is especially true for people with lung disease. However, for people with asthma, swimming may be the preferred exercise, as the moisture helps reduce shortness of breath. People with heart disease who have severely irregular heartbeats and have had an implantable defibrillator (AICD) should avoid swimming. For most people with chronic illness, however, swimming is excellent exercise. It uses the whole body. If you haven't been swimming for a while, consider a refresher course.

To make swimming an aerobic exercise, you will eventually need to swim continuously for 10 minutes. Try different strokes, changing strokes after each lap or two. This lets you exercise all joints and muscles without overtiring any one area.

Note that although swimming is an excellent aerobic exercise, it does not improve balance, nor does it provide essential weight-bearing exercise for healthy bones. Incorporating swimming as one part of your overall fitness regime is recommended.

Swimming tips

- The breast stroke and crawl normally require a lot of neck motion and may be uncomfortable. To solve this problem, use a mask and snorkel so that you can breathe without twisting your neck.

- Chlorine can be irritating to the eyes. Consider a good pair of goggles. You can even have swim goggles made in your eyeglass prescription.

- A hot shower or soak in a hot tub after your workout helps reduce stiffness and muscle soreness. Remember not to work too hard or get too tired. If you're sore for more than 2 hours, go easier next time.

- Always swim where there are qualified lifeguards, if possible, or with a friend. Never swim alone.

Aquacize

If you don't like to swim or are uncomfortable learning strokes, you can walk laps in the pool or join the millions who are "aquacizing"—exercising in water.

Aquacize is comfortable, fun, and effective as a flexibility, strengthening, and aerobic activity. The buoyancy of the water takes weight off the hips, knees, feet, and back. Because of this, exercise in water is generally better tolerated than walking by people who have pain in the hips, knees, feet, and back. Exercising in a pool allows you a degree of privacy in doing your own routine in that no one can see you much below shoulder level.

Getting started

Joining a water exercise class with a good instructor is an excellent way to get started. The Arthritis Foundation and the Y sponsor water exercise classes and train instructors to teach them. The heart and lung associations can refer you to exercise programs that include aquacize classes. Contact your local chapter or branch office to see what is available. Many community and private health centers also offer water exercise classes, some geared to older adults.

If you have access to a pool and want to exercise on your own, there are many water exercise books available that can guide you. Water temperature is always a concern when people talk about water exercise. The Arthritis Foundation recommends a pool temperature of 84°F (29°C), with the surrounding air temperature in the same range. Except in warm climates, this means a heated pool. If you're just starting to aquacize, find a pool around this temperature. If you can exercise more vigorously and don't have cold sensitivity, you can probably aquacize in cooler water. Many pools where people swim laps are about 80–83°F (27–28°C). It feels quite cool when you first get in, but starting off with water walking, jogging, or another whole-body exercise helps you warm up quickly.

The deeper the water you stand in, the less stress there is on joints; however, water above the chest can make it hard to keep your balance. You can let the water cover more of your body just by spreading your legs apart or bending your knees a bit.

Aquacize tips

- Wear something on your feet to protect them from rough pool floors and to provide traction in the pool and on the deck. There is footgear especially designed to wear in the water. Some styles have Velcro straps to make them easier to put on. Beach shoes with rubber soles and mesh tops also work well.

- If you are sensitive to cold or have Raynaud's phenomenon, wear a pair of disposable latex surgical gloves. Boxes of gloves are available at most pharmacies. The water trapped and warmed inside the glove seems to insulate the hand. If your body gets cold in the water, wear a T-shirt or full-leg Lycra exercise tights for warmth.

- If the pool does not have steps and it is difficult for you to climb up and down a ladder, suggest that pool staff position a three-step kitchen stool in the pool by the ladder rails. This is an inexpensive way to provide steps for easier entry and exit, and the steps are easy to remove and store when not needed.

- Wearing a flotation belt or life vest adds extra buoyancy and comfort by taking weight off hips, knees, and feet.

- As on land, moving slower makes your exercise easier. Another way to regulate exercise intensity is to change how much water you push when you move. For example, when you move your arms back and forth in front of you under water, it is hard work if you hold your palms facing each other and clap. It is easier if you turn your palms down and slice your arms back and forth with only the narrow edge of your hands pushing against the water.

- Be aware that additional buoyancy allows for greater joint motion than you are probably used to, especially if you are exercising in a warm pool. Start slowly and do not overextend your time in the pool because it feels good until you know how your body will react or feel the next day.

- If you have asthma, exercising in water can help you avoid the worsening of asthma symptoms that occurs during other types of exercise. This is probably due to the beneficial effect of water vapor on the lungs. Remember, though, that for many people with lung disease, exercises involving the arms can cause more shortness of breath than leg exercises. You may want to focus most of your aquacizing, therefore, on exercises involving mainly the legs.

- If you have had a stroke or have another condition that may affect your strength and balance, make sure that you have someone to help you in and out of the pool. Finding a position close to the wall or staying close to a buddy who can lend a hand if needed are ways to add to your safety and security. You may even wish to sit on a chair in fairly shallow water as you do exercises. Ask the instructor to help you design the best exercise program, equipment, and facilities for your specific needs.

Stationary Bicycling

Stationary bicycles offer the fitness benefits of bicycling without the outdoor hazards. They're better for people who don't have the flexibility, strength, or balance to be comfortable pedaling and steering on the road. Some people

with paralysis of one leg or arm can exercise on stationary bicycles with special attachments for their paralyzed limb. Indoor use of stationary bicycles may also be preferable to outdoor bicycling for people who live in a cold or hilly area.

The stationary bicycle is a particularly good alternative exercise. It doesn't put excess strain on your hips, knees, and feet; you can easily adjust how hard you work; and weather doesn't matter. Use the bicycle on days when you don't want to walk or do more vigorous exercise or when you can't exercise outside.

Making it interesting

The most common complaint about riding a stationary bike is that it's boring. If you ride while watching television, reading, or listening to music, you can become fit without becoming bored. One woman keeps interested by mapping out tours of places she would like to visit and then charts her progress on a map as she rolls off the miles. Other people set their bicycle time for the half hour of soap opera or news that they watch every day. There are also videocassettes and DVDs of exotic bike tours that put you in the rider's perspective. Book racks that clip onto the handlebars make reading easy.

Riding tips

- Stationary bicycling uses different muscles than walking. Until your leg muscles get used to pedaling, you may be able to ride for only a few minutes. Start off with no resistance. Increase resistance slightly as riding gets easier. Increasing resistance has the same effect as bicycling up hills. If you

Stationary-Bicycle Checklist

- The bicycle is steady when you get on and off.

- The resistance is easy to set and can be set to zero.

- The seat is comfortable and can be adjusted for full knee extension when the pedal is at its lowest point.

- Large pedals and loose pedal straps allow the feet to move slightly while pedaling.

- There is ample clearance from the frame for the knees and ankles.

- The handlebars allow good posture and comfortable arm position.

use too much resistance, your knees are likely to hurt, and you'll have to stop before you get the benefit of endurance.

- Pedal at a comfortable speed. For most people, 50 to 70 revolutions per minute (rpm) is a good place to start. Some bicycles tell you the rpm rate, or you can count the number of times your right foot reaches its lowest point in a minute. As you get used to bicycling, you can increase your speed. However, faster is not necessarily better. Listening to music at the right tempo makes it easier to pedal at a consistent speed. Experience will tell you the best combination of speed and resistance.

- Set your goal at 20 to 30 minutes of pedaling at a comfortable speed. Build up your time by alternating intervals of brisk pedaling with less exertion. Use your heart rate or the perceived exertion talk test to make sure you aren't working too hard. If you're alone, reciting poems or telling a story to yourself as you pedal can make the time pass more quickly. If you get out of breath, slow down.

- Keep a record of the times and distances of your bike trips. You'll be amazed at how much you can do.

- On bad days, maintain your exercise habit by pedaling with no resistance, at a lower rpm, or for a shorter period of time.

Other Exercise Equipment

If you have trouble getting on or off a stationary bicycle or don't have room for a bicycle where you live, you might try a restorator or arm crank. Ask your therapist or doctor, or call a medical supply house.

A restorator is a small piece of equipment with foot pedals that can be attached to the foot of a bed or placed on the floor in front of a chair. It allows you to exercise by pedaling. Resistance can be varied, and placement of the restorator lets you adjust for leg length and knee bend. A restorator can be a good alternative to an exercise bicycle for people who have problems with balance, weakness, or paralysis. People with other chronic illnesses, such as lung disease, may find the restorator to be an enjoyable way to start an exercise program.

Arm cranks or arm ergometers are bicycles for the arms. They are mounted on a table. People who are unable to use their legs for active exercise can improve their cardiovascular fitness and upper body strength by using the arm crank. It's important to work closely with a physical therapist to set up your program, because using only your arms for endurance exercise requires different intensity monitoring than using the bigger leg muscles. As mentioned previously, many people with lung disease may find arm exercises to be less enjoyable than leg exercises because they may experience shortness of breath.

There are many other types of exercise equipment. These include treadmills, self-powered and motor-driven rowing machines, cross-country skiing machines, mini-trampolines, and stair-climbing and elliptical machines. Most are available in both commercial and home models. If you're thinking about exercise equipment, know what you want to achieve. For cardiovascular fitness and endurance, you want equipment that will help you exercise as much of your body at one time as possible. The motion should be rhythmic, repetitive, and smooth. The equipment should be comfortable, safe, and not stressful on joints. If you're interested in a new piece of equipment, try it out for a week or two before buying.

Exercise equipment that requires you to use weights usually does not improve cardiovascular fitness unless individualized circuit training can be designed. Most people will find that the flexibility and strengthening exercises in this book will help them safely achieve significant increases in strength as well as flexibility. Be sure that you consult with your doctor, therapist, or trained fitness instructor if you want to add strengthening exercises involving weights or weight machines to your program.

Low-Impact Aerobics

Most people find low-impact aerobic dance a fun and safe form of exercise. "Low impact" means that one foot is always on the floor and there is no jumping. However, low impact does not necessarily mean low intensity, nor do the low-impact routines protect all joints. If you participate in a low-impact aerobics class, you'll probably need to make some changes to suit your needs. You can also get low-impact aerobic exercise in classes that include dancing such as Zumba or Jazzercise. Regular dancing such as salsa, ballroom, and square dancing also provide good aerobic exercise.

Getting Started

Let the instructor know who you are, that you may modify some movements to meet your needs, and that you may need to ask for advice. It's easier to start off with a newly formed class than it is to join an ongoing class. If you don't know people, try to get acquainted. Be open about why you may sometimes do things a little differently. You'll be more comfortable and may find others who also have special needs.

Most instructors use music or count to a specific beat and do a set number of repetitions. You may find that the movement is too fast or that you don't want to do as many repetitions. Modify the routine by moving to every other beat or keeping up with the beat until you start to tire and then slowing down or stopping. If the class is doing an exercise that involves arms and legs and you get tired, try resting your arms and doing only the leg movements or just walking in place until you are ready to go again. Most instructors will be able to instruct you in "chair aerobics" if you need some time off your feet.

Some low-impact routines use a lot of arm movements done at or above shoulder level to raise the heart rate. Remember that for people with lung disease, hypertension, or shoulder problems, too much arm exercise above shoulder level can worsen shortness of breath, increase blood pressure, or cause pain. Modify the exercise by lowering your arms or taking a rest break.

Being different from the group in a room walled with mirrors takes courage, conviction, and a sense of humor. The most important thing you can do for yourself is to choose an instructor who encourages everyone to exercise at her or his own pace and a class where people are friendly and having fun. Observe classes, speak with instructors, and participate in at least one class session before making any financial commitment.

Aerobics tips

- **Wear shoes.** Many studios have cushioned floors and soft carpet that might tempt you to go barefoot. Don't! Shoes help protect the small joints and muscles in your feet and ankles by providing a firm, flat surface on which to stand.

- **Protect your knees.** Stand with knees straight but relaxed. Many low-impact routines are done with bent, tensed knees and a lot of bobbing up and down. This can be painful and is unnecessarily stressful. Avoid this by remembering to keep your knees relaxed (aerobics instructors call this "soft knees"). Watch in the mirror to see that you keep the top of your head steady as you exercise. Don't bob up and down.

- **Don't overstretch.** The beginning (warmup) and end (cool-down) of the session will have stretching and strengthening exercises. Remember to stretch only as far as you comfortably can. Hold the position, and don't bounce. If the stretch hurts, don't do it. Instead, ask your instructor for a less stressful substitute, or choose one of your own.

- **Change movements.** Do this often enough that you don't get sore muscles or joints. It's normal to feel some new sensations in your muscles and around your joints when you start a new exercise program. However, if you feel discomfort doing the same movement for some time, change movements or stop for a while and rest.

- **Alternate kinds of exercise.** Many exercise facilities have a variety of exercise opportunities: equipment rooms with cardiovascular machines, pools, and aerobics studios. If you have trouble with an hour-long aerobics class, see if you can join the class for the warm-up and cool-down and use a stationary bicycle or treadmill for your aerobics portion. Many people have found that this routine gives them the benefits of both an individualized program and group exercise.

Self-Tests for Endurance (Aerobic Fitness)

For some people, just the feelings of increased endurance and well-being are enough to indicate progress. Others may need proof that their exercise program is making a measurable difference. You can use one or both of these endurance or aerobic fitness tests. Not everyone will be able to do both tests, so pick one that works best for you. Record your results. After 4 weeks of exercise, repeat the test and check your improvement. Measure yourself again after 4 more weeks.

Testing by Distance

- **Use a pedometer.** One of the least expensive pieces of equipment is a pedometer. Because distance can be difficult to set, the best pedometers measure your steps. If you get in the habit of wearing a pedometer, it is easy to motivate yourself to add a few extra steps each day. You will be surprised at how these add up.

- **Measure distance.** Find a place to walk, bicycle, swim, or water-walk where you can measure distance. A running track works well. On a street you can measure distance with a car. A stationary bicycle with an odometer provides the same measurement. If you plan on swimming or water-walking, you can count lengths of the pool. After a warm-up, note your starting point and then bicycle, swim, or walk as briskly as you comfortably can for 5 minutes. Try to move at a steady pace for the full time. At the end of 5 minutes, mark your spot or note the distance or number of laps, and immediately take your pulse or rate your perceived exertion from 0 to 10. Continue at a slow pace for 3 to 5 more minutes to cool down. Record the distance, your heart rate, and your perceived exertion.

- **Repeat the test** after several weeks of exercise. There may be a change in as soon as 4 weeks. However, it often takes 8 to 12 weeks to see improvement.

  Goal: To cover more distance, to lower your heart rate, or to lower your perceived exertion.

Testing by Time

- **Set a time.** Measure a given distance to walk, bike, swim, or water-walk. Estimate how far you think you can go in 1 to 5 minutes. You can pick a number of blocks, actual distance, or lengths in a pool. Spend 3 to 5 minutes warming up. Start timing and begin moving steadily, briskly, and comfortably. At the finish, record how long it took you to cover your course, your heart rate, and your perceived exertion.

- **Repeat the test** after several weeks of exercise, as you would for distance.

  Goal: To complete the distance in less time, at a lower heart rate, or at a lower perceived exertion.

Suggested Further Reading

Fortmann, Stephen P., and Prudence E. Breitrose. *The Blood Pressure Book: How to Get It Down and Keep It Down*, 3rd ed. Boulder, Colo.: Bull, 2006.

Karpay, Ellen. *The Everything Total Fitness Book*. Avon, Mass.: Adams Media, 2000.

Knopf, Karl. *Make the Pool Your Gym: No-Impact Water Workouts for Getting Fit, Building Strength and Rehabbing from Injury*. Berkeley, Calif.: Ulysses Press, 2012

Nelson, Miriam E, Alice H. Lichtenstein, and Lawrence Lindner. *Strong Women, Strong Hearts: Proven Strategies to Prevent and Reverse Heart Disease Now*. New York: Putnam, 2005.

White, Martha. *Water Exercise: 78 Safe and Effective Exercises for Fitness and Therapy*. Champaign, Ill.: Human Kinetics, 1995.

Other Resources

☐   Sit and Be Fit (chair exercise): http://www.sitandbefit.org

CHAPTER 9

Communicating with Family, Friends, and Health Care Professionals

"You just don't understand!"

HOW OFTEN HAS THIS STATEMENT summed up a frustrating discussion? Whenever we talk with someone, our goal is that the person understands. And we are frustrated when we feel we have not been understood. Failure to communicate effectively can lead to anger, helplessness, isolation, and depression. Such feelings can be even worse when we have a long-term health problem. When communication breaks down, symptoms may go up. Pain can increase, blood sugar and blood pressure levels may rise, and there is increased strain on the heart. Worry caused by conflict and misunderstanding can make us irritable, interfere with concentration, and sometimes lead to accidents. Clearly, poor communication is bad for our physical, mental, and emotional health.

141

Healthy communication is the lifeblood of relationships, and relationships are a lifeline to healthy coping. Poor communication is the biggest reason for poor relationships between spouses or partners or with family members, friends, coworkers, or members of our health care team.

Good communication is a necessity when you have a long-term condition. Your health care team, in particular, must understand you. And when you don't understand advice or recommendations from your doctor, the results can be life-threatening. As a self-manager, effective communication skills are essential.

In this chapter we discuss tools to improve communication. Specifically, these are tools to help you express your feelings in a positive way, to minimize conflict, to ask for help, and to say no. We will also discuss how to listen, how to recognize body language and different styles of communication, and how to get more information from others.

Keep in mind that communication is a two-way street. As uncomfortable as you may feel about expressing your feelings or asking for help, chances are that others are also feeling the same way. It may be up to you to make sure the lines of communication are open. Here are two keys to better communication:

- Do not make assumptions regarding others because "they should know." People are not mind readers. If you want to be sure they know something, tell them.

- You cannot change the communication of others. What you can do is change your communication to be sure you are understood.

Expressing Your Feelings

When communication is difficult, take the following steps. First, review the situation. Exactly what is bothering you? What are you feeling? Here is an example.

John and Steve had agreed to go to a football game. When John came to pick him up, Steve was not ready. In fact, he was not sure he wanted to go because he was having trouble with his arthritic knees. The following conversation took place.

Steve: *You just don't understand. If you had pain like I do, you wouldn't be so quick to criticize. You don't think of anyone but yourself.*

John: *Well, I can see that I should just go by myself.*

In this conversation, neither John nor Steve had stopped to think about what was really bothering him or how he felt about it. Each blamed the other for an unfortunate situation.

The following is the same conversation but with both people using more thoughtful communications.

John: *When we have made plans and then at the last minute you are not sure you can go, I feel frustrated and angry. I don't know what to do—go on without you, stay here and change our plans, or just not make future plans.*

Steve: *When this arthritis acts up at the last minute, I am also confused. I keep hoping I can go and so I don't call you because I don't want to disappoint you and I really want to go. I keep hoping that my knees will get better as the day wears on.*

John: *I understand.*

Steve: *Let's go to the game. You can let me off at the gate before parking so I won't have to walk as far. Then I can do the steps slowly and be in our seats when you arrive. I really want to go to the game with you. In the future, I will let you know sooner if I think my arthritis is acting up.*

John: *Sounds good to me. I really do like your company and knowing how I can help. It is just that being caught by surprise sometimes makes me angry.*

In this dialogue, John and Steve talked about the situation and how they felt about it. Neither blamed the other.

Unfortunately, we are often in situations where the other person uses blaming communications. Maybe we are not listening, get caught, and then we blame the other person. Even in this situation, thoughtful communication can be helpful. Look at the following example.

Jan: *Why do you always spoil my plans? At least you could have called. I am really tired of trying to do anything with you.*

Sandra: *I understand. When my anxiety acts up at the last minute, I am confused. I keep hoping I can go and so I don't call you because I don't want to disappoint you. I really want to go. I keep hoping that I will feel less anxious as the day wears on.*

Jan: *Well, I hope that in the future you will call. I don't like being caught by surprise.*

Sandra: *I understand. If it is OK with you, let's go shopping now. If I start feeling too anxious, I'll take a break in the coffee shop with my book while you continue to shop. I do want us to keep making plans. In the future, if I am too anxious, I will let you know sooner.*

In this example, only Sandra is using thoughtful communication. Jan continues to blame. The outcome, however, is still positive. Both people got what they wanted.

The following are some suggestions for using good communications and creating supportive relationships.

- **Show respect.** Always show respect and regard for the other person. Try not to preach or be excessively demanding. Avoid demeaning or blaming comments such as "Why do you always spoil my plans?" The use of the word *you* is a clue that your communication might be blaming. A bit of tact and courtesy can go a long way in defusing situations (see "Anger" in Chapter 4, page 56).

- **Be clear.** Describe a specific situation or your observations using the facts. Avoid words like *always* and *never*. For example, Sandra said, "When anxiety acts up at the last minute, I am confused. I keep hoping I can go and so I don't call you because I don't want to disappoint you and I really want to go. I keep hoping that I will feel better as the day wears on."

- **Don't make assumptions.** Ask for more detail. Jan did not do this. She assumed that Sandra was rude because she did not call. It would have been better if she asked Sandra why she hadn't called earlier. Assumptions are the enemy of good communication. Many arguments arise from one person expecting the other person to be a mind reader. One sign that you are making assumptions is thinking, "This person should know . . ." Don't rely on mind reading; express your own needs and feelings directly and clearly, and ask questions if you don't understand something.

- **Open up.** Try to express your feelings openly and honestly. Don't make others guess what you are feeling—chances are they may be off-base. Sandra did the right thing. She talked about wanting to go, not wanting to disappoint Jan, and hoping that her anxiety would get better.

- **Accept the feelings of others.** Try to understand them. This is not always easy.

Sometimes you need to think about what was said instead of answering at once. You can always stall a bit by saying "I understand" or "I'm not sure I understand; could you explain some more?"

- **Use humor—sparingly.** Sometimes gently introducing a bit of humor works wonders. But don't use sarcasm or demeaning humor, and know when to be serious.

- **Avoid the role of victim.** You become a victim when you do not express your needs and feelings or expect that someone else should act in a certain way. Unless you have done something to hurt another person, you should not apologize. Apologizing all the time is a sign that you view yourself as a victim. You deserve respect, and you have a right to express your wants and needs.

- **Listen first.** Good listeners seldom interrupt. Wait a few seconds when someone is finished talking before you respond. He or she may have more to say.

"I" Messages

Many of us are uncomfortable expressing our feelings, especially when it may seem that we are being critical of someone else.

If emotions are high, attempts to express frustration can be full of "you" messages. These suggest blame, causing the other person to feel under attack. Suddenly, the other person is on the defensive, and barriers go up. The situation just escalates from there, leading to anger, frustration, and bad feelings.

"I" statements are direct, assertive expressions of your views and feelings; whereas "you" sentences are accusative and confrontational. For example, "I try very hard to do the best work I can," not "You always criticize me." Or "I appreciate it when you turn down the television while I talk," not "You never pay attention." Notice that "I feel that you are not treating me fairly" is actually a disguised "you" statement. A true "I" statement would be, "I feel angry and hurt." Here are some more examples:

"You" message: *"Why are you always late? We never get anywhere on time."*

"I" message: *"I get really upset when I'm late. It's important to me to be on time."*

"You" message: *"There's no way you can understand how lousy I feel."*

"I" message: *"I'm not feeling well. I could really use a little help today."*

Watch out for hidden "you" messages. These are "you" messages with "I feel . . ." stuck in front of them. Here's an example:

"You" message: *"You always walk too fast."*

Hidden "you" message: *"I feel angry when you walk so fast."*

"I" message: *"I have a hard time walking fast."*

The trick to "I" messages is to avoid the use of the word *you* and instead report your personal feelings using the word *I*. Of course, like any new skill, crafting "I" messages takes practice. Start by really listening, to yourself and to others. (Grocery stores are a good place to here

lots of "you" messages as parents talk to their children.) In your head, take some of the "you" messages and turn them into "I" messages. You'll be surprised at how fast "I" messages become a habit. If using "I" statements seems difficult, try adopting this format:

"I notice . . ." (state just the facts)

"I think . . ." (state your opinion)

"I feel . . ." (state what your feelings are)

"I want . . ." (state exactly what you'd like the other person to do)

For example, you make a special bread to bring as a gift to a friend. Somebody comes along in the kitchen, sees it on the counter, and cuts out a large slice. You're upset because, with a piece missing, the gift is ruined. You might say to the bread eater: "You cut into my special bread (observation). You should have asked me about it first (opinion). I'm really upset and disappointed because I can't give it as a gift now (feeling). I'd like an apology, and I'd like for you to ask me first next time (want)."

Here are some "I" message cautions. First, they are not a cure-all. Sometimes the listener has to have time to hear them. This is especially

---

Exercise: "I" Messages

Change the following statements into "I" messages. (Watch out for hidden "you" messages.)

1. "You expect me to wait on you hand and foot!"

2. "Doctor, you never have enough time for me. You're always in a hurry."

3. "You hardly ever touch me anymore. You haven't paid any attention to me since my heart attack."

4. "Doctor, you didn't tell me the side effects of all these drugs or why I have to take them."

Ensuring Clear Communication

Words That Aid Understanding	Words That Hinder Understanding
I	You
Right now, at this time, at this point	Never, always, every time, constantly
Who, which, where, when	Obviously . . .
What do you mean, please explain, tell me more, I don't understand	Why?

true if the person is used to hearing blaming "you" messages. If using "I" messages do not work at first, continue to use them. Things will change as you gain skill and old patterns of communication are broken.

Second, some people use "I" messages as a means of manipulation. They may often express that they are sad, angry, or frustrated in order to gain sympathy from others. If used in this way, problems can escalate. Effective "I" messages must report honest feelings.

Finally, note that "I" messages are an excellent way to express positive feelings and compliments. For example, "I really appreciate the extra time you gave me today, doctor."

Good communication skills help make life easier for everyone, especially those with long-term health problems. The table above summarizes some words that can help or hinder this communication.

Minimizing Conflict

Besides "I" messages, there are other ways to reduce conflict.

- **Shift the focus.** If a discussion gets off topic and emotions are running high, shift the focus of the conversation. That is, bring the discussion back to the agreed topic. For example, you might say something like "We're both getting upset now and drifting away from the topic we agreed to discuss." Or "I feel like we are bringing up other things than what we agreed to talk about, and I'm getting upset. Can we discuss these other things later and just talk about what we originally agreed on?"

- **Buy time.** For example, you might say, "I think I understand your concerns, but I need more time to think about it before I can respond." Or "I hear what you are saying, but I am too frustrated to respond now. I need to find out more about this before I can respond."

- **Make sure you understand each other's viewpoints.** You do this by summarizing what you heard and asking for clarification. You can also switch roles. Try arguing the other person's position as thoroughly and thoughtfully as possible. This will help you understand all sides of an issue, as well as convey that you respect and value the other's point of view. It will also help you develop tolerance and empathy for others.

- **Look for compromise.** You may not always find the perfect solution to a problem or reach total agreement. Nevertheless, it may be possible to compromise. Find something on which you can both agree. For example, you can do it your way this time and the other person's way the next time. Agree to part of what you want and part of what the other person wants. Or decide what you'll do and what the other person will do in return. These are all forms of compromise that can help you through some difficult times.

- **Say you're sorry.** We have all said or done things that have, intentionally or unintentionally, hurt others. Many relationships are hurt—sometimes for years—because people have not learned the powerful social skill of apologizing. Often all it takes is a simple, sincere apology to restore a relationship.

Rather than a sign of weak character, an apology shows great strength. To be effective, an apology must do all of the following:

Admit the specific mistake and accept responsibility for it. You must name the offense; no glossing over with just "I'm sorry for what I did." Be specific. You might say, for example, "I'm very sorry that I spoke behind your back." Explain the particular circumstances that led you to do what you did. Don't offer excuses or sidestep responsibility.

Express your feelings. A genuine, heartfelt apology involves some suffering. Sadness shows that the relationship matters to you.

Acknowledge the impact of wrongdoing. You might say, "I know that I hurt you and that my behavior cost you a lot. For that I am very sorry."

Offer to make amends. Ask what you can do to make the situation better, or volunteer specific suggestions.

Making an apology is not fun, but it is an act of courage, generosity, and healing. It brings the possibility of a renewed and stronger relationship, and it can also bring peace within yourself.

Asking for Help

Getting and giving help is a part of life but one that can cause many problems. Even though most of us sometimes need help, few of us like to ask for it. We may not want to admit that we are unable to do things for ourselves. We may not want to be a burden on others. We may hedge or make a very vague request: "I'm sorry to have to ask this . . ." "I know this is asking a lot . . ." "I hate to ask this, but . . ." Hedging tends to put the other person on the defensive: "Gosh, what's he going to ask that's so much, anyway?" To avoid this response, be specific. A general request can lead to misunderstanding. The person being asked to help may react negatively if the request is not clear. This leads to a further breakdown in communication and no help. A specific request is more likely to have a positive result.

> General request: *"I know this is the last thing you want to do, but I need help moving. Will you help me?"*
>
> Reaction: *"Uh . . . well . . . I don't know. Um . . . can I get back to you after I check my schedule?"* (probably next year!)
>
> Specific request: *"I'm moving next week, and I'd like to move my books and kitchen stuff*

ahead of time. Would you mind helping me load and unload the boxes in my car Saturday morning? I think it can be done in one trip."

> Reaction: *"I'm busy Saturday morning, but I could give you a hand Friday night."*

People with health problems sometimes deal with offers of help that are not needed or desired. In most cases, these offers come from important people in your life. These people care for you and genuinely want to help. A well-worded "I" message allows you to decline the help without embarrassing the other person. "Thank you for being so thoughtful, but today I think I can handle it myself. I hope I can take you up on your offer another time."

Saying No

Let's look at the other side: you are the one being asked for help. It is probably best not to answer right away. You may need more information. If a request leaves you feeling negative, trust your feelings.

The example of helping a person move is a good one. "Help me move" can mean anything from moving furniture up stairs to picking up the pizza for the hungry troops. Using skills that get at the specifics will avoid problems. It is important to understand any request fully before responding. Asking for more information or restating the request will often bring more clarity: "Before I answer, . . ." will not only clarify the request but also prevent the person from assuming that you are going to say yes.

If you decide to say no, it is important to acknowledge the importance of the request. In this way, the person will see that you are rejecting the request rather than the person. Your turndown should not be a putdown. "That sounds like a worthwhile project you're doing, but it's beyond what I can do this week." Again, specifics are the key. Try to be clear about the conditions of your turndown: will you always turn down this request, or is it just that today or this week or right now is a problem? If you are feeling overwhelmed and put upon, saying no can be a useful tool. You may wish to make a counteroffer such as "I won't be able to drive today, but I will next week." But remember, you always have the legitimate right to decline a request, even if it is a reasonable one.

Accepting Help

We often hear "How can I help?" Our answer is often "I don't know" or "Thank you, but I don't need any help." All the time we are thinking, "They should know . . ." Be prepared to accept help by having a specific answer. For example, "It would be great if we could go for a walk together once a week" or "Could you please take out the garbage? I can't lift it." Just remember that people cannot read your mind, so you'll need to tell them what help you want and thank them for it. Think about how each person can help. If possible, give people a task that they can easily accomplish. You are giving them a gift. People like being helpful and feel rejected when they cannot assist someone for whom they care. It is also beneficial to be grateful for the help you receive (see "Practice Gratitude," page 86, in Chapter 5).

Listening

Good listening is probably the most important communication skill. Most of us are much better at talking than we are at listening. When others talk to us, we are often preparing a response instead of just listening. There are several steps to being a good listener:

1. **Listen to the words and tone of voice, and observe body language** (see page 142). There may be times when the words being used don't tell the whole story. Is the voice wavering? Is the speaker struggling to find the right words? Do you notice body tension? Does he or she seem distracted? Do you hear sarcasm? What is the facial expression? If you pick up on some of these signs, the speaker probably has more on his or her mind.

2. **Let the person know you heard what he or she said.** This may be a simple "uh huh." Many times the only thing the other person wants is acknowledgment or just someone to listen. Sometimes it is helpful just to talk to a sympathetic listener.

3. **Let the person know you heard both the content and the emotion behind what he or she said.** You can do this by restating the content. For example, "Sounds like you are planning a nice trip." Or you can respond by acknowledging the emotions: "That must be difficult" or "How sad you must feel." When you respond on an emotional level, the results are often startling. These responses tend to open the gates for more expression of feelings and thoughts. Responding to either the content or the emotion can help communication. It discourages the other person from simply repeating what has been said. But don't try to talk people out of their feelings. They are real to them. Just listen and reflect.

4. **Respond by seeking more information** (see page 142). This is especially important if you are not completely clear about what was said or what is wanted.

Getting More Information

Getting more information is a bit of an art. It can involve both simple and more complicated techniques.

The simplest way to get more information is to ask. "Tell me more" will probably get you more, as will "I don't understand; please explain," "I would like to know more about . . . ," "Would you say that another way?" "How do you mean?" "I'm not sure I got that," and "Could you expand on that?"

Another way to get more information is to paraphrase (repeat what you heard in your own words). This is a good tool if you want to make sure you understand what the other person meant (the actual meaning behind what he or she said). Paraphrasing can either help or hinder effective communication. This depends on the way the paraphrase is worded. It is important to remember to paraphrase in the form of a question, not a statement. For example, someone says:

"I don't know. I'm really not feeling up to par. This party will be crowded, there'll probably be smokers, and I really don't know the hosts very well."

Provocative paraphrase:

"Obviously, you're telling me you don't want to go to the party."

This response might provoke an angry response such as "No, I didn't say that! If you're going to be that way, I'll stay home for sure." Or the response might be no response—a total shutdown because of either anger or despair ("he just doesn't understand"). People don't like to be told what they meant.

Here's a better paraphrase, expressed as a question:

"Are you saying that you'd rather stay home than go to the party?"

The response to this paraphrase might be:

"That's not what I meant. Now that I'm using oxygen, I'm feeling a little nervous about meeting new people. I'd appreciate it if you'd stay near me during the party. I'd feel better about it, and I might have a good time."

As you can see, the second paraphrase helps communication. You have discovered the real reason for expressing doubt about the party. In short, you get more information when you paraphrase with questions.

Be specific. If you want specific information, you must ask specific questions. We often speak in generalities. For example:

Doctor: *"How have you been feeling?"*

Patient: *"Not so good."*

The doctor has not gotten much information. "Not so good" isn't very useful. Here's how the doctor gets more information:

Doctor: Are *you still having those sharp pains in your right shoulder?*

Patient: *Yes. A lot.*

Doctor: *How often?*

Patient: *A couple of times a day.*

Doctor: *How long do they last?*

Patient: *A long time.*

Doctor: *About how many minutes would you say?*

. . . and so on.

Health care providers are trained to get specific information from patients, although they sometimes ask general questions. Most of us are not trained, but we can learn to ask specific questions. Simply asking for specifics often works: "Can you be more specific about . . . ?" "Are you thinking of something special?"

Avoid asking, "Why?" This is far too general a question. "Why?" makes a person think in terms of cause and effect and can put people on the defensive. A person may respond at an entirely different level than you had in mind.

Most of us have had the experience of being with a 3-year-old who just keeps asking "Why?" over and over again. This goes on until the child gets the wanted information (or the parent runs from the room, screaming). The poor parent doesn't have the faintest idea what the child has in mind and answers "Because . . ." in an increasingly specific order until the child's question is answered. Sometimes, however, the parent's answers are very different from what the child really wants to know, and the child never gets the information she or he wanted. Rather than using *why*, begin your responses with *who*, *which*, *when*, or *where*. These words promote a specific response.

We should point out that sometimes we do not get the correct information because we do not know what question to ask. For example, you may be seeking legal services from a senior center. You call and ask if there is a lawyer on staff and hang up when the answer is no. If instead you had asked where you might get low-cost legal advice, you might have gotten some referrals.

Body Language and Conversational Styles

Part of listening to what others are saying includes observing how they say it. Even when we say nothing, our bodies are talking; sometimes they are even shouting. Research shows that our body language is more than half of what we communicate. If we want to communicate really well, we must be aware of body language, facial expressions, and tone of voice. These should match what we say in words. If we do not do this, we are sending mixed messages and creating misunderstandings. For example, if you want to make a firm statement, look at the other person, and keep your expression friendly. Stand tall and confident; relax your legs and arms, and breathe. You may even lean forward to show your interest. Try not to sneer or bite your lips; this might indicate discomfort or doubt. Don't move away or slouch, as these communicate disinterest and uncertainty.

When you notice that the body language and words of others do not match, gently point this out. Ask for clarification. For example, you might say, "Dear, I hear you saying that you would like to go with me to the family picnic, but you look tired and you're yawning as you speak. Would you rather stay home and rest while I go alone?"

In addition to reading people's body language, it is helpful to recognize and appreciate that we all express ourselves differently. "Our conversational styles vary according to where we were born, how we were raised, our occupations, our cultural backgrounds, and especially our genders."

For example, women tend to ask questions that are more personal. These show interest and help form relationships. Men are more likely to offer opinions or suggestions and to state facts. They tend to discuss problems just to find solutions, whereas women want to share their feelings and experiences. No one style is better or worse; they're just different. By acknowledging and accepting these differences, we can reduce some of the misunderstanding, frustration, and resentment we feel in our communications with others.

Communicating with Members of Your Health Care Team

One of the keys to getting good health care is to communicate well with our health care providers. This can be a challenge. We may be afraid to talk freely, or we feel that there is not enough time. Health professionals may use words we do not understand; we may not want to share personal and possibly embarrassing information. These fears and feelings can block communications with our providers and harm our health.

Providers share the responsibility for poor communication. They sometimes feel too busy or important to take the time to talk with and know their patients. They may ignore or tune out our questions. Their actions or inaction might offend us.

Although we do not have to become best friends with our providers, we should expect them to be attentive, caring, and able to explain things clearly. This is especially important if we have an ongoing health condition. We may think that we can only get the best care by going to specialists. This may sometimes be true, but it can also greatly complicate the care you receive. You may be seeing several specialists. They may not get to really know you and may not be aware of what the other care providers are doing, thinking, or prescribing. These are good reasons to have a primary provider or a medical "home." A relationship with a provider is much like a business partnership or even a marriage. Establishing and maintaining this long-term relationship may take some effort, but it can make a large difference to your health.

Your provider probably knows more intimate details about you than anyone else, except perhaps your spouse, partner, or parents. You, in turn, should feel comfortable expressing your fears, asking questions that you may think are "stupid," and negotiating a treatment plan to satisfy you both.

Two things will help keep the lines of communication open. First, we must be clear about what we want from our providers. Many of us would like them to be like warmhearted computers—gigantic brains, stuffed with knowledge about the human body and mind (especially ours). We want our providers to analyze the situation, read our minds, make a perfect diagnosis, come up with a treatment plan, and tell us what to expect. At the same time, we want them to be warm and caring and to make us feel as though we are their most important patient.

Most providers wish they were just that sort of person. Unfortunately, no one provider can be all things to all patients. Providers are human. They have bad days, they get headaches, they get tired, and they get sore feet. They have families who demand their time and attention, and they may get frustrated by paperwork, electronic record keeping, and large bureaucracies.

Most doctors and other health care professionals endured grueling training. They entered the health care system because they wanted to help sick people. They are frustrated when they cannot cure someone with a chronic condition. Many times they must take their satisfaction from improvements rather than cures or even from slowing the decline of some conditions. Undoubtedly, you have been frustrated, angry, or depressed from time to time about your illness, but bear in mind that your doctor has probably felt similar emotions about his or her inability to make you well. In this, you are truly partners.

Time is the second threat to a good patient-provider relationship. If you or your provider had a fantasy about the best thing to happen in your relationship, it would probably involve more face-to-face time. When time is short, the resulting anxiety can bring about rushed communication. "You" messages, and misunderstandings are common.

Most doctors and other providers are on very tight schedules. This becomes painfully clear when you have had to wait in the doctor's office

because of an emergency or a late patient that has delayed your appointment. Doctors try to stay on schedule. This sometimes causes both patients and doctors to feel rushed. One way to help you to get the most from your visit is to take PART (Prepare, Ask, Repeat, Take action).

> **Take P.A.R.T.**
>
> **P**repare
> **A**sk
> **R**epeat
> **T**ake action

Prepare

Before visiting or calling your health care provider, prepare an agenda. What are the reasons for your visit? What do you expect from your doctor?

Take some time to make a written list of your concerns or questions. Have you ever thought to yourself, after you walked out of the doctor's office, "Why didn't I ask about . . . ?" or "I forgot to mention . . . " Making a list beforehand helps ensure that your main concerns get addressed. Be realistic. If you have 13 different problems, your provider probably cannot deal with all of them in one visit. Star or highlight your two or three most important items.

Give the list to your doctor at the beginning of the visit, and explain that you have starred your most important concerns. By giving your doctor the whole list, you let the doctor know which items are the most important to you; it also lets the doctor see everything in case there is something medically important that is not starred. If you wait until the end of your appointment to bring up concerns, there will not be time to discuss them.

Here is an example. The provider asks, "What brings you in today?" and you might say something like "I have a lot of things I want to discuss this visit" (looking at his or her watch and thinking of the appointment schedule, the doctor immediately begins to feel anxious), "but I know that we have a limited amount of time. The things that most concern me are my shoulder pain, my dizziness, and the side effects from one of the medications I'm taking" (the doctor feels relieved because the concerns are focused and potentially manageable within the appointment time available).

There are two other things to prepare before your visit. Bring a list of all your medications and the dosage. If this is difficult, put all your meds in a bag and bring them with you. Do not forget vitamins and over-the-counter medications and supplements.

The final thing to prepare is your story. Visit time is short. When the provider asks how you are feeling, some people will go on for several minutes about this and that symptom. It is better to say, "I think that overall my anxiety is less, but now I have more trouble sleeping." You should be prepared to describe your symptoms:

When they started

How long they last

Where they are located

What makes them better or worse

Whether you have had similar problems before

Whether you have changed your diet, exercise, or medications in a way that might contribute to the symptoms

What worries you most about the symptoms

What you think might be causing the symptoms

If you were on a new medication or treatment, be ready to report how it went. If you are going to several providers, bring with you all the tests that you have had in the past 6 months.

In telling your story, talk about trends (are you getting better or worse, or are you the same?). Also talk about tempo (are your symptoms more or less frequent or intense?). For example, "In general, I am slowly getting better, although today I do not feel well."

Be as open as you can in sharing your thoughts, feelings, and fears. Remember, your provider is not a mind reader. If you are worried, explain why: "I am worried that I may not be able to work," or "My father had similar symptoms before he died." The more open you are, the more likely it is that your provider can help. If you have a problem, don't wait for the provider to "discover" it. State your concern immediately. For example, "I am worried about this mole on my chest."

The more specific you can be (without overdoing it with irrelevant details), the clearer a picture the doctor will have of your problem, and the less time will be wasted for both of you.

Share your hunches or guesses about what might be causing your symptoms, as they often provide vital clues to an accurate diagnosis. Even if it turns out that your guesses are not correct, it gives your doctor the opportunity to reassure you or address your hidden concerns.

Ask

Your most powerful tool in the doctor-patient partnership is the question. You can fill in vitally important missing pieces of information and close critical gaps in communication with your questions. And asking all your questions reflects your active participation in the process of care, a critical ingredient to restoring your health. Getting answers and information you understand is a cornerstone of self-management. Be prepared to ask questions about diagnosis, tests, treatments, and follow-up.

- **Diagnosis.** Ask what's wrong, what caused it, if it is contagious, what the future outlook (prognosis) is, and what can be done to prevent or manage it.

- **Tests.** If the doctor wants to do tests, ask how the results are likely to affect treatment and what will happen if you are not tested. If you decide to have a test, find out how to prepare for the test and what it will be like. Also ask how and when you will get the results.

- **Treatments.** Ask if there are any choices in treatments and the advantages and disadvantages of each. Ask what will happen if you have no treatment (see Medications, page 217).

- **Follow-up.** Find out if and when you should call or return for a follow-up visit. What symptoms should you watch for, and what should you do if they occur?

Repeat

One way to check that you have really gotten everything is to briefly report back key points. For example, "You want me to take this three times a day." Repeating back also gives the provider a chance to quickly correct any misunderstandings and miscommunications.

If you don't understand or remember something the provider said, admit that you need to go over it again. For example, "I'm pretty sure you told me some of this before, but I'm still confused about it." Don't be afraid to ask what you may consider a stupid question. Such questions are important and may prevent misunderstanding.

Sometimes it is hard to remember everything. You may want to take notes or bring another person to important visits. You can even tape-record the visit if the medical professional grants permission.

Take Action

At the end of a visit, you need to clearly understand what to do next. This includes treatments, tests, and when to return. You should also know any danger signs and what you should do if they occur. If necessary, ask your provider to write down instructions, recommend reading material, or indicate other places you can get help.

If for some reason you can't or won't follow the provider's advice, let her or him know. For example, "I didn't take the aspirin. It gives me stomach problems" or "My insurance doesn't cover that much therapy. I can't afford it" or "I've tried to exercise, but I can't seem to keep it up." If your provider knows why you can't or won't follow advice, she or he may be able to make other suggestions. If you don't share the barriers to taking actions, it's difficult for your provider to help.

Asking for a Second Opinion

Sometimes you may want to see another provider or have a second opinion. Asking for this can be hard. This is especially true if you have had a long relationship with your provider. You may worry that asking for another opinion will anger your provider or that your provider will take your request in the wrong way. Providers are seldom hurt by requests for a second opinion. If your condition is complicated or difficult, the doctor may have already consulted with another doctor (or more than one). This is often done informally. However, if you find yourself asking for third, fourth, and fifth opinions, this may be unproductive.

Asking for a second opinion is perfectly acceptable, and providers are taught to expect such requests. Ask for a second opinion by using a nonthreatening "I" message:

"I'm still feeling confused and uncomfortable about this treatment. I feel that another opinion might reassure me. Can you suggest someone I could see?"

In this way, you have expressed your own feelings without suggesting that the provider is at fault. You have also confirmed your confidence in your provider by asking for his or her recommendation. (However, you are not bound by this suggestion; you may choose to see anyone you wish.)

Giving Positive Feedback to Your Providers

Let your provider know how satisfied you are with your care. If you do not like the way you have been treated by any of the members of your health care team, let them know. Likewise, if you are pleased with your care, let your providers know. Everyone appreciates compliments and positive feedback, especially members of your health care team. They are human, and your praise can help nourish and console these busy, hardworking professionals. Letting them know that you appreciate their efforts is one of the best ways to improve your relationship with them—plus it makes them feel good!

Your Role in Medical Decisions

Many decisions in medical care are not clear-cut, and often there is more than one option. The best decisions, except in life-threatening emergencies, depend on your values and preferences and should not be left solely to your doctor. For example, if you have high blood pressure, you might say, "I'm very conservative about taking medications. What's a reasonable period of time for me to try exercise, diet, and relaxation first, before I start taking the medication?"

To make an informed choice about any treatment, you need to know what the cost and risks of the proposed treatment are. This includes the likelihood of possible complications such as drug reactions, bleeding, infection, injury, or death. It also includes the personal costs, such as absences from work, and financial considerations, such as how much of the proposed treatments your insurance will cover.

You also need to understand how likely it is that the proposed treatments will benefit you in terms of prolonging your life, relieving your symptoms, or improving your ability to function.

Sometimes the best choice may be to delay a decision about treatment in favor of "watchful waiting."

No one can tell you which choice is right for you. But to make an informed choice, you need information about the treatment options. Informed choice, not merely informed consent, is essential to quality medical care. The best medical care for you combines your doctor's medical expertise with your own knowledge, skills, and values.

Making decisions about treatments can be difficult. For some suggestions on how to make decisions, see page 18, and see Chapter 14 for help on how to evaluate new treatments.

Working with the Health Care System

So far we have discussed communication with providers. Today most providers work in larger systems such as clinics. Appointments, billing, and telephone and e-mail use are usually decided by someone other than your provider.

If you are unhappy with your health care system, don't just suffer in silence. Do something about it. Find out who is running the organization and who makes decisions. Then share your feelings in a constructive way by letter, phone, or e-mail. Most health care systems want to keep you as a patient and therefore usually respond. The problem is that the people who make the decisions tend to isolate themselves. It is easier to express our feelings to the receptionist, nurse, or doctor. Unfortunately, these people have little or no power in the system. However, they can tell you whom to write to. The more closely you can form a partnership with your providers, the better able all of you together will be to make the system more responsive.

If you do decide to write or e-mail, here are some suggestions. Keep your letter short and factual. Tell what actions you would find helpful. For example:

Dear Mr. Brown:

Yesterday I had a 10:00 A.M. appointment with Dr. Zim. She did not see me until 12:15 P.M., and my total time with the doctor was eight minutes. I was told to make another appointment so I could get my questions answered.

I know that sometimes there are emergencies. I would appreciate being called if my doctor is running late or told when to return. I would also like 15 or more minutes with my doctor.

I would appreciate a reply within two weeks.

The following are a few hints for working with the health care system. Not all of these problems and suggestions will apply to all systems, but most do.

■ **"I hate the phone system."** Often when we call for an appointment or information, we reach an automated system. This is frustrating. Unfortunately, we cannot change this. However, phone systems do not change often. If we can memorize the numbers or keys to press, we can move more quickly from one part of the system to another. Sometimes pressing the pound key (#) or 0 will get us to a real person. Once you do get through, ask if there is a way to do this faster next time.

■ **"It takes too long to get an appointment."** Ask for the first available appointment. Take it. Then ask how you can learn about cancellations. Some systems are happy to call you when they have an empty spot. In others, you may have to call them once or twice a week to check on cancellations. Ask the person making the schedule what you can do to get an earlier appointment. Ask for a telephone number so you can reach the person making appointments directly. Some systems are now setting time aside each day for same-day appointments. If this is available, know when to call. It is usually early in the morning. If you are in pain or believe that you must see a doctor soon, tell the scheduler. If nothing is available, ask how you can see someone soon. No matter how frustrated you are, be nice. The scheduler has the power to either give you an appointment or not.

- **"I have so many providers; I do not know whom to ask for what."** One of those providers has to be in charge. Your job is to find out which one. Ask each provider who is in charge of coordinating your care. When you get a name, it is most likely your primary care doctor or GP. Call the doctor to confirm that he or she is coordinating your care. Ask how you can help. One way is to let this doctor know when someone else orders a test or new medication. Keeping the doctor informed is especially important when your providers are not in the same system and are not sharing their electronic medical records.

- **"What is an electronic medical record (EMR) anyway?"** Most of your medical information is on a secure computer. Your information can be seen by any provider in the same system. You should know what

information is on the system. Sometimes the EMR has just test results, other times it has test results and medication information, and sometimes it has everything that is known about you. An electronic medical record is just like a paper record: it does no good if your providers don't read it. For example, when you have a test, the doctor ordering the test will know when the test results are ready. However, your other doctors will not know anything about the test unless you tell them to read the results. In short, learn about the medical records system so you can help all your providers use it more effectively.

In the United States and many other countries, you have the right to a copy of almost everything in your record. Ask for copies of all your test results so that you can carry them with you from one provider to the next. In this way, you know that they will not get lost.

- **"I can never talk to my doctor."** It is hard to get a provider on the phone, but you might be able to e-mail. Many systems now have ways that doctors and patients can communicate by text or e-mail. The next time you see your provider, ask about this. One good thing about systems is that there is usually a way to get routine things like medication refills done quickly. It may mean calling a special number or talking to the nurse. Learn how to do this.

A medical emergency is important. Do not waste time trying to contact your doctor; rather, call 911 (in the United States), go to a hospital emergency department, or call the rescue squad.

- **"I have to wait too long in the waiting room or the examination room."** Emergencies happen sometimes, and this can cause a wait. More often the system is not efficient. If your schedule is tight and may cause a problem if you are delayed at your appointment, you might try calling your doctor's office and asking how long you will have to wait. If you learn that your doctor is running late, you can decide whether to go with a book to read or ask to reschedule. You can also show up with your book and ask about the wait. Rather than getting upset, let the receptionist know that you are going to step out for a little while to run a short errand nearby or for a cup of coffee or some shopping and that you will return within a specified amount of time.

- **"I don't have enough time with the provider."** This may be a system problem since someone else often decided how many patients to schedule and for how long. The decision is sometimes based on what you tell the scheduler. If you say you need a blood pressure check, you will be given a short visit. If you say you are very depressed and cannot function, you may be given a longer appointment. When making the appointment, ask for the amount of time you want, especially if this is more than 10 or 15 minutes. Be prepared to make

a case for more time. You can also ask for the last appointment in the day. You may have to wait a while, but at least the provider will not be pressured because there are more patients to see.

- Once you are with a provider and you request more time than is allotted, you make other people wait. An extra 5 minutes may not seem like much. However, a doctor often sees 30 patients a day. If each one takes 5 extra minutes, this means that the doctor has to work an extra 2½ hours that day! Those little bits of extra time add up.

Parting Words of Advice

- If something in the health care system is not working for you, ask how you can help make it work better. Very often, if you learn how to navigate the system, you can solve or at least partially solve your problems.

- Be nice—or at least as nice as possible. If the system or your provider sees you as a difficult patient, life will become more difficult.

If you think that things should not be this way and that it is not fair to place this burden on the patient, we wholeheartedly agree. Health systems should change to be more responsive and patient-friendly. A few health care systems are already doing this. In the meantime, we offer these suggestions to help you deal with a difficult situation.

Suggested Further Reading

Beck, Aaron T. *Love Is Never Enough: How Couples Can Overcome Misunderstandings, Resolve Conflicts, and Solve Relationship Problems Through Cognitive Therapy.* New York: HarperCollins, 1989.

Davis, Martha, Kim Paleg, and Patrick Fanning. *The Messages Workbook: Powerful Strategies for Effective Communication at Work and Home.* Oakland, Calif.: New Harbinger, 2004.

Gottman, John M., and Joan DeClaire. *The Relationship Cure : A 5-Step Guide to Strengthening Your Marriage, Family, and Friendships.* New York: Three Rivers, 2001.

Gottman, John M., and Nan Silver. *The Seven Principles for Making Marriage Work: A Practical Guide from the Country's Foremost Relationship Expert.* New York: Three Rivers, 1999.

Hendrix, Harville. *Getting the Love You Want: A Guide for Couples.* New York: Henry Holt, 1988.

Jones, J. Alfred, Gary L. Kreps, and Gerald M. Phillips. *Communicating with Your Doctor: Getting the Most Out of Health Care.* Cresskill, N.J.: Hampton Press, 1995.

McKay, Matthew, Martha Davis, and Patrick Fanning. *Messages: The Communication Skills Book.* Oakland, Calif.: New Harbinger, 2009.

Tannen, Deborah. *"You Just Don't Understand": Women and Men in Conversation.* New York: HarperCollins, 1990.

Other Resources

☐ Medline Plus, *Talking with Your Doctor,* 2012, http://www.nlm.nih.gov/medlineplus/talkingwithyourdoctor.html

CHAPTER **10**

Sex and Intimacy

LOVING RELATIONSHIPS WITH PHYSICAL INTIMACY and sexual
pleasure are basic human needs. However, many indi-
viduals and couples with chronic physical or mental health problems are challenged
in maintaining this important part of their lives. Emotions, including fear of injury, of
being unable to perform, or of causing a health emergency, can dampen desire in one or
both partners. Likewise, fear of increasing symptoms can frustrate couples, even if the
symptoms occur only during sex itself. Sex, after all, is supposed to be joyful and pleasurable, not scary or uncomfortable!

For humans, sex is more than the act of sexual intercourse or achieving orgasm; it is
also the sharing of our physical and emotional selves. There is a special intimacy when
we make love. Believe it or not, then, having a chronic health problem may actually offer
the opportunity to improve your sex life by encouraging you to experiment with new
types of physical and emotional stimulation. This process of exploring sensuality with

161

your partner can open communication and strengthen your relationship. Furthermore, when we have sex, natural "feel-good" hormones, including endorphins, are released into our bloodstream. These help us achieve a deep sense of relaxation and feeling of well-being.

For many people with chronic conditions, intercourse is difficult because of the physical demands. Intercourse increases the heart rate and breathing and can tax someone with limited energy or with breathing or circulatory problems. Therefore, it is helpful to spend more time on sensuality or foreplay and less on actual intercourse. By concentrating on ways to arouse your partner and give pleasure while in a comfortable position, your intimate time together can last longer and be very satisfying. Many people enjoy climax without intercourse; others may wish to climax with intercourse. For some, climax may not be as important as sharing pleasure. There are many ways to enhance sensuality during sexual activity. In sex, as in most things, our minds and bodies are linked. By recognizing this, we can increase the sexual pleasure we experience through both physical and mental stimulation.

Emotional concerns can also be a serious factor for someone with health problems. Someone who has had a heart attack or a stroke is often concerned that sexual activity will bring on another attack. People with breathing difficulties worry that sex is too strenuous and will trigger coughing and wheezing or worse. Their partners may fear that sexual activity might cause these problems or even death and that they would be responsible. Some diseases such as diabetes can make erections difficult or cause vaginal dryness. These worries can certainly hurt the relationship.

Loss of self-esteem and a changed self-image can be subtle and devastating sexual barriers. Many people with chronic conditions believe that they are physically unattractive. This may be because of paralysis, shortness of breath, weight gain from medications, the changing shape of their joints, or the loss of a breast or other body part. Mental health problems also damage people's sense of self, which causes them to avoid sexual situations; they "try not to think about it." Ignoring the sexual part of the relationship or physically and emotionally distancing themselves from their partner leads to depression, which in turn leads to lack of interest in sex and more depression—a vicious cycle. Depression can be treated, and you can feel better. For more on depression and how to help yourself overcome it, see Chapter 4. If self-management techniques are not enough, talk to your doctor or therapist.

Even good sex can get better. Thankfully, there are ways you and your partner can explore sensuality and intimacy, as well as some ways to overcome fear during sex.

Overcoming Fear During Sex

Anyone who has experienced a chronic condition has experienced fear that it will get worse or that any worsening could be life-threatening.

Health problems can really get in the way of the activities that we want and need to do. When sex is the activity that fear affects, we have a

Misconceptions About Sex

Many of our sexual attitudes and beliefs are learned—they are not automatic or instinctual. We begin learning these when we are young. They come from friends, older children, parents, and other adults. We also learn them through jokes, magazines, TV, and movies. Much of what we learn about sex is mixed with inhibitions, "shoulds," "musts," "should nots," "must nots," and misconceptions.

To maximize your sexual enjoyment, you often have to break down your misconceptions so that you are free to discover and explore your own sexuality. For example, many people believe a number of things that simply aren't true:

- Older people can't enjoy sex.
- Sex is for people with beautiful bodies.
- A "real man" is always ready for sex.
- A "real woman" should be sexually available whenever her partner is interested.
- Lovemaking has to involve sexual intercourse.
- Sex must lead to orgasm.
- Orgasm should occur simultaneously in both partners.
- Kissing and touching should only be done when they lead to sexual intercourse.

difficult problem: not only are we denying ourselves an important, pleasurable part of life, but we probably also feel guilty about disappointing our partner. On the other hand, our partner may feel more fearful and guilty than we do—afraid that he or she might hurt us during sex and guilty for perhaps feeling resentful. This dynamic can cause serious relationship problems. The resulting stress and depression can produce even more symptoms. We don't have to allow this to happen!

For successful sexual relationships, the most important thing is communication. The most effective way to address the fears of both partners is to confront them and find ways to alleviate them through good communication and problem solving. Without effective communication, learning new positions and ways to increase sensuality are not going to be enough. This is particularly important for people who

may worry about how their health problem may make them look physically to others. Often they find that their partner is far less concerned about their looks than they are.

When you and your partner are comfortable with talking about sex, you can go about finding solutions. Start by sharing what kinds of physical stimulation you prefer and which positions you find most comfortable. Then you can share the fantasies you find most arousing. It's difficult to dwell on fears when your mind is occupied with a fantasy.

To get this process started, you and your partner may find some help with communication skills in Chapter 9 and problem-solving techniques in Chapter 2. Remember, if these techniques are new, give them time and practice. As with any new skill, it takes patience to learn to do them well.

Sensual Sex

In our society sexual attraction has become almost solely dependent on the visual experience. This leads to an emphasis on our physical image. Sight, however, is only one of our five senses. Therefore, when we think about being sensual, we must also appreciate the seductive qualities of our partner's voice, scent, taste, and touch. Sensual sex is about connecting with our partner through all the senses, making love not only with the eyes but with our ears, nose, mouth, and hands as well.

Sensual touch is particularly important because the largest sensual organ of our bodies is the skin; it is rich with sensory nerves. The right touch on almost any area of our skin can be very erotic. Fortunately, sexual stimulation through touch can be done in just about any position and can be enhanced with the use of oils, flavored lotions, scents, feathers, fur gloves—whatever the imagination desires. Just about any part of the body is an erogenous zone. The most popular are the mouth, ear lobes, neck, breasts and nipples (for both genders), navel area, hands (fingertips if you are giving pleasure, palms if you are receiving pleasure), wrists, small of the back, buttocks, toes, and insides of the thighs and arms. Experiment with the type of touch—some people find a light touch arousing; others prefer a firm touch. Many people also become very aroused when touched with the nose, lips, and tongue or even sex toys.

Sensuality with Fantasy

What goes on in our mind can be extremely arousing. If it weren't, there would be no strip clubs, pornography, or romance novels. Most people engage in sexual fantasy at some time or another. There are probably as many sexual fantasies as there are people. It is OK to mentally indulge in fantasy. If you discover a fantasy that you and your partner share, you can play it out in bed, even if it is as simple as a particular saying you or your partner like to hear during sex.

Engaging the mind during sexual activity can be every bit as arousing as the physical stimulation. It is also useful when symptoms during sex interfere with your enjoyment. But you also want to be careful—sometimes fantasy leads to unrealistic expectations. Your real partner might not compare favorably to your dream lover. You may find decreased sexual satisfaction if you regularly fire up your imagination with explicit photos or videos of young, hard bodies.

Overcoming Symptoms During Sex

Some people are unable to find a sexual position that is completely comfortable. Others find that pain, shortness of breath, fatigue, or even negative thoughts (self-talk) during sex are so distracting that they interfere with the enjoyment of sex or the ability to have an orgasm. This can pose some special problems. If you are unable to climax, you may feel resentful of your partner.

If he or she is unable to climax, you may feel guilty about it. If you avoid sex because you are frustrated, your partner may become resentful and you may feel guilty. Your self-esteem may suffer. Your relationship with your partner may suffer. Everything suffers.

One thing you can do to help deal with this situation is to time the taking of medication so that it is at peak effectiveness when you are ready to have sex. Of course, this involves planning ahead. The type of medication may be important too. If you take a narcotic-type pain reliever, for example, or one containing muscle relaxants or tranquilizers, you may find that your sensory nerves are dulled along with your pain. Obviously, it would be counterproductive to dull the nerves that will give you pleasure. Your thinking may also be muddled due to the medication, making it more difficult to focus. Some medications can make it difficult for a man to achieve an erection; others can help with an erection. Ask your doctor or pharmacist about possible timing or alternatives if this is a problem for you.

Another way to deal with uncomfortable symptoms is to become an expert at fantasy. To be really good at something, you have to train for it, and this is no exception. The idea here is to develop one or more sexual fantasies that you can indulge in when needed, making it vivid in your mind. Then, during sex, you can call up your fantasy and concentrate on it. By concentrating on the fantasy or on picturing you and your partner making love while you actually are, you are keeping your mind consumed with erotic thoughts rather than your symptoms or negative thoughts. However, if you have not had experience in visualization and imagery

techniques, generally used for relaxation exercises such as those in Chapter 5, you will need to practice several times a week to learn them well. All of this practice need not be devoted to your chosen sexual fantasy, however. You can start with any guided imagery tape or script such as the ones in Chapter 5, working to make it more vivid each time you practice. Start with just picturing the images. When you get good at that, add and dwell on colors; then, in your mind, look down to your feet as you walk; then listen to the sounds around you; then concentrate on the smells and tastes in the image and feel your skin being touched by a breeze or mist; finally, feel yourself touch things in the image. Work on one of the senses at a time. Become good at one before going on to another. Once you are proficient at imagery, you can invent your own sexual fantasy and picture it, hear it, smell it, and feel it. You can even begin your fantasy by picturing yourself setting your symptoms aside. The possibilities are limited only by your imagination.

Learning to call on this level of concentration can also help you focus on the moment. Really focusing on your physical and emotional sensations during sex can be powerfully erotic. If your mind wanders (which is normal), gently bring it back to the here and now. ***IMPORTANT: Do not try to overcome chest pain or sudden weakness on one side of the body in this way. These symptoms should not be ignored, and a physician should be consulted right away.***

If you decide that you wish to abstain from sexual activity because of your chronic health problem or if it is not an important part of your life, that's OK—but it is important that your partner be in agreement with your decision. Good communication skills are essential in this situation, and you may even benefit from discussing the situation with a professional therapist present. Someone trained to deal with important interpersonal situations can help facilitate the discussion.

Sexual Positions

Finding a comfortable sexual position can minimize symptoms during sex. They can also minimize fear of pain or injury for both partners. Experimentation may be the best way of finding the right positions for you and your partner. Everybody is different; no one position is good for everyone. We encourage you to experiment with different positions, possibly before you and your partner are too aroused. Experiment with placement of pillows or with using a sitting position on a chair. Experimentation itself can be erotic.

No matter which position you try, it is often helpful to do some warm-up exercises before sex. Look at some of the stretching exercises in Chapter 7. Exercise can help your sex life in other ways as well. Becoming more fit is an excellent way to increase comfort and endurance during sex. Walking, swimming, bicycling, and other activities can benefit you in bed as well as elsewhere by reducing shortness of breath, fatigue, and pain. They also help you learn your limits and how to pace yourself, just as in any other physical activity.

During sexual activity, it may be advisable to change positions once in a while. This is especially true if your symptoms come on or increase when you stay in one position too long. This can be done in a playful fashion, whereby it becomes fun for both of you. As with any exercise, stopping to rest is OK.

Special Considerations

People with certain health problems have specific concerns about sex and intimacy. For example, people who are recovering from a heart attack or stroke are often afraid to resume sexual relations for fear of not being able to perform or of bringing on another attack or even death. This fear is even more common for their partners. Fortunately, there is no basis for this fear, and sexual relations can be resumed as soon as you feel ready to do so. Studies show that the risk of sexual activity contributing to a heart attack is less than 1%. And this risk is even lower in individuals who do regular physical exercise. After a stroke, in particular, any remaining paralysis or weakness may require a little more attention to finding the best positions for support and comfort and the most sensitive areas of the body to caress. There may also be concerns about bowel and bladder control. The American Heart Association (http://www.heart.org) has some excellent guides about sex after a heart attack or stroke.

People with diabetes sometimes report problems with sexual function. Men may have difficulty achieving or maintaining an erection, which can be caused by medication side effects or other medical conditions associated with diabetes. Women and men can have reduced feeling (neuropathy) in the genital area. Women's most common complaint is not enough vaginal lubrication. For people with diabetes, the most effective ways to prevent or lessen these problems is to maintain tight management of blood sugar, exercise, keep a positive outlook, and generally take care of themselves. Lubricants can help with sensitivity for both men and women. If you are using condoms, be sure to use a water-based lubricant; petroleum-based lubricants destroy latex. The use of a vibrator can be very helpful for individuals with neuropathy, and concentrating on the most sensual parts of the body for stimulation can help make sex pleasurable. There are new therapies for men with erectile problems. The American Diabetes Association (http://www.diabetes.org) has more detailed information about sex and diabetes.

Chronic or recurring pain can put a big damper on sexual interest. It can be difficult to feel sexy when you are hurting or are afraid that sex will make you hurt. Pain is often the main symptom of arthritis, migraine headaches, bowel disease, and many other disorders. People with these conditions have the challenge of overcoming pain in order to become sexually aroused or to have an orgasm. This is one area where concentration and focus, as discussed earlier in this chapter, are helpful skills. Learning to focus on the moment or on sexual fantasy can distract you from the pain and allow you to concentrate on sex and your partner. Time your

pain medication to have maximum effect during sex, find a comfortable position, take it slow and easy, relax, and enjoy extended foreplay.

People who are missing a breast, testicle, or another body part as a result of their treatment for cancer or some other medical condition, or people with surgical scars or swollen or disfigured joints from arthritis, may also have fears about sex and intimacy. In these cases, people may worry about what their partner will think. Will their partner or potential partner find them undesirable? Although this may happen sometimes, it actually occurs less often than you think. Usually when we fall in love with someone, we fall in love with who the person is, not that person's breast, testicle, or other body part. Here again, good communication and the sharing of your concerns and fears with your partner can help. If this is difficult to do alone, perhaps talking with a couples counselor may help you. Often what you think will be a problem really is not.

Fatigue is another symptom that can kill sexual desire. In Chapter 4 we talked a lot about how to deal with fatigue. Here we will add one more hint: plan your sexual activities around your fatigue; that is, try to engage in sex during the times you are less tired. This might mean that mornings are better than evenings.

Many mental health conditions and the medications used to treat their symptoms can also interfere with sexual function and desire. Therefore, it is important to talk with your doctor about these side effects so that together you can find alternatives. Sometimes the doctor may find another medication, change the dosage and timing of the medication, or refer you to a therapist who may help you and your partner learn other coping strategies to decrease or eliminate symptoms. Individual or couples therapy can also help in dealing with other non-medication-related personal relationship, intimacy, and sexual problems.

No matter what your chronic health problem, your doctor should be your first consultant on chronic-condition-related sexual problems. It's unlikely that your problem is unique; your doctor has probably heard about it many times before and may have some solutions. Remember, this is just another problem associated with your chronic condition, just like fatigue, pain, and physical limitations, and it is a problem that can be addressed. Chronic health problems need not end sex. Through good communication and planning, satisfying sex can prevail. By being creative and willing to experiment, both the sex and the relationship can actually be better.

Suggested Further Reading

Agravat, Pravin. *A Guide to Sexual and Erectile Dysfunction in Men*. Leicester, England: Troubador, 2010.

American Heart Association. *Sex and Heart Disease*. Dallas, Tex.: American Heart Association, 2008.

American Heart Association and American Stroke Association. *Sex After Stroke: Our Guide to Intimacy After Stroke*. Dallas, Tex.: American Heart Association and American Stroke Association, 2011.

Ford, Vicki. *Overcoming Sexual Problems*. London: Constable & Robinson, 2010.

Garrison, Eric Marlowe. *Mastering Multiple-Position Sex: Mind-Blowing Lovemaking Techniques That Create Unforgettable Orgasms*. Beverly, Mass.: Quiver Books, 2009.

Hall, Kathryn. *Reclaiming Your Sexual Self: How You Can Bring Desire Back into Your Life*. Hoboken, N.J.: Wiley, 2004.

Kaufman, Miriam, Cory Silverburg, and Fran Odette. *The Ultimate Guide to Sex and Disability: For All of Us Who Live with Disabilities, Chronic Pain, and Illness*. Berkeley, Calif.: Cleis Press, 2007.

Klein, Marty. *Beyond Orgasm: Dare to Be Honest About the Sex You Really Want*. Berkeley, Calif.: Celestial Arts, 2002.

McCarthy, Barry W., and Michael E. Metz. *Men's Sexual Health: Fitness for Satisfying Sex*. New York: Routledge, Taylor & Francis, 2008.

Schnarch, David. *Intimacy and Desire: Awaken the Passion in Your Relationship*. New York: Beaufort Books, 2009.

Schnarch, David. *Resurrecting Sex: Solving Sexual Problems and Revolutionizing Your Relationship*. New York: HarperCollins, 2002.

Other Resources

☐   American Diabetes Association: http://www.diabetes.org/

☐   American Heart Association: http://www.heart.org/

☐   Arthritis Foundation: http://www.arthritis.org/

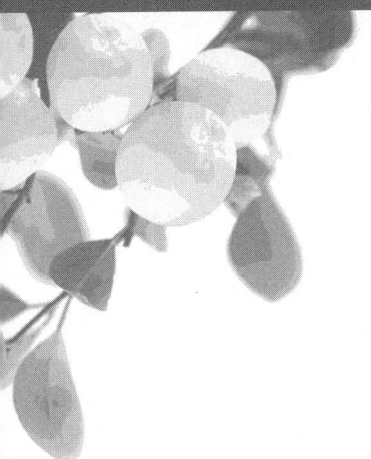

CHAPTER **11**

Healthy Eating

HEALTHY EATING IS ONE OF YOUR BEST personal investments. It is a central player that influences your health. No matter what the media or your friends say, there is no one best way of eating that fits everyone; there is no perfect food.

Eating healthy means that most of the time you make good and healthful food choices. It does not mean being rigid or perfect. It can mean finding new or different ways to prepare your meals to make them tasty and appealing. If you have certain health conditions, it may mean that you have to be choosier. Eating well does not usually mean you can never have the foods you like most.

Unfortunately, thanks to the Internet, books, other media, friends, and relatives, we can get overloaded with information about what we should and should not eat. The

Special thanks to Bonnie Bruce, DrPH, RD, for her help with this chapter.

169

whole eating thing gets very confusing. In this chapter we give you basic science-based nutrition and diet information. We are not going to tell you what to eat or how to eat. That is your decision. We will tell you what is known about nutrition for adults and some ways to help you fit that information to your specific likes and needs. On pages 192–194 we give information for individuals with the most common long-term health conditions. We hope that this chapter will help you start making changes on your way to healthier eating.

Why Is Healthy Eating So Important?

The human body is a very complex and marvelous machine, much like an automobile. Autos need the proper mix of fuel to run right. Without it, they may run rough and may even stop working. The human body is similar. It needs the proper mix of good food (fuel) to keep it running well. It does not run right on the wrong fuel or on empty.

Healthy eating cuts across every part of your life. It is linked to your body and your mind's well-being, including how your body responds to some illnesses.

When you give your body the right fuel and nourishment, here's what happens:

- You have more energy and feel less tired.

- You increase your chances of potentially preventing or lessening further problems from health conditions such as heart disease, diabetes, and cancer.

- You feed your brain, which can help you handle life's challenges as well as its emotional ups and downs.

What Is Healthy Eating?

At the heart of healthy eating are the choices we make over the long run. Healthy eating is being flexible and allowing yourself to occasionally enjoy small amounts of foods that may not be so healthy. There is no such thing as a perfect eating style. Being too strict or rigid and not allowing yourself ever to have a treat will likely cause your best efforts to fail.

For some of us, healthy eating means having to be somewhat choosy about the foods we eat. For example, people with diabetes need to watch their carbohydrate intake to manage their blood sugar levels. They do best each day by deciding which carbohydrate foods, such as fruit, breads, beans, cereals, and rice, they will eat. Others, who have heart disease or are at risk for heart disease, find that watching the amount and kinds of fat they eat can help control their blood cholesterol levels. Those with high blood pressure find that they can help lower their blood pressure by eating lots of fruits, vegetables, low-fat dairy foods, and for some people cutting back on salt. To lose or gain weight, we need to pay attention to how many calories we eat.

We have come a long ways since meat and potatoes were thought of as the backbone of a great diet. Today, vegetables, fruits, whole grains, low-fat milk and low-fat milk products, lean meats, poultry, and fish are at the core of a great diet. There is still a place for meat and potatoes; it is just not the most important place.

The real issue for most of us is not the healthy foods we choose but the less healthy ones. One-third of most American diets is made up of foods that are high in added sugars, solid fats (butter, beef fat [tallow, suet], pork fat [lard], chicken fat, stick margarine, shortening), and sodium (salt). We also eat a lot of food that is made from white flour and other refined grains. These added sugars, fats, and sodium contribute to such health problems as high blood pressure, diabetes, and obesity.

Trade-offs are a big part of healthy eating. This means learning how food affects you and then deciding when you can treat yourself and when you should pass. For instance, it may be important for you to have a very special meal on your birthday, but then you can trade off and make healthier choices when you are out for a casual lunch. Trading off is a tool that can help you stay on the path of healthy eating. As you get better at this, you will find it gets easier and even becomes part of your everyday life.

Most dietary guidelines suggest that a good starting place is to move toward eating more plant foods: whole grains, fruits, vegetables, cooked dry beans and peas, lentils, nuts, and seeds. This does not mean giving up meats and other foods high in sugar, fat, or sodium but rather eating them in smaller amounts or less often. Many current dietary guidelines recommend moderate amounts of lean meats, poultry, and eggs. Balance in the kinds of foods you eat and how much you eat are the primary elements. (We'll have more to say about this a little later in this chapter.)

This all sounds simple, but every day we are faced with hundreds of food choices. It is often easier and quicker to grab something less healthful than to think about what we will eat, much less cook the food. So how do we put together meals that are tasty and enjoyable yet healthful? Let's try to make it as simple as possible.

Key Principles of Healthy Eating

- **Choose foods as nature originally made them.** This means the less processed the better. By *processed* we mean foods that have been changed from their original state by having ingredients added (often sugar or fat) or removed (often fiber or nutrients) to make them tastier—for example, whole grains made into white flour for bakery products or animal foods made into luncheon or deli meats. Foods that are least or minimally processed include a grilled chicken breast instead of fried breaded chicken nuggets, a baked potato (with skin) rather than French fries, and whole grains, such as whole-grain bread and pasta and brown rice, instead of refined grains such as white bread and white rice.

- **Get your nutrients from food, not supplements.** We know that for most people, vitamin, mineral, and other dietary supplements cannot completely take the place of food. Foods as nature makes them contain nutrients and other healthy compounds (such as fiber) in the right combinations and amounts to do the body's work properly. When we remove nutrients from their natural state in food, they may not work the way they should. They may even have harmful side effects.

For instance, take beta carotene, an important source of vitamin A, found in plant foods such as carrots and winter squash. It helps our vision and enhances our immune system. However, artificial beta-carotene supplements have been shown in some people to increase some cancer risks. This same risk does not happen when beta carotene is eaten as it is naturally found in food.

Another reason to get your nutrition from foods as close as possible to how nature made them is that these choices could contain as yet unknown healthful compounds. When you take a supplement such as a vitamin pill, you could be missing out on many other helpful substances that are naturally packaged with the food from which the vitamin was removed.

In most of the world, including the United States, diet and nutrition supplements do not have to follow government rules for quality or goodness. Unlike over-the-counter medications, with supplements there is no guarantee that you are getting what you pay for or that you are not getting harmful substances.

Is there ever a place for dietary supplements? Yes, sometimes we cannot get enough of one or more of the nutrients we need. For example, older men and women need a large amount of calcium to help prevent or slow osteoporosis. Although we could get enough calcium from milk and milk products such as yogurt or cheese, getting the amount needed can be difficult. If you are thinking of taking a supplement, talk to your health care professional or a registered dietitian first.

- **Eat a wide variety of colorful and minimally processed foods.** The more variety in your foods, the better; the more colors on your plate, the better; and the less processed your food, the better.

  By following these three simple rules, your body will probably get all the good things it needs. This means a plate that contains minimally processed meat, fish, or poultry and a lot of colorful fruits and vegetables—think blue and purple for grapes and blueberries; yellow and orange for pineapple, oranges, and carrots; red for tomatoes, strawberries, and watermelon; and green for spinach and green beans—along with the white and warm brown tones from mushrooms, onions, and cauliflower and whole grains such as brown rice.

- **Eat foods high in phytochemicals.** Phytochemicals are compounds that are found only in plant foods—fruits, vegetables, whole grains, nuts, and seeds (*phyto* means "plant"). There are hundreds of health-promoting and disease-fighting phytochemicals. These include compounds that give fruits and vegetables their bright colors. Whenever a food is refined or processed, as when whole wheat is made into white flour, phytochemicals are lost. The more often you choose foods that are not refined, and as close as possible to how nature made them, the better.

■ **Eat regularly.** A gas-fueled vehicle will not run without the gas, and a fire eventually burns out without more wood. Your body is much the same. It needs refueling regularly to work at its best. Eating something, even a little bit, at regular intervals helps keep your "fire" burning.

Eating at regular times during the day, preferably evenly spaced over the day, also helps maintain and balance your blood sugar level. Blood sugar is a key player in supplying the body, especially the brain, with energy. Usually, the brain can only use blood sugar for energy. If you do not eat regularly, your blood sugar drops, and depending on how low it gets, low blood sugar can cause weakness, sweating, shaking, mood changes (irritability, anxiety, or anger, for example), nausea, headaches, or poor coordination. Low blood sugar (hypoglycemia) can be dangerous for many people.

Eating regularly helps you get the nutrients you need and helps your body use those nutrients. Of course, not skipping meals or not letting too many hours go between meals also helps keep you from getting overly hungry. Being overly hungry often leads to overeating. This can in turn lead to such problems as indigestion, heartburn, and weight gain.

Finally, eating regularly does not mean that you must stick to the same routine every day. Nor does it mean that you must follow the "normal" pattern of eating three meals a day. Allow yourself room for give and take.

If you have certain health conditions, such as cancer, you may find that sometimes several small meals over the day while at other times fewer, bigger meals work best. For people with diabetes, spacing meals regularly and balancing what you eat is important, but this could mean several small meals a day, three meals mixed with a snack, or just three meals, based on what is best for you.

■ **Eat what your body needs (not more or less).** This is easy to say but more difficult to put into action. How much you should eat depends on things like the following:

Your age (we need fewer calories as we get older)

If you are a man or woman (men usually need more calories than women)

A Note About Breakfast

Breakfast is just that: "breaking the fast." It refuels your body after going without eating for many hours and helps you resist the urge to eat extra snacks or overeat the rest of the day.

We know that you may not want to eat breakfast, not only because you don't have the time or aren't hungry but maybe because you do not like the usual breakfast foods. There are no set rules about what you should eat in the morning. Breakfast can be anything—fruit, beans, rice, bread, broccoli, even leftovers. The important thing is to kick-start your body each day by refueling it.

Your body size and shape (in general, if you are taller or have more muscle, you can eat more)

Your health needs (some conditions affect how your body uses calories)

Your activity level (the more you move or exercise, the more calories you can eat)

Tips to Help You Manage How Much You Eat

- **Stop eating when you first feel full.** This helps you control the amount you eat and helps prevent overeating. Pay attention to your body so you can learn what this feels like. Like all new skills, it takes some practice. If it is hard to stop eating when you begin to feel full, remove your plate or get up from the table, if you can.

- **Eat slowly.** Eating slowly gives you more enjoyment and helps prevent overeating. Make your meals last at least 15 to 20 minutes. It takes this much time for the brain to catch up and tell your stomach that it is getting full. If you finish quickly, wait at least 15 minutes before getting more food. If this is difficult, there are some more tips on pages 198-199.

- **Pay attention to what you eat.** If you are not aware of what you are doing, it is easy to eat an entire bag of chips or cookies or eat too much of any bite-sized pieces of food without even knowing it. This can happen easily when we are with friends, using the computer, or watching television. In these situations, try portioning out what you want to eat or keeping food out of reach or out of sight.

- **Know a serving size when you see one.** To do this, you need to know a little about what a serving size or portion looks like. A ½-cup portion is about the size of a tennis ball or a closed fist. A 3-ounce portion of cooked meat, fish, or poultry is about the size of a deck of playing cards or the palm of your hand. The end of your thumb to the first joint is about 1 teaspoon; three times that is a tablespoon. (*Tip:* Using a measuring cup is a great way to see what a serving size looks like.)

- **Watch out for supersizing and portion inflation.** In recent years, serving sizes have literally "beefed up." The typical adult cheeseburger used to have about 330 calories; now it has a whopping 590 calories. Twenty years ago, an average cookie was about 1½ inches wide and had 55 calories; now it is 3½ inches wide and has 275 calories—*five times* the calories! Soda typically came in 6½-ounce bottles with 85 calories; today it's 20 ounces to a bottle, with 250 calories.

  It takes an extra 3,500 calories more than we need to gain a pound of body fat. This means that over one year's time, only an extra 100 calories a day will cause you to put on 10 pounds. This is equal to each day eating only an extra third of a bagel! There are many published ranges of recommended serving sizes for different foods. In the food guide on pages 186–192, we list some common serving sizes for a variety of foods along with selected nutrients.

■ **When practical, select single-size portions.** Foods that come prepackaged as single servings can help you see what a suggested serving should look like. If that serving size seems too small compared to what you would usually eat, we suggest that you start slowly by cutting how much you now

eat by just a small amount at a time. For example, if you usually eat 1 cup of rice, try eating ½ cup instead.

■ **Make your food attractive.** We really do eat with our eyes! Compare the mouth-watering appeal of a plate with white fish, white rice, and white cauliflower with one of golden brown chicken, grilled sweet potato, and bright green spinach. Which of these two meals seems more appetizing?

An Easy Map for Healthy Eating

A map will help you along your path and get you to where you are going. The U.S. Department of Agriculture's Map for Healthy Eating in Figure 11.1 helps you see what a healthy meal should look like. Put your meal together so that one-fourth of the plate is covered with colorful fruit, one-fourth with vegetables, one-fourth with a protein source (lean meat, fish, or poultry, or better yet, plant foods such as tofu, cooked dry beans, or lentils), and the remaining one-fourth with grains (preferably at least half from whole grains) or other starches such as potatoes, rice, yams, or winter squash. Finish off your plate with calcium-rich foods. These could be milk or foods made from milk (preferably fat-free or low-fat), such as cheese, yogurt, frozen yogurt, puddings, or calcium-fortified soy foods such as soymilk. Of course, your food choices and amounts will depend on what you like and need. If you would like more information about this way of eating, check out the USDA's MyPlate Web site at http://www.chooseMyPlate.gov.

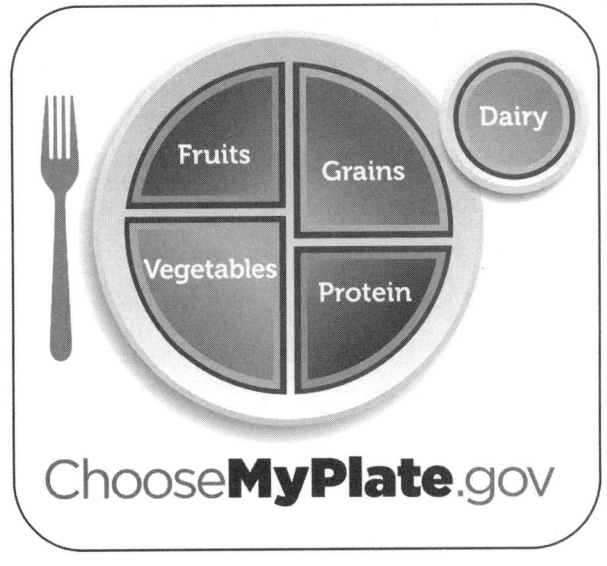

Figure 11.1 **MyPlate: A Map for Healthy Eating**

For people with diabetes, the American Diabetes Association recommends a similar plate, shown on page 193.

Even with this map, calories and portion sizes are important. Plate sizes are now larger, making it is easier to get more calories than you want or need. Table 11.1 on page 180 can help you plan. It gives you examples of recommended daily portions from different food groups. Note that these amounts are general recommendations and may be different if you have special dietary needs. If you have questions, check with your doctor or a registered dietitian.

Note, too, when you go to the Internet, you will find many people who say they are nutrition experts, but they may not be. If you want a real expert, look for a registered dietitian (RD). These health professionals are specially trained and are the best sources for diet and nutrition advice and information.

Nutrients: What the Body Needs

Earlier we talked about the need to get nutrients from food. In the following sections, we talk about carbohydrates, fats, protein, water, and a few vitamins and minerals. In addition, although it is technically not a nutrient, we also talk about fiber. Fortunately, it is quite easy to get everything that we need from healthy eating.

First, take a look at Table 11.1, Daily Recommended Servings, with Examples for Healthy Meal Planning. It shows the number of recommended servings for adult women and men along with examples of serving sizes. These recommendations are for people who do less than 30 minutes of moderate exercise a day and eat 1,000 to 3,000 calories. If you have a special health problem or condition, such as diabetes, you may need to change how much you eat of certain foods. Even so, you can still follow the Map for Healthy Eating. We discuss some special dietary issues such as diabetes later in this chapter.

Carbohydrates: Your Body's Chief Energy Source

With few exceptions, carbohydrates are your body's go-to fuel for the brain, central nervous system, and red blood cells. Carbohydrates largely determine your blood glucose (sugar) level—more so than protein or fat. But carbohy-

drates do a great deal more. They also provide us with basic materials to help make other vital parts for the body. Nearly every part of your body, from your toenails to the top of your head, probably used some part of a carbohydrate in its construction. These include hormones, fats, cholesterol, and even some vitamins and proteins.

Carbohydrates are found mostly in plant foods. Milk and yogurt are about the only animal foods with more than a very small amount of carbohydrate. Foods with carbohydrates can be categorized by whether they are high in sugar or high in starch. Foods that are high in sugar usually break down faster, get into your blood faster, and give you energy faster than high-starch foods. Many minimally processed plant foods also contain fiber. Although fiber is essentially not absorbed into the body and does not have calories, it helps you in important ways.

Sugary carbohydrates are found in fruit and juice, milk, yogurt, table sugar, honey, jellies, syrups, and sugar-sweetened drinks. There are also a lot of other sugars (maltose and dextrose among them) that are found naturally in foods and are often added to processed foods.

Starchy carbohydrates are found in vegetables such as corn, green peas, potatoes, winter squash, dried beans and peas, lentils, and grains such as rice. Pasta, tortillas, and bread are also high in carbohydrates. The amount of carbohydrate in whole grains, brown rice, and whole wheat bread is similar to that in refined grains, such as white bread and white rice. The big difference between them is that the refined grains have lost nutrients, phytochemicals, and fiber during processing.

Fiber is found naturally in whole and minimally processed plant foods with "skins, seeds, and strings." For example, whole grains, dried beans, peas, lentils, fruits, vegetables, nuts, and seeds all have some fiber. Some foods have added fiber (as when pulp is added to juice). Animal foods and refined and processed foods (white flour, bread, many baked and snack foods) have little or no fiber unless it was added by the manufacturer.

Different types of fiber help your body in different ways. Wheat bran, some fruits and vegetables, and whole grains act as "nature's broom"; they keep your digestive system moving and help prevent constipation. The fiber in oat bran, barley, nuts, seeds, beans, apples, citrus fruits, carrots, and psyllium seed can help manage your blood sugar because they help slow the amount of time it takes for sugar to get into the bloodstream. They can also help lower blood cholesterol. High fiber diets are also thought to help reduce the risk of rectal and colon cancers.

Oils and Solid Fats: The Good, the Bad, and the Deadly

Most of us think that all fat is bad for us. But we need some fat for survival and for your body to work properly. The body needs about a tablespoon of fat a day. Fat can also be used almost without limit by our bodies to store energy as body fat.

Tips for Choosing Healthier Carbohydrates and Increasing Fiber

- Fill at least half of your plate with different kinds of vegetables and whole fruits.

- At least half of the grains you eat should be whole grains (brown rice, whole-grain breads and rolls, whole-grain pasta, and tortillas).

- Choose foods with whole wheat or a whole grain (such as oats) listed first on the ingredients list on the food label.

- Choose dried beans and peas, lentils, or whole-grain pasta instead of meat or as a side dish at least a few times a week.

- Choose whole fruit rather than fruit juice. Whole fruit contains fiber, takes longer to eat, fills you up better than juice, and can help keep you from overeating.

- Choose higher-fiber breakfast cereals such as shredded wheat, Grape-Nuts, or raisin bran.

- Eat higher-fiber crackers, such as whole-rye or multigrain crackers and whole-grain flatbread.

- Snack mostly on whole-grain crackers or breads, whole fruit, or nonfat yogurt rather than sweets, pastries, or ice cream.

- When you add fiber to your diet, do it gradually over a period of a few weeks. Drink plenty of water to process the fiber and prevent constipation.

Although all fats for the same portion size have the same number of calories, some fats are more healthful than others (we call these good fats), and some can be harmful when we eat too much (bad fats).

Good fats (also called unsaturated fats) are by and large oils that are usually liquid at room temperature. They help keep our cells healthy, and some can help reduce blood cholesterol. Good fats include soybean, safflower, corn, peanut, sunflower, canola, and olive oils. Nuts, seeds, and olives (and their oils), as well as avocados, are also rich in good fats.

There is another group of good fats, the omega-3s, which can be helpful for some people in reducing the risk of heart disease and may help with rheumatoid arthritis symptoms. These fats are found in fatty deepwater fish such as salmon, mackerel, trout, and tuna. Other sources of omega-3s include wheat germ, flaxseed, and walnuts, although the body may not use omega-3s from plants as well as it does the omega-3s from fish.

Tips for Choosing Good Fats and Healthier Fats

The following tips will help you eat less bad fat and more good fat. Just be sure that if you decide to choose more good fats, you are eating less bad fat. You do not want to increase the amount of fat you eat.

When Choosing Foods

- Keep cooked portions of meat, fish, and poultry to 2 to 3 ounces. This is about the size of a deck of cards or the palm of your hand.

- Do not eat the skin on poultry.

- Eat more deep-water fish, such as salmon, tuna, and mackerel.

- Choose leaner cuts of meat (round, sirloin, or flank).

- Trim off all the fat you can see from meat before cooking.

- Use low-fat or fat-free milk and dairy foods (cheese, sour cream, cottage cheese, yogurt, and ice cream).

- In cooking and baking, use oil (such as olive or canola oil) and soft (tub) margarines instead of shortening, lard, butter, or stick margarine.

When Preparing Foods

- Use a nonstick pan or a pan with small amounts of cooking oil spray.

- Broil, barbecue, or grill meats.

- Avoid frying or deep frying foods.

- Skim the fat from stews and soups during cooking. (If you refrigerate them overnight, the solid fat lifts off easily.)

- Use less butter, margarine, gravies, meat-based and cream sauces, spreads, and creamy salad dressings.

The bad fats (also called saturated fats) are usually solid at room temperature (think shortening, butter, lard, and bacon grease). They can increase blood cholesterol and the risk of heart disease. Most bad fats are found in animal foods such as butter, beef fat (tallow, suet), chicken fat, and pork fat (lard). Other foods high in bad fats include stick margarines, red meat, regular ground meat, processed meats (sausage, bacon, luncheon and deli meats), poultry skin, whole- and low-fat milk, whole-milk and low-fat cheeses including cream cheese and sour cream. Palm kernel oil, coconut oil, and cocoa butter are also considered bad fats because they are high in saturated fat.

The fats classed as "deadly" are the trans fats. They have more harmful effects on our blood cholesterol and risk of heart disease than the bad fats. Trans fats are found in many processed foods, including pastries, cakes, cookies, crackers, icing, margarine, and most microwave popcorn. They are listed on food labels as "partially hydrogenated" or "hydrogenated" oils. Be warned! Food companies can legally claim "no" or "0" trans fats on the label even when the food has up to half a gram (0.5 g) per serving. The best advice is to eat as little trans fats as possible.

There are no specific daily recommendations for how much fat you should eat. Most people get more than enough. The best recommendation is to eat very little bad and deadly fats and to replace them with the good fats, without increasing the amount of fat you eat.

There is one more thing you should know about fat. All fats contain twice the calories per teaspoon as protein or carbohydrate. Calories from fat add up quickly. For instance, 1 teaspoon of sugar has about 20 calories, but 1 teaspoon of oil or solid fat has about 35 calories. When we eat more calories than we need—no matter where they come from—the extra calories get stored as body fat, which leads to weight gain.

Protein: Muscle Builder and More

Protein is vital for hundreds of activities that keep you alive and healthy. Protein is part of your red blood cells and the enzymes and hormones that help regulate the body, as well as your muscles. It helps your immune system fight infection and builds and repairs damaged tissues. Protein can also give you some energy. But like fat, protein is not as good a source of energy for the body as carbohydrate.

There are two types of proteins, based on how they are built. Complete proteins have all the right parts in the right amounts. Your body uses them just as they are. Complete proteins are found in animal foods—meat, fish, poultry, eggs, milk and other dairy products—as well as in soy foods such as soybeans, tofu, and tempeh. Incomplete proteins are low in one or more parts. They are found in plant foods such as grains, dried beans and peas, lentils, nuts, and seeds. Most fruits and vegetables contain much less, if any, protein. For your body to be able to use incomplete proteins best, eat them with at least one other incomplete protein or along with a complete protein.

Over centuries, people have learned to survive by eating protein combinations. Two of the most plentiful and commonly eaten incomplete protein pairs are beans and rice and peanut butter and bread. Although nearly all plant proteins are incomplete proteins, they are at the heart of eating healthy. By eating a small amount of an animal protein (such as chicken) with a plant food such as lentils or black beans, you get all the benefits of a complete protein. In addition, some plant foods, such as nuts and seeds, are sources of the good fats, and many plants foods are good sources of fiber. Plant foods have no cholesterol and little to no trans fats.

Table 11.1 **Daily Recommended Servings, with Examples for Healthy Meal Planning**

These recommendations are for average adults (19 years and older) who exercise less than 30 minutes daily and eat 1,000 to 3,000 calories. They are based on the United States Dietary Guidelines.

If you have a special condition, you may need to modify portion sizes of certain foods but should aim for an overall balance.

	Recommended Servings per Day		
Protein-Rich Foods	**Women**	**Men**	**Examples**
Animal (meat, fish, poultry) and plant sources (beans, nuts, seeds)	5–5½ ounces	5½–6½ ounces	What counts as a 1-ounce serving: *Contains Little to No Carbohydrate* 1 ounce cooked lean meat, poultry, or fish 1 egg 1 tablespoon nut butter (peanut, almond, soy, etc.) About 2 tablespoons (½ ounce) nuts (12 almonds, 7 walnut halves) *Contains Carbohydrates* ½ cup cooked dry beans, peas, or lentils ½ cup baked or refried beans 1 ounce cooked tempeh 2 tablespoons hummus ½ cup roasted soybeans 4-ounce falafel patty
Milk, cheese (except cream cheese), yogurt, milk-based desserts (Choose fat-free or low-fat most of the time)	3 cups	3 cups	What counts as a 1-cup serving: *Contains Little to No Carbohydrate* 1½ ounces cheese ⅓ cup shredded cheese 2 cups cottage cheese *Contains Carbohydrates* 1 cup milk, yogurt, or kefir 1 cup pudding or frozen yogurt 1½ ounces ice cream 2 ounces processed cheese or cottage cheese

The good news is that most people eat more than enough protein. Unless you have a special medical condition, there is no need to be concerned. Unfortunately, many people get most of their protein from meat, which tends to be high in the bad fats. The best way to get protein is mainly from plant foods along with small amounts of lean meat, poultry, or fish.

Table 11.1 **Daily Recommended Servings (*continued*)**

	Recommended Servings per Day		
Carbohydrate-Rich Foods	**Women**	**Men**	**Examples**
Grains (At least half should be whole grains)	5–6 ounces	6–8 ounces	What counts as a 1-ounce serving: 1-ounce slice of bread ½ English muffin 1 cup ready-to-eat flaked cereal ½ cup cooked rice, cooked pasta, or cooked cereal 6-inch flour or corn tortilla
Vegetables	2–2½ cups	2½–3 cups	What counts as a 1-cup serving: *Low in Starch* 1 cup cooked vegetables (greens, broccoli family, green beans) or vegetable juice 2 cups raw leafy greens 12 medium baby carrots *High in Starch* 1 cup cooked sweet potato, white potato, or winter squash 1 cup cooked dry beans, peas, or lentils 1 cup (8 ounces) tofu 1 cup corn or green peas
Fruit	1½–2 cups	2 cups	What counts as a 1-cup serving: 1 cup fruit 1 cup 100% juice ½ cup dried fruit 1 banana (8–9 inches) 8 large strawberries
Oils and Solid Fats	5–6 teaspoons	6–7 teaspoons	What counts as a 1-teaspoon serving: About 1-teaspoon salad or cooking oil, margarine, mayonnaise, or salad dressing 1 teaspoon butter or margarine

Vitamins and Minerals

Vitamins help regulate the body's inner workings. Minerals are part of many cells and cause important reactions to happen in the body. All vitamins and minerals are essential for survival and health, and most of us can get what we need from healthy eating. But the minerals, sodium, potassium, and calcium stand out because they are related to current health problems, and many of us eat either too much or too little of these nutrients.

Sodium

For some people, too much sodium can raise blood pressure. This can lead to heart disease, stroke, and kidney failure. Cutting back on sodium can help lower blood pressure, and it can help prevent high blood pressure.

It is easy to get enough sodium to meet our bodies' needs, but most of us get way too much. We need only about 500 milligrams a day (in terms of table salt, this is less than a fifth of a teaspoon). Yet most people eat 8 to 12 times that much. Adults should limit sodium intake to 2,300 mg a day, which is about the amount in 1 teaspoon of table salt. People who have high blood pressure, kidney disease, or diabetes, are African American, and who are middle-aged or older should not have more than 1,500 mg of sodium a day.

We get sodium from most foods we eat—from teeny amounts in some plant foods to higher amounts in some animal foods. But the real culprits are processed foods, which typically have a lot of different forms of sodium added to them.

Our love of sodium is learned. It is not something we are born with. Cutting down takes some getting used to, but over time you will learn to enjoy the natural flavors of food. Here are some tips to help you keep your sodium intake in check:

- Always taste your food before salting it; many times, it is good as is.

- Don't add salt to food when cooking; season with spices, herbs, pepper, garlic, onion, or lemon.

- Use fresh or frozen minimally processed poultry, fish, and lean meat, instead of canned, breaded, or prepared packaged food.

- Choose foods labeled "low sodium" or those with 140 mg or less per serving. (Check out the Nutrition Facts label for this information.)

- Save high-sodium food for special occasions. Serve bacon, luncheon or deli meats, frozen dinners, packaged mixes, salted nuts, salad dressings, and high-sodium canned soups as part of celebrations, not as everyday fare.

- In restaurants, ask that your food not be salted during preparation.

Potassium

This mineral helps regulate our heartbeat, among other important jobs in the body. In contrast to sodium, which raises blood pressure, potassium can help lower blood pressure. When you follow the Map for Healthy Eating, it is easy to get enough potassium. Lots of vegetables are good sources. These include broccoli, peas, lima beans, tomatoes, potatoes, sweet potatoes, and winter squash; fruits, including citrus fruits, cantaloupe, bananas, kiwifruit, prunes, and apricots; and nuts. Meat and poultry, some fish (salmon, cod, flounder, and sardines), and milk, buttermilk, and yogurt also contain some potassium.

Calcium

You probably know that calcium helps build bones, but did you know that it is also needed for blood clotting and helps with blood pressure? It may also help protect against colon cancer, kidney stones, and breast cancer.

Unfortunately, most people, especially women and young children, do not get enough calcium. Most women under 60 should get the amount of calcium found in 3 cups of milk every day. Other good sources of calcium are yogurt and kefir (a beverage similar to yogurt); calcium-fortified soy, rice, and almond milks and orange juice; seaweed; and leafy greens (bok choy, kale, brussels sprouts, broccoli, kohlrabi, collards, and some other leafy greens). But our bodies cannot use the calcium in spinach, Swiss chard, and rhubarb. Most fruits are low in calcium, except for dried figs (there's not much in fig cookies, though) and the tropical cherimoya (custard apple).

Water

Water is your most important nutrient. Like the air you breathe, you cannot live without it. More than half of your body is made up of water, and each cell is bathed in it. Water helps keep our kidneys working, helps prevent constipation, and helps us eat less by making us feel full. It also helps prevent some medication side effects.

Although most people can last weeks without food, you cannot typically live longer than a week or so without water. Most adults lose about 10 cups of water a day. However, we usually have no problem getting the six to eight glasses each day many experts recommend. This is especially true when you consider that most liquids and foods we eat contain some water. Remember, you get water from what you drink as well as the food you eat. Even the driest cracker has a tiny bit of water.

To see if you are drinking enough, check your urine. If it is light-colored, you are fine. When you start to get thirsty, you need more water. Milk, juice, and many fruits and vegetables are good sources of water. Beware, though: coffee, tea, and other drinks with caffeine, as well as alcohol, can cause you to lose water. Do not depend on these drinks for your water.

If you have kidney disease or congestive heart failure or are taking special medications, your needs for water may be different. Talk to a registered dietitian or your health care provider.

Eating for Specific Long-Term Conditions

The Map for Healthy Eating is a general plan designed to work for most of us. However, some people have different needs and likes. These depend on age, sex, body size, activity level, health, and even availability and affordability of food. Here we present some information and guidelines for selected long-term health problems.

The Nutrition Facts Label: "What's in That Package of Food?"

Food labels help us find out what is in the packaged foods we eat. The Nutrition Facts panel and the ingredients list are two important parts. They tell you what you will be eating, which can help you make better choices. Reading and understanding the information on food labels can be overwhelming. We will focus on the serving size, calories, total fat, trans fat, cholesterol, sodium, and total carbohydrates.

Serving Size

This is the first thing to look at because all of the other information on the label is based on the serving size, and many packages contain more than one serving. But the serving size on the package may not be what you usually eat. If you would usually have less or more than the stated serving size, you have to change all the amounts. For example, if a serving size is ½ cup cooked rice and you eat 1 cup, which is 2 servings, you will need to double all the values. Most serving sizes are stated in cups, ounces, or pieces of the food.

Calories

Total calories are given for the stated serving size. So if you eat more or less than one serving, you will have to do a little arithmetic. On the same line you will see a number for calories from fat. If you want, you can figure out the percentage of calories you will get from fat. This is important if you are interested in how much fat you are eating, but it doesn't tell you the kind of fat. Divide the calories from fat by the calories in the serving size and then multiply by 100. In this example, divide the 45

Nutrition Facts	
Serving Size	1 package (28 g)
Servings Per Container	1

Amount Per Serving

Calories 280   Calories from Fat 45

	% Daily Value*
Total Fat 5 g	7%
Saturated Fat 2 g	10%
Trans Fat 0 g	
Polyunsaturated Fat 1 g	
Monounsaturated Fat 2 g	
Cholesterol 20 mg	7%
Sodium 540 mg	22%
Total Carbohydrate 49 g	16%
Dietary Fiber 3 g	12%
Sugars 7 g	
Protein 10 g	

Vitamin A 4%	Vitamin C 4%
Calcium 15%	Iron 4%

*Percent Daily Values are based on a 2,000 calorie diet. Your daily values may be higher or lower depending on your calorie needs.

	Calories:	2000	2500
Total fat	Less than	65 g	80 g
Sat fat	Less than	20 g	25 g
Cholesterol	Less than	300 mg	300 mg
Sodium	Less than	2,400 mg	2,400 mg
Potassium	Less than	3,500 mg	3,500 mg
Total Carbohydrate		300 g	375 g
Fiber		25 g	30 g

fat calories by the 280 in the serving and you get 0.16. Then multiply by 100 to get 16%.

Total Fat, Cholesterol, and Sodium

The total fat number includes good fats (polyunsaturated and monounsaturated), bad fat (saturated), and trans fat in grams (a unit of weight). You can change grams to calories by multiplying by 9. In the example, multiply the 5 g (total fat) by 9 to get 45 calories. This is the same number of calories as shown in the calories from fat line. The amount of calories in all the fats should add up to the calories for total fat. If they don't, they will be close (due to the arithmetic).

Remember our warning about trans fats! Due to the way food companies are allowed to do the arithmetic, any food with up to ½ (0.5) g per serving of trans fat can be listed as having no trans fat, but you still could be getting some. If the ingredients list has the words *partially hydrogenated* or *hydrogenated,* the product contains trans fat (even if the amount of trans fats per serving is 0 g). So trans fats could add up, especially if you have more than one serving.

The cholesterol line tells you the amount of cholesterol by serving size. Because cholesterol is found only in animal foods, this line may be missing or show 0 g for foods not made with animal products. If you are watching the amount of cholesterol you eat, you need to be especially careful because even if a food does not have any cholesterol, it may have bad or trans fat, particularly if it is a processed food. Trans fats can raise your blood cholesterol level more than the cholesterol from food.

To tell if the fat, cholesterol, or sodium is high or low, look at the "% Daily Value" column. Any value of 20% or more is high. If you want to eat less or want to eat more than one serving, look for values of 5% or less. You can see in this example that the values for total fat, saturated fat, and cholesterol are low but sodium is high. Note that % values are not available for trans fats and protein, as there are no recommended Daily Values for them. If you want to learn more about these recommended Daily Values, go to the MyPlate Website, http://www.choosemyplate.gov.

Total Carbohydrate, Dietary Fiber, and Sugars

This section breaks out values for dietary fiber and sugars and is important for people who want to watch or count their carbohydrates. You will also be able to see if a food is high or low in fiber. Most of us should be eating more fiber. Note that there is no % Daily Value for sugar. However, for many people with diabetes, it's the total amount of carbohydrate that matters, not the specific kind. A general guideline is to keep this amount between 45 to 60 g per meal, assuming three meals a day.

Ingredients List

Always check a package's ingredients list. It will show you what is in the food you will be eating. Ingredients are listed in order *by weight.* If you see sugar listed first, then the food contains more sugar than anything else. Remember, too, when you see the words *partially hydrogenated* or *hydrogenated,* the product contains trans fats (even if the amount for trans fats is 0 g).

Food Guide for Healthy Meal Planning

Nutritional values are based on data from the United States Department of Agriculture and the American Diabetes Association.

Abbreviations: g = grams, mg = milligrams, oz = ounce, c = cup, Tbsp = tablespoon, tsp = teaspoon

Protein Foods

Animal Protein Sources with Little or No Carbohydrate

BEEF, PORK, LAMB, VEAL, POULTRY, and FISH

Serving Size: 3–4 oz, cooked, NOT breaded, fried, or cooked with added fat unless noted. This portion is the size of the palm of your hand and ½ to 1 inch (1.0 to 2.5 cm) thick.

Per Serving: approx. 21–28 g protein; fat and calories vary

Lean (up to 9 g fat, 135–180 calories)

Beef, fat trimmed, from the round, sirloin, and flank, tenderloin sirloin, ground round

Pork, fresh, cured, boiled ham, Canadian bacon, tenderloin, center loin chop

Lamb and veal, rib roast, chop, leg

Chicken and turkey, white or dark meat, no skin

Duck and goose, drained of fat, no skin

Game, buffalo, ostrich, rabbit, venison

Fish (fresh or frozen), catfish, cod, flounder, haddock, halibut, orange roughy, salmon, tilapia

Fish (canned), tuna, in water or oil, drained; herring, uncreamed or smoked, 6–8 sardines

Shellfish, clams, crab, lobster, scallops, shrimp, imitation shellfish

Oysters (fresh or frozen), 18 medium

Processed meats (luncheon meat, deli meat), turkey ham, kielbasa, pastrami, chipped beef, shaved meats

Medium-fat (12–21 g fat, 150–300 calories)

Beef, ground, meatloaf, corned beef, short ribs, prime rib, tongue

Pork, shoulder roast, Boston butt (picnic), cutlets

Lamb, rib roast and chops, roasts, ground

Veal, cutlet

Chicken, turkey, with skin, fried, ground

Pheasant, dove, wild duck, wild goose

Fish, all fried

High-fat (24 g or more fat, 300–400 calories)

Pork, spareribs, ground

Sausage, pork, bratwurst, chorizo, Italian, Polish, smoked, summer

Processed meats, luncheon meat and deli meats, bologna, salami

Bacon, 6 slices

Organ Meats

Serving Size: 2–3 oz

Per Serving: 14–21 g protein; fat and calories vary; high in cholesterol

Kidney (1–3 g fat, 70–105 calories)

Liver, heart (6–9 g fat, 55–100 calories)

Eggs

Per Serving: 7 g protein

Whole egg, 1 large, cooked (5 g fat, 75 calories)

Egg whites, 2 large, cooked (0–1 g fat, 35 calories)

Cheese

Per Serving: 7 g protein; fat and calories vary

Fat-free and low-fat (0–1 g fat, 35 calories)

Fresh (Mexican) and nonfat cheese, 1 oz

Cottage cheese, fat-free, ¼ c

Medium-fat (4–7 g fat, 75 calories)

Feta, skim-milk mozzarella, string cheese, reduced-fat and processed cheese spreads, 1–2 oz

Ricotta, ¼ c (2 oz)

Grated parmesan, 2 Tbsp

High-fat (8 g fat per oz, 100+ calories)

All regular cheese: American, blue, brie, Swiss, cheddar, Monterey jack, Swiss, provolone, whole-milk mozzarella, goat, queso, 1–2 oz

Meat Substitutes

Per Serving: Little to no carbohydrate; fat and calories vary

Nuts and seeds* (5 g fat, 45 calories)

Almonds, cashews, mixed nuts, 6 nuts

Peanuts, 10 nuts

Pecans, walnuts, 4 halves

Tahini (sesame paste), 1 Tbsp

Pumpkin seeds (pepitas), sunflower seeds, 1 Tbsp

Nut butters (peanut, almond, etc.), 2 Tbsp (8 g fat)

Egg substitute, plain, ¼ c (1 g fat, about 50 calories)

*These foods contain good fats (see page 178).

Protein Foods

Animal Protein Foods with Carbohydrate

Milk

Serving Size: 1 c

Per Serving: 8 g protein, 12 g carbohydrate; fat and calories vary

Nonfat, fresh or evaporated 1%, nonfat or low-fat buttermilk (0–3 g fat, 100 calories)

Low-fat (2%) sweet acidophilus (5 g fat, 120 calories)

Whole, fresh or evaporated goat, buttermilk (8 g fat, 160 calories)

Yogurt

Per Serving: 8 g protein, 12 g carbohydrate; fat and calories vary

Nonfat, plain or flavored with artificial sweetener, 2/3 c (6 oz) (0–3 g fat, 90–100 calories)

Low-fat, sugar-sweetened, with fruit, 2/3 c (6 oz) (5 g fat, 120 calories)

Plain whole milk, kefir, 3/4 c (8 g fat, 150 calories)

Nonfat fruit-flavored, sweetened with sugar, 1 c (30+ g carbohydrate, 0–3 g fat, 100–150 calories)

Nonfat or low-fat fruit-flavored, sweetened with sugar substitute, 1 c (0–3 g fat, 90–130 calories)

Protein Substitutes

Per Serving: as noted

Soymilk, regular, 1 c (4 g fat, 100 calories)

Dried beans and peas, lentils, cooked, 1/2 c (15 g carbohydrate, 7 g protein, 0–1 g fat, 80 calories)

Edamame (soybeans), 1/2 c (8 g carbohydrate, 7 g protein, 0–1 g fat, approx. 60 calories)

Hummus (garbanzo bean spread), 1/3 c (15 g carbohydrate, 7 g protein, approx. 8 g fat, 100 calories)

Refried beans, canned, 1/2 c (15 g carbohydrate, 7 g protein, 0–3 g fat, approx. 100 calories)

Tofu, regular, 1/2 c (4 oz) (3 g carbohydrate, 8 g protein, 5 g fat, 75 calories)

Carbohydrate Foods

Per Serving: 15 g carbohydrate, 3 g protein, 0–1 g fat, 80 calories
Tip: Choose whole grains as often as you can.

Breads, Rolls, Muffins, and Tortillas

Bagel, large, ¼ (1 oz)

Buns, hot dog or hamburger, ½

English muffin, plain, ½

Roll, regular, ½

Pancake, 4 inches across, 1

Pita bread, 6 inches across, ½

Tortilla, corn or flour, 6 inches across, 1

Waffle, 4½ inches square, reduced-fat, 1

Bread, white, whole grain,* rye, pumpernickel, 1 slice (1 oz)

Cereals

Bran flakes, spoon-size shredded wheat,* ½ c

Granola,* low-fat or regular, Grape-Nuts* ¼ c

Puffed, unfrosted, 1½ c

Oats,* cooked, ½ c

Grains

Bulgur wheat,* grits, cooked, tabbouleh, prepared, ½ c

Pasta, barley, couscous, quinoa, cooked, ⅓ c

Rice, white, or brown,* cooked, ⅓ c

Wheat germ,* dry, 3 Tbsp

Wild rice,* cooked, ½ c

*Good source of fiber

Crackers and Snacks

Graham crackers, 2½ inches square, 3

Matzo, ¾ oz

Melba toast (2 inches by 4 inches), 4

Pretzels, ¾ oz

Rice cakes, 4 inches across, 2

Saltines, 6

Whole-wheat crackers, no fat added, 3–4 oz (2–5 crackers)

Low-Starch Vegetables

Per Serving: approx. 5 g carbohydrate, 2 g protein, no fat, 25 calories
Serving Size: ½ c cooked or vegetable juice, 1 c raw fresh, frozen, or canned (frozen or canned may be high in sodium)

Amaranth	Beets	Carrots	Chicory
Artichoke	Broccoli	Cauliflower	Chilies, spicy
Asparagus	Brussels sprouts	Celery	Cucumber
Bamboo shoots	Cabbage, Chinese cabbage	Chayote (vegetable pear)	Eggplant (aubergine)
Bean sprouts			Garlic

Low-Starch Vegetables (*continued*)

Green beans

Green onion, scallions

Greens (collard, kale, mustard, turnip)

Jicama

Kohlrabi

Nopales (cactus)

Mushrooms

Okra

Onions

Pea pods

Radishes

Rutabaga

Salad greens

Snap peas

Spinach

Summer squash (yellow squash, zucchini)

Sweet peppers

Tomatoes (raw, canned, sauce)

Turnips

Watercress

Vegetable juice (usually high in sodium)

Starchy Vegetables

Per Serving: 15 g carbohydrate, 0–3 g protein, 0–1 g fat, 80 calories

Corn, ½ c or ½ large cob (5 oz)

Mixed vegetables with corn, peas, or pasta, 1 c

Parsnips, ½ c

Plantain, ripe, ⅓ c

Potato, baked or boiled, large, with skin, 1 (3 oz)

Succotash (lima beans and corn), ½ c

Winter squash (acorn, butternut, pumpkin), 1 c

Yam, sweet potato, ½ c

Yautia, yuca (cassava), ½ c

Fruit

Per Serving: 15 g carbohydrate, no protein, 0–1 g fat, approx. 80 calories

Fresh

Apple, small, 2 inches, 1 (4 oz)

Apricots, 4

Banana, extra small, 1 (4 oz)

Berries, strawberries, blueberries, raspberries, ¾–1 c

Cherries, ½ c (approx. 12)

Coconut, fresh (shredded), ½ c

Dates, 3

Figs, large, 2

Fruit cocktail, ½ c

Grapefruit, small, ½

Grapes, small, ½ c

Guava, medium, 2

Kiwifruit, large, 1

Lemon, lime, large, 1

Mango, cubed, ½ c

Melon (honeydew, cantaloupe), ¼

Orange, small, 1

Papaya, small, cubed, 1 c

Pineapple, cubed, ¾ c

Peach, nectarine, 1

Pear, ½

Persimmon, medium, 1

Plum, small, 2

Tangerine, small, 2

Watermelon, cubed, ½ c

Canned

Unsweetened, ¼–½ c

In sugar syrup, ¼ c

Dried

Apricots, 8 halves

Figs, 2

Prunes, 3

Fruit (*continued*)

Juice, unsweetened (if the label doesn't say 100% juice, it usually contains added sugar)

Apple, grapefruit, orange, pineapple, ½ c

Apricot nectar, ½ c Grape, prune, juice blends, ⅓ c

Juice drinks, sweetened

Carbonated juice drinks, ½ c

Cranberry cocktail, ⅓ c

Raisins, 1 Tbsp

Tamarind, ½ c

Oils and Solid Fats

Per Serving: little or no carbohydrate, 5 g fat, 45 calories

Tip: Choose good fats as often as you can.

Good fats (unsaturated fats) (see page 178)

Salad and cooking oils (corn, olive, safflower, soybean, etc.), 1 tsp

Avocado, medium, ¼

Olives, all types, large, 5

Margarine (soft), reduced-fat, 1 tsp

Mayonnaise, regular, 1 tsp

Mayonnaise, reduced-fat, 1 Tbsp

Salad dressing, 1 Tbsp

Bad fats (saturated fats) (see page 178)

Butter, regular, 1 tsp

Butter, reduced-fat, 1 Tbsp

Bacon fat, 1 tsp

Cream, liquid nondairy creamer, 1 Tbsp

Cream, half-and-half, whipped, 2 Tbsp

Cream cheese, 1 Tbsp

Margarine (stick), regular, made with hydrogenated fat, 1 tsp

Sour cream, regular, 1 Tbsp

Shortening, lard, 1 tsp

Extras

Tip: These foods are high in fat or sugar or both; they're best saved for special occasions.

Cake with frosting, 1 small slice or 2-inch square

Cookies, small, 2

Danish, small, 1

Flan, with milk, ½ c

Fruit tart or pie, 1 slice

Honey, 1 Tbsp

Ice cream (regular), ½ c

Jam or jelly (regular), 1 Tbsp

Jam or jelly (low-sugar or light), 2 Tbsp

Juice bar (frozen, 100% juice), 1

Pudding, ½ c

Sherbet, sorbet, ½ c

Syrup (regular), 1 Tbsp

Syrup (sugar-free), 2 Tbsp

Alcoholic Beverages

Per Serving: no protein or fat; carbohydrate and calories vary

Distilled spirits, 80 proof, 1½ oz
(0 carbohydrate, 80–110 calories)

Liqueurs, 1½ oz (approx. 20 g carbohydrate,
125 calories)

Wine, red, white, dry, sparkling, 4 oz
(1–2 g carbohydrate, 80 calories)

Wine, sweet or dessert, 4 oz
(approx. 14 g carbohydrate, 120 calories)

Beer, regular, 12 oz.
(approx. 13 g carbohydrate, about
160 calories)

Beer, lite or nonalcoholic, 12 oz (approx.
5 g carbohydrate, 60–120 calories)

Mixed drinks (margarita, mojito, gin and tonic,
etc.), 1 drink (approx. 12 g carbohydrate,
150–250 calories)

Free Foods

*Per Serving: up to 5 g carbohydrate, up to 20 calories; enjoy moderate servings as often
as you like*

Atol (cornmeal drink) 1 c

Bouillon, broth, consommé

Candy, hard (sugar-free)

Chewing gum (sugar-free)

Club soda, mineral water

Coffee or tea, unsweetened or with sugar
substitute

Gelatin (sugar-free or unflavored)

Herbs, spices

Horchata (rice drink)

Hot pepper sauces

Soft drinks (sugar-free)

Soy sauce

Worcestershire sauce

Sugar substitutes (approved by the United States Food and Drug Administration)

Equal (aspartame)

Splenda (sucralose)

Sprinkle Sweet (saccharin)

Sweet One (acesulfame K)

Sweet-10 (saccharin)

Sugar Twin (saccharin)

Sweet'N Low (saccharin)

Diabetes

When you eat a meal, the body breaks down the carbohydrates into glucose, the basic fuel for the body's cells, which is then absorbed into the bloodstream. Protein and fat usually contribute little to the body's blood sugar. The hormone insulin takes the glucose (blood sugar) into the cells. In people with diabetes, cells do not absorb or use glucose very well. Glucose then builds up in the bloodstream, which can lead to other health problems. Managing blood sugar levels is one of the prime goals in diabetes and involves many different things. These include taking medication, exercising, and keeping a careful eye on diet (for more on diabetes, see Chapter 18).

In years past, people with diabetes were told that they could not eat sweets and that they could only eat certain types of carbohydrates. As we learn more, things change. We now know that people with diabetes do not have to avoid any specific food. However, they do need to watch what and how much they eat. These things will vary from person to person.

The American Diabetes Association recommends "Create My Plate" to plan meals. Looking at your plate, divide it in half. Then take one of those halves and divide it in half again. You should have 3 sections on the plate now.

- Half of the plate should be non-starchy vegetables, such as spinach, greens, carrots, lettuce, cabbage, bok choy, broccoli, green beans, tomatoes, cauliflower, salsa, cucumber, okra, peppers, mushrooms, beets, turnip

- One small section should be starchy food, such as whole grain breads, whole grain cereal, rice, pasta, tortillas, dal, oatmeal hominy, grits, cooked beans and peas, potatoes, corn, lima beach, green peas, sweet potatoes, fat-free popcorn, low fat crackers, pretzels

- The other small section should be meat or meat substitute, such as chicken or turkey (without the skin), fish, lean cuts of beef or pork, eggs, low-fat cheese, tofu

    Add to that one 8-ounce glass of non- or low-fat milk, or 6 ounces of light yogurt, and a small piece of fruit or ½ cup fruit salad

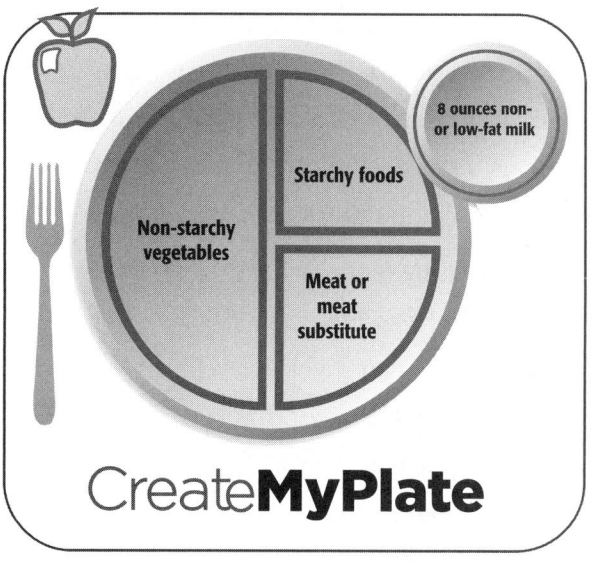

Figure 11.2 **"Create My Plate" from the American Diabetes Association**

Here are some general points about healthy eating for people with diabetes:

- Follow the Map for Healthy Eating (page 175). People with diabetes are at higher risk for heart disease and other chronic health conditions. Following the Map is especially important to help prevent future problems.

- Start each day with something to eat. Eating something in the morning is truly "breaking the fast." It helps fuel the body after a long night of resting and not having any food; it gives us energy to start the day's activities.

- Regularly space meals and snacks over the day, and don't skip meals. Spacing your meals at usual times gives your body the chance to produce and use its insulin or time for your medication to work to keep up your energy level. The number of meals you eat and the time between your meals will vary depending on your personal health and lifestyle. Many of us eat three meals a day, while others may prefer or need to eat smaller meals more often.

■ Eat the same amount of food at each meal. This helps you maintain an even energy flow and blood sugar level throughout the day. Skipping meals or mixing large meals with small meals can throw off your energy level. It can also lead to overeating or making poorer, less healthy food choices. This can in turn cause swings in your blood sugar and result in symptoms such as irritability, shakiness, and mood swings, pain or difficulties breathing due to stomach bloating, heartburn, indigestion, or even poor sleep.

It is important that you learn to manage the carbohydrates you eat. Nearly all carbohydrates break down into glucose, so they have the greatest effect on your blood sugar. Too much carbohydrate causes blood sugar to increase; too little makes your blood sugar low. General guidelines suggest eating between 45 and 60 g of carbohydrates per meal, but this amount may vary widely from person to person.

For most people with diabetes, there is no such thing as a bad carbohydrate or one that is off limits. What matters most is the total amount of carbohydrate, not the specific kind, although some people may feel that certain foods affect them differently. Carbohydrates are found mostly in plant foods (milk and yogurt are exceptions) in the form of sugars (honey, jelly, table sugar, and the like) and starches (dried beans, winter squashes, and grains such as rice and flour). You get the most benefit by getting the majority of your carbohydrates from whole grains (brown rice, oats, whole-wheat bread), fruits (preferably whole fruit rather than juice), vegetables, and dried beans, peas, and lentils. These foods are high in vitamins, minerals, fiber, and other good things that help keep the body healthy and protect it from disease. Also, foods such as barley, dried beans, oats, apples, citrus fruits, carrots, and psyllium seed are absorbed by the body more slowly and can help you manage your blood sugar level. They can also help lower blood cholesterol, which helps lower heart disease risk.

Because of the increased risk of heart disease and stroke, it very important to eat fewer bad fats (saturated and trans fats; see page 178). Instead, replace them (not add to them) with good fats (such as olive and canola oils). In addition, eat more plant foods and fewer animal foods. Get less sodium by eating fewer processed and prepared foods, and use the salt shaker sparingly, if at all. If you are carrying some extra weight, losing some weight can help lower your blood sugar. Even a small weight loss of 5 to 10 pounds (2–4 kg) can make a big difference in your blood sugar level. (See the tips for healthier eating in the boxes on pages 177 and 178, and find tips for choosing healthy fats on page 178).

Heart Disease and Stroke

Healthy eating for people with heart disease or those who have had a stroke usually involves keeping arteries from hardening or getting clogged (for details on heart disease, see Chapter 16). So it is important to watch the amount and kind of fat you eat. Most of the fat you eat should come from the good fats (unsaturated fats) and very little from the bad (saturated) fats. You should eat little to no trans fat. Also, increasing the amount of fiber you eat, especially from oats, barley, dried beans and peas, lentils, apples, citrus fruits, carrots, and psyllium seed can be helpful in managing high blood cholesterol, a major risk factor for heart disease. Eating less salt and sodium can help prevent or control high blood pressure. Try to limit the daily total amount of sodium you get to no more than that found in 1 teaspoon of table salt (about 2,300 mg). Use herbs, spices, lemon, and vinegar for flavor. The tips on page 177 also provide suggestions for ways to make healthy fat choices and increase fiber in your eating plan.

Lung Disease

For people with lung disease, especially emphysema, it is sometimes necessary to increase the amount of protein you eat. This helps increase energy, strength, and the ability to fight lung infections. When it is hard for you to eat enough food, as when you have little or no appetite, try eating higher-calorie foods—fruit nectars instead of juice, dried fruit instead of fresh fruit, sweet potato instead of white potato—or try nibbling on a small handful of nuts over the course of the day. Our discussion of the common challenges of gaining weight in Chapter 12 (page 214) gives you some tips to help you increase how much you eat.

If you have specific concerns about what to eat, talk to your doctor or a registered dietitian. These professionals can tell you what's best for you as well as help you fit our general recommendations to your unique health needs.

Osteoporosis

Osteoporosis makes bones brittle and easily broken. It has been called a silent disease because its first symptom can be a bone fracture, especially in the spine, hip, or wrist. However, it is never too late to help slow its progress. You can help by getting enough calcium and vitamin D, regularly doing muscle-strengthening and weight-bearing exercise (such as walking; see Chapter 7), and following your health care professional's recommendations, such as taking prescribed medications for bone loss.

Osteoporosis is technically not a calcium deficiency disease, and after bone has been lost, getting more calcium will not fix it. But getting vitamin D along with enough calcium can help the body absorb the calcium. Everybody needs some calcium every day. The best sources are milk and foods made from milk. But some people avoid milk products because they don't like them, do not eat animal products, or have problems digesting milk sugar (lactose intolerance). You can get enough calcium from your diet even if you have problems with milk sugar. Many people can enjoy milk products if they take them in small amounts or eat other foods at the same time, like cereal with milk; if they use lactase tablets to help digest the lactose; or if they find that they can eat foods like kefir or yogurt. There are also some fruits and vegetables that are high in calcium, including kale, collard greens, bok choy, and broccoli; calcium-treated tofu; cooked dried beans; and foods with added calcium, such as soymilk, juices, cereals, and pasta. If you think you may not be getting enough calcium, talk to your doctor or a registered dietitian about your diet and whether calcium supplements are needed to meet your calcium needs.

Eating and Your Thoughts

Do you eat when you're bored, down in the dumps or sad, or feeling lonely? Many people find comfort in food or just eating as something to do when they need to take their minds off something or have nothing else to do. Some eat when they are feeling angry, anxious, or depressed. At these times, it is easy to lose track of what and how much you eat. These are also the times when celery sticks, apples, or popcorn just won't do. Here are some ways to help control these urges:

- Keep a food-mood diary.. Every day, list what, how much, and when you eat. Note how you are feeling when you have the urge to eat. Try to spot patterns so you can anticipate when you will want to eat without really being hungry.

- If you catch yourself feeling bored and are thinking about eating, ask yourself, "Am I really hungry?" If the answer is no, make yourself do something else for 2 to 3 minutes—go for a short walk around the house or around the block, work on a jigsaw puzzle, or play a computer game.

- Keep your mind and hands busy. Getting your hands dirty is helpful (as with gardening).

- Write down action plans for when these situations arise. Sometimes it is easier to refer to the written word than to remember what you said you would do.

Common Challenges to Making Healthier Food Choices

"Healthy food doesn't taste the same as food I am used to. When I eat, I want something with substance, like meat and potatoes or a piece of apple pie! The healthy stuff just doesn't fill me up!"

Making healthier food choices does not mean that you cannot have something you want or crave. It means trading off to fit in favorites while making the better choices most of the time. Some of these tips are discussed in Chapter 12, and more information is available at the end of this chapter. There are also many excellent cookbooks with healthy recipes, as well as Internet sites with good, healthful recipe ideas.

"But I love to cook!"

If you love to cook, you are in luck. Take a new cooking class, begin watching one on television, buy a new cookbook on healthy cooking, or find an Internet site with healthy recipes. If you have odds and ends, even leftovers, in your kitchen, do a computer search to see what recipes you can find. Play around with ways to modify your favorite recipes, making them lower in fat, sugar, and sodium.

"I'm living alone now, and I'm not used to cooking for one. I find myself overeating so that food isn't wasted."

This can be a problem, particularly when the situation is new. You may be overeating or eating a "second dinner" to fill in time. Maybe you are one of those people who will eat for as long as food is in front of you. Whatever the reason, here are some ways to help you deal with the extra food:

▪ Don't eat "family style" by putting serving dishes on the table. Put as much as you feel you can comfortably eat on a plate, and bring only that plate to the table.

▪ As soon as you have finished eating, or even right after you have served your portion, immediately put leftovers in the refrigerator or freezer. This will also give you leftovers for the next day or whenever you don't feel like fixing a meal.

▪ Have company over for dinner once in a while so that you can share food and other people's company. Plan a potluck supper with neighbors, relatives, or members of your house of worship, clubs, or other groups.

"Food doesn't taste as good as before."

Many things can affect how food tastes. Having surgery, taking certain medications, being on oxygen, and even the common cold can make food taste off, bad, or funny. When this happens, you tend to eat less. Many people automatically add extra salt to their food to try to make it taste better. Unfortunately, this can cause you to retain water or feel bloated, which can increase blood pressure. Here's how you can make foods taste better:

▪ Use herbs (basil, oregano, tarragon), spices (cinnamon, cumin, curry, ginger, nutmeg) in cooking or even sprinkled on top.

▪ Squirt fresh lemon juice on foods.

▪ Use a small amount of vinegar in or on top of hot or cold foods. There are dozens of different kinds, from balsamic to berry- and fruit-flavored varieties; experiment with new flavors.

▪ Add healthy ingredients to the foods you usually eat (carrots or barley to soup, for example, or dried fruits and nuts to salads) to give them more texture and make them tastier.

▪ Chew your food slowly and well. This will allow the food to remain in your mouth longer and release more flavor.

If the lack of taste is keeping you from eating enough, you may need to add more calories to your meals or snacks. Tips for doing this are given on page 215.

"It takes so long to prepare meals. By the time I'm done, I'm too tired to eat."

This is common, especially when you do not have much energy. This situation calls for planning to help make sure that you do eat. Here are some hints to help:

▪ When you do have some energy, cook enough for two, three, or even more servings or meals, especially if it is something you really like.

▪ Do a meal exchange with friends or family, and freeze what you get in single-serving sizes for times when you are tired.

▪ Break your food preparation into steps, resting in between.

▪ Ask for help, especially for big holiday meals or family gatherings.

"Sometimes eating causes discomfort."

"I'm afraid I'll become short of breath while I'm eating."

"I really have no appetite."

People who experience shortness of breath or who find it difficult and physically uncomfortable to eat meals tend to eat less. For some, eating a large meal causes stomach problems such as indigestion, discomfort, or nausea. Indigestion, along with a full stomach, reduces the space your breathing muscles have to expand and contract. This can aggravate breathing problems.

If these are challenges you sometimes face, try the following:

- Eat four to six small meals a day, rather than the usual three large meals. You will be using less energy for each meal.

- Avoid foods that produce gas or make you feel bloated. Many foods can produce gas, although foods affect people differently. Among the more common foods that can cause discomfort are cabbage, broccoli, brussels sprouts, onions, beans, and certain fruits, including bananas, apples, melons, and avocados.

- Eat slowly, take small bites, and chew your food well. You should also pause occasionally during a meal. Eating quickly to avoid an episode of shortness of breath can actually cause shortness of breath. Slowing down and breathing evenly reduces the amount of air you swallow while eating.

- Do a relaxation exercise about half an hour before mealtime, or take time out for a few deep breaths during the meal.

- Choose food that is easy to eat, such as yogurt or pudding, or to drink, like a shake or fruit nectar.

"I can't eat very much in one sitting."

There is no rule that says we must eat only three meals a day. In fact, many people find that four to six smaller meals work better. If you choose to eat more frequently, include no-fuss, high-calorie snacks such as shakes, muffins and other baked products, and protein or meal bars as part of these extra meals. If you still can't finish a whole meal, eat the portion of your meal that is highest in calories first.

Common Challenges to Eating Healthy

"I love to eat out, so how do I know if I'm eating well?"

Whether it is because you don't have time, you hate to cook, or you just don't have the energy to shop for groceries or fix meals, eating out may suit your needs. This is not necessarily bad if you know how to make the best choices possible. Here are some tips on eating out:

- Select restaurants that have a variety of menu items prepared in healthy ways (for example, grilled or steamed dishes in addition to or instead of fried foods).

- Ask what is in a dish and how it is prepared, especially if you are eating in a restaurant where the dishes are new to you.

■ Before you go out, decide what type of food you will eat and how much. Many restaurants post their menus on the Internet or at the front of the restaurant.

■ Order small plates or appetizers instead of main courses.

■ When you are with a group, order first so that you aren't tempted to change your mind after hearing what others have selected.

■ See if you can split an entree with a dining companion, or order a half portion. You could also plan to eat only half of what you are served and take the rest home for another meal. Ask to have the take-home container brought to you with your food, and box it up before you start eating.

■ If you don't mind wasting food, heavily (really heavily) salt or pepper half of your food so you won't be able to eat it.

■ Choose menu items that are low in fat, sodium, and sugar, or ask if they can be prepared that way.

■ Whenever possible, order broiled, barbecued, baked, grilled, or steamed dishes rather than breaded, fried, sautéed, creamed, or covered in cheese.

■ Ask for vegetables steamed or raw without butter, sauces, or dips.

■ Eat bread without butter, or ask that no butter or dipping oil be served with it.

■ Request salad with dressing on the side, and dip your fork into the dressing before spearing each mouthful.

■ For dessert, select fruit, nonfat yogurt, sorbet, or sherbet.

■ Share an entrée or a dessert with at least one other person.

"I snack while I am doing other things— watching TV, working on the computer, or reading."

If this is a problem for you, plan ahead by keeping a list of healthier snacks to grab. Here are some examples:

■ Rather than snack crackers, chips, and cookies, munch on fresh fruit, raw vegetables, or fat-free or plain popcorn.

■ Measure out your snack in a single-portion size so you won't be tempted to eat more.

■ Make specific places at home and work "eating areas," and don't eat anywhere else.

Healthy eating is about the food choices you make most of the time. It is not about never being able to eat certain foods. There is no such thing as a perfect food or a bad food. Healthy eating means enjoying a moderate amount of a wide variety of minimally processed foods in the proper amounts for your body while allowing for occasional treats. Eating this way can help you maintain your health, help prevent future health problems, and help you manage your disease symptoms as best possible. Eating healthy, however, may mean making some changes to what you are now doing. These could include making more food choices that are higher in good fats and fiber and fewer food choices that are high in bad and trans fats, sugar, and sodium. Healthy is equally important to whether you want to lose weight and keep it off, maintain your weight, or gain weight (see Chapter 12).

If you choose to make some of the changes suggested in this chapter, think of this as doing something positive and wonderful for yourself, not as punishment. As a self-manager, it's up to you to find the changes that are best for you. And if you experience setbacks, identify the problems and work at resolving them. You can do it!

Suggested Further Reading

Center for Science in the Public Interest, *Nutrition Action Healthletter:* http://www.cspinet.org/

Duyff, Roberta Larson. *American Dietetic Association's Complete Food and Nutrition Guide.* Hoboken, N.J.: Wiley, 2006.

Environmental Nutrition [newsletter]: http://www.environmentalnutrition.com/

Gaines, Fabiola Demps, and Roniece Weaver. *The New Soul Food Cookbook for People with Diabetes.* Alexandria, Va.: American Diabetes Association, 2006.

Mayo Clinic, "Nutrition and Healthy Eating": http://www.mayoclinic.com/health/nutrition-and-healthy-eating/MY00431

Tufts University Health & Nutrition Letter: http://www.healthletter.tufts.edu/

University of California, Berkeley, Wellness Letter, http://www.wellnessletter.com/

U.S. Department of Health and Human Services, "Heart Healthy Home Cooking, African American Style": http://www.nhlbi.nih.gov/health/public/heart/other/chdblack/cooking.pdf

Warshaw, Hope. *Eat Out, Eat Right: The Guide to Healthier Restaurant Eating,* 3rd ed. Chicago: Surrey Books, 2008.

Woodruff, Sandra, and Leah Gilbert-Henderson. *Soft Foods for Easier Eating Cookbook: Easy-to-Follow Recipes for People Who Have Chewing and Swallowing Problems.* Garden City Park, N.Y.: Square One, 2010.

Other Resources

☐ American Cancer Society: http://www.cancer.org/

☐ American Diabetes Association: http://www.diabetes.org/

☐ American Dietetic Association: http://www.eatright.org

☐ American Heart Association: http://www.heart.org/nutrition

☐ Center for Science in the Public Interest: www.cspinet.org/

☐ Food and Nutrition Information Center: http://www.nal.usda.gov/fnic

☐ Harvard School of Public Health: http://www.hsph.harvard.edu/

☐ International Food Information Council: http://www.ific.org/

☐ U.S. Department of Agriculture, Agricultural Research Service: http://www.ars.usda.gov/Services/docs.htm?docid=7783

☐ U.S. Department of Agriculture: http://www.choosemyplate.gov/

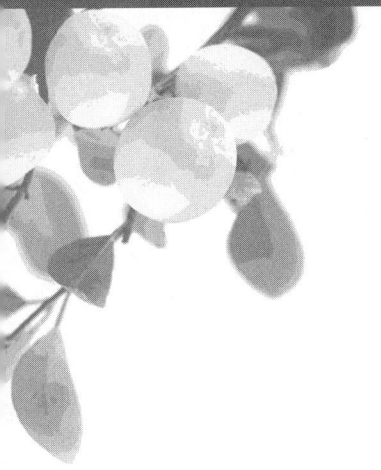

CHAPTER 12

Healthy Weight Management

OUR WEIGHT AFFECTS OUR HEALTH, how we look, and our ability to move; and it can affect how we feel about ourselves. Too much weight contributes to arthritis from too much joint stress, diabetes from high blood sugar, and high blood pressure. Being underweight can weaken our immune system and make us less able to fight infection. Being underweight can also increase our likelihood of developing osteoporosis (thin bones), and in younger women it could affect fertility and result in menstrual problems. Thus being either overweight or underweight can have major effects on your life.

Special thanks to Bonnie Bruce, DrPH, RD, for her help with this chapter.

Why Is Body Weight Important?

Being at a healthy weight can help us have better health and a better quality of life. It can help us manage symptoms such as lack of energy, joint pain, and shortness of breath. It can help us prevent or hold off related health problems such as diabetes and high blood pressure. In addition, maintaining a healthy weight can help you be more active and sleep better. In general, it can help you be able to do the things you want and need to do. In this chapter we spell out the truth about what defines a healthy weight, how to make changes, how to decide whether you should lose or gain weight, and how to maintain changes you make.

What Is a Healthy Weight?

Most people's weight tends to shift up and down over time, even over the course of a few days. So a healthy weight is not just one specific number on the scale or some sort of "ideal" number. There is no such thing as an "ideal" weight. A healthy weight is a range of pounds that is unique and personal. It is a range that will help you lower your risk of developing or further

Table 12.1 **Body Mass Index**

BMI	Normal						Overweight				
	19	20	21	22	23	24	25	26	27	28	29
Height (feet-inches)	Weight (pounds)										
4'10"	91	96	100	105	110	115	119	124	129	134	138
4'11"	94	99	104	109	114	119	124	128	133	138	143
5'0"	97	102	107	112	118	123	128	133	138	143	148
5'1"	100	106	111	116	122	127	132	137	143	148	153
5'2"	104	109	115	120	126	131	136	142	147	153	158
5'3"	107	112	118	124	130	135	141	146	152	158	163
5'4"	110	116	122	128	134	140	145	151	157	163	169
5'5"	114	120	126	132	138	144	150	156	162	168	174
5'6"	118	124	130	136	142	148	155	161	167	173	179
5'7"	121	127	134	140	146	153	159	166	172	178	185
5'8"	125	131	138	144	151	158	164	171	177	184	190
5'9"	128	135	142	149	155	162	169	176	182	189	196
5'10"	132	139	146	153	160	167	174	181	188	195	202
5'11"	136	143	150	157	165	172	179	186	193	200	208
6'0"	140	147	154	162	169	177	184	191	199	206	213
6'1"	144	151	159	167	174	182	189	196	204	212	219
6'2"	148	155	163	171	179	186	194	202	210	218	225
6'3"	152	160	168	176	184	192	200	208	216	224	232
6'4"	156	164	172	180	189	197	205	213	221	230	238

worsening health problems and help you feel good in your mind and your body.

Pinpointing your healthy weight range and deciding whether you want or need to change your weight depend on several things. These include your age, your activity level, your health, how much and where your body fat is located, and your family history of weight-related health problems, such as high blood pressure or diabetes.

How to Figure Out Your Healthy Weight

To get a sense of a healthy weight range for you, look at Table 12.1 from the National Institutes of Health. It will give you your body mass index (BMI). Although not a perfect tool, the BMI is a useful, quick, and general guide for adults based on weight and height. For many people it relates to total body fat and health risks. In the table, simply find your height and follow that line to your weight. The heading on that column above your weight will give you your BMI. Then refer to Table 12.2, which tells you in BMI units the range where your current weight falls.

Another way to judge your weight is to use this rough rule of thumb. Give or take 10%, women should weigh about 105 pounds for the first 5 feet of height and another 5 pounds per inch after

Table 12.1 **Body Mass Index (*continued*)**

						Obese						Extreme Obesity	
BMI	**30**	**31**	**32**	**33**	**34**	**35**	**36**	**37**	**38**	**39**	**40**	**41**	**42**
Height (feet-inches)	**Weight (pounds)**												
4'10"	143	148	153	158	162	167	172	177	181	186	191	196	201
4'11"	148	153	158	163	168	173	178	183	188	193	198	203	208
5'0"	153	158	163	168	174	179	184	189	194	199	204	209	215
5'1"	158	164	169	174	180	185	190	195	201	206	211	217	222
5'2"	164	169	175	180	186	191	196	202	207	213	218	224	229
5'3"	169	174	180	186	191	197	203	208	214	220	225	231	237
5'4"	175	180	186	191	197	204	209	215	221	227	232	238	244
5'5"	180	186	192	198	204	210	216	222	228	234	240	246	252
5'6"	186	192	198	204	210	216	223	229	235	241	247	253	260
5'7"	191	198	204	211	217	223	230	236	242	249	255	261	268
5'8"	197	204	210	216	223	230	236	243	249	256	262	269	276
5'9"	203	210	216	223	230	236	243	250	257	263	270	277	284
5'10"	209	216	222	229	236	243	250	257	264	271	278	285	292
5'11"	215	222	229	236	243	250	257	265	272	279	286	293	301
6'0"	221	228	235	242	250	258	265	272	279	287	294	302	309
6'1"	227	235	242	250	257	265	275	280	288	295	302	310	318
6'2"	233	241	249	256	264	272	280	287	295	303	311	319	326
6'3"	240	248	256	264	272	279	287	295	303	311	319	327	335
6'4"	246	254	263	271	279	287	295	304	312	320	328	336	344

Table 12.2 **Weight Classifications Based on Body Mass Index**

Body Mass Index	Weight Classification	What It Means
Less than 18.5	Underweight	Unless you have other health problems, being in this weight class may not be an issue if you are small or petite.
18.5 to 24.9	Normal weight	This is the healthy range to aim for.
25 to 29.9	Overweight	This range suggests that you are carrying extra pounds. But it may not be of much concern if you are healthy and have few or no other health problems or risk factors or are physically active and have a lot of muscle.
30 to 39.9	Obese	This range signals that it is likely you have a large amount of body fat. It puts you at increased risk for weight-related health problems.
40 and over	Extremely (morbidly) obese	This weight class pinpoints that a high proportion of your body weight is fat. It puts you at very high risk of developing or complicating serious health problems.

that; men should weigh about 106 pounds for the first 5 feet and an added 6 pounds per inch. For example, for a woman who is 5 foot 5 inches tall a healthy weight would be 125 pounds, and her healthy weight range would be roughly 112–138 pounds. Note that this weight range places her in the BMI "normal weight" class.

Another way to judge your weight is to measure the distance around your waist (your "waist circumference"). If you are overweight and most of your body fat is around your waist (rather than on hips and thighs), you are at higher risk for heart disease, high blood pressure, and type 2 diabetes. For non-pregnant women, this means that health risks go up with a waist size that is more than 35 inches (88 cm). For men, this is a waist circumference that is greater than 40 inches (100 cm). To measure your waist correctly, stand and place a tape measure (one that is not old and stretched out) around your bare middle, just above your hipbone. Measure your waist just after you breathe out.

The Decision to Change Your Weight

Reaching and maintaining a healthy weight may mean that you will need to make some changes in your eating habits and lifestyle. This is true whether you want to gain or lose weight. Now for an important bit of advice: you must decide to do this for yourself—not for friends or family.

Make changes that you believe you can stick with for a long time. If you decide to make changes for someone other than yourself or plan for only short-term changes, you probably won't succeed.

To get started, review the information about action planning in Chapter 2. If you think that you want to change your weight, consider asking your doctor to refer you to a registered dietitian for help. This is not something you need to do alone.

When making this decision, you must ask yourself two primary questions:

- **Why do I want to change my weight?** The reasons for losing or gaining weight are personal and different for each of us. The most important reason for some may be physical health, but for others there may be personal or emotional reasons for wanting to change. To help you begin and to increase your chances of success, think about the reasons that make you want to gain or lose weight. Here are some examples:

  To improve my symptoms (pain, fatigue, shortness of breath, and so on)

  To manage my blood sugar

  To have more energy to do the things I want to do

  To feel better about myself

  To change the way others think of me

  To feel more in control of my health or my life

Jot your important reasons here:

_____

_____

_____

_____

_____

- **Am I ready to make lifelong changes?** The next step is to find out whether this is a good time for you to start making changes in your eating and exercise. If you are not ready, you may be setting yourself up for failure. But the truth is that there will likely never be a "perfect" time. So take a look at your situation to see how things can work for you.

  Consider the following:

  Is there someone or something that can be supportive and make it easier for you to begin and continue with your changes?

  Are there problems or obstacles that will keep you from becoming more active or changing the way you eat?

  Will worries or concerns about family, friends, work, or other commitments affect your ability to carry out your plans successfully at this time?

Use Table 12.3 on page 206 to help you identify some of these factors. If you find barriers, use some of the problem-solving tools found in Chapter 2.

After you have thought about these issues, you may find that now is not the best or right time to start. If it is not, set a future date to revisit things. In the meantime, accept that this is the right decision for you at this time, and focus your attention on other goals. If you do decide that now is the right time, start by changing the things that are simplest, easiest, and most comfortable for you, using "baby steps." This means working on only one or two things at a time; do not try to do too much too quickly. Remember, slow and steady wins the race.

Table 12.3 Factors Affecting the Decision to Gain or Lose Weight *Now*

Things That Will Enable Me to Make My Desired Changes	Things That Will Make It Difficult for Me to Change
Example: I have the support of family and friends.	*Example:* The holidays are coming up, and there are too many gatherings to prepare for.

Where to Start

A good starting point is to keep a diary of what you eat now and how much you exercise. Do this for a week. It will help you learn where you need to make changes. Write down:

- What you eat and where you are eating
- Why you are eating (are you hungry or just eating because you are bored?)
- How you feel when eating (your mood or emotions)

- Your exercise (what you are doing or not doing now)

You might also have a section in your diary for ideas about what you would like to do differently. Don't worry; if all your ideas don't work out right away, you can always go back to them. Our sample lifestyle tracking diary (see Table 12.4 on page 208) may be useful.

How to Make Changes

Two important ingredients for successfully changing your weight are to start small by taking "baby steps" and to make changes that you know will work. Whether you want to lose or gain weight, there is no getting around it; most people will need to change the amount and perhaps the way they eat. This may seem scary or even impossible, but by starting with things that are doable, you will be successful. This could mean that if you want to lose weight you will need to eat a little less or if you want to gain weight eat a little more. For instance, instead of eating ½ cup of rice, eat a few tablespoons less or a few tablespoons more. To help you eat less, try slowing down how fast you eat; to help you increase calories, spread out your eating over several small meals a day.

When you find things you want to change, start by choosing only one or two things at a time. Yes, we said this before but it is really important. Allow yourself time to get used to these changes and then slowly add more things you want to change. If you tell yourself you are going to walk 5 miles a day every day of the week and never eat potatoes or bread again, you won't be able to stick with that for very long. It is likely you won't lose weight, and you will feel frustrated and discouraged. But if you make a plan to have only one piece of toast at breakfast instead of two pieces and take two 10-minute walks 4 times a week and stick to it, you will be making good, long term changes that will lead you to success.

When you change your weight slowly over time, you have a better chance of maintaining that change. This is partly because your brain begins to recognize the changes you are slowly making as part of your regular routine or habit and not just a passing fad. The goal-setting and action-planning skills discussed in Chapter 2 will help with this. Remember, the best plan combines healthy eating and exercise and is a slow, steady plan that feels right to you.

The 200 Plan

A simple and practical plan to get you started is the 200 Plan. It involves making small daily changes in what you eat and in the amount of

Table 12.4 **Lifestyle Tracking Diary**

Date	Time	What I Ate	Where I Ate	Why I Ate	My Mood or Emotions	My Exercise

physical activity you do. You change what you do by 200 calories a day, which can add up to a 20-pound weight change over a year. The 200 Plan is a good way to balance eating and exercise and helps you make a long term change in your weight.

In a few words, to lose weight, eat 100 fewer calories a day than you do now and burn off 100 calories a day more with extra exercise. If you would like to gain weight, add 100 calories while keeping your exercise level at the recommended 20 to 40 minutes most days of the week. Sticking to this kind of plan on a daily basis is essential for success.

How to change what you eat by 100 calories a day

Start by checking out the food guide on pages 186–192 which gives estimated serving sizes and calories. For example, you can see that a 1-ounce slice of bread has close to 100 calories. By not eating one of the slices of bread on your sandwich, right there you have cut out close to 100 calories. To easily eat 100 calories more, add about 2 tablespoons of nuts to your food intake over the day.

How to burn an extra 100 calories a day

Add 20 to 30 minutes to your regular exercise routine, which could be walking, bicycling, dancing, or gardening. Take the stairs more and park farther away from the store or work. If time is an issue, doing your exercise in three 5 to 10-minute chunks of time over the day works just as well as doing it all at once.

Exercise and Weight Loss

Exercise can help you lose weight and keep it off. But it is very difficult to exercise enough to lose weight without also changing what you eat. Adding aerobic or cardio exercise is the best for weight loss. This is the kind of exercise that gets your heart pumping: walking, jogging, bicycling, swimming, and dance all do the trick. These kinds of exercises help you lose weight because they use the large muscles in the body that burn the most calories. The exercise guidelines (see Chapter 8) to get 150 minutes of moderate or brisk aerobic activity a week are the same for general health, weight loss, and keeping the weight off. Exercising in 10-minute bouts works as well as longer workouts. If you can add more minutes, that is even better.

It is true that the more calories you burn up with exercise, the more weight you can lose. However, that is only one part of the story. It is important to understand that the most success comes from making exercise and eating changes that become part of your daily life.

When you add more exercise to your routine, be honest with yourself about what you can do and what is safe and enjoyable for you. If you try to exercise too hard or too long for your body and health, you are more likely to have to stop because of an injury, fatigue, frustration, or loss of interest. The truth is that whatever you do to increase your physical activity to burn more calories will be helpful only if you do it regularly and at a pace that is good for you.

Some people become discouraged after awhile. The pounds may not melt off right away, or weight loss may stop. This may be true even if someone is still exercising and being careful about what they eat. There are many reasons why weight loss slows. Exercise may be building muscle as well as reducing fat. Muscle weighs more than fat, so you could be losing fat but the scale is not showing it. If you keep track of body measurements such as waist and hips or notice that your clothes fit better or are looser, this can be a signal that exercise is working. And remember, when you exercise regularly, even if you don't lose weight, you are doing good things for your body. Regular aerobic exercise can help give you more energy and help a person who is pre-diabetic avoid diabetes. It can reduce blood glucose and blood fat (triglyceride) levels, increase good cholesterol, reduce risk of heart disease, and help with depression and anxiety.

Pointers for Losing Weight

Many studies show that eating fewer calories and being physically active are both important for successful weight loss. Just eating less is usually not enough. Being active will not only help you burn calories, but it will also help you build muscle (which burns more calories than fat) and give you more strength and zip. You will be able to move and breathe better, and your energy level will increase. You will find more information about exercise and tips for choosing activities that suit your needs and lifestyle in Chapters 6 through 8.

- **Set small, gradual weight loss goals.** Break the total amount of weight you want to lose into small, reachable goals. Think in terms of, say, 1 to 2 pounds a week or 5 to 7 a month instead of looking at the total number, especially if you have a lot of weight you would like to lose. For most people, aiming to lose 1 to 2 pounds (0.5–1 kg) a week is realistic and doable. When you set small goals rather than large ones—say 5 pounds instead of 20 pounds—your goals become more possible and practical.

- **Identify the exact steps you will take to lose your weight.** For example, walking 20 minutes a day 5 days a week, not eating between meals, and eating more slowly.

- **Keep on top of what is happening.** Keep track of your weight on a schedule that works for you. Some people decide that when they regain say, 3 pounds, it is a signal to get back into action.

- **Think long-term.** Instead of "I really need to lose 10 pounds right away," tell yourself, "Losing this weight gradually will help me keep it off for good."

- **Be "in the present" when you eat.** By focusing on what you are eating and not what you are doing (such as watching television), you will more likely really enjoy the food, become satisfied sooner, and eat less.

- **Eat more slowly.** If you take less than 15 or 20 minutes to eat a meal, you are probably eating too fast and not allowing yourself to feel the enjoyment of eating. You may be surprised to learn that many of us can both enjoy food more and eat less simply by eating more slowly. If you find it hard to slow down how fast you eat, try putting your fork down on the table between bites, and pick it up only after you have swallowed the food.

■ **Become keenly aware of your stomach.** Learn to become aware of when your stomach is just starting to feel full and to stop eating as soon as you get that signal. This will take attention and practice. When you do recognize the feeling of becoming full, remove your plate immediately or get up from the table if you can.

■ **Portion out your food.** Especially when first starting to make changes, measure out your portions—and do this frequently over time. It is amazing just how easily ½ cup of rice can "grow" to a 1-cup serving. When you can, use food products that are already in single-size portions.

■ **Choose smaller portions.** When eating away from home, select appetizers or first courses over main entrees, or order a child's meal. This will help you eat fewer calories. Over a year, it takes only an extra 100 calories a day to put on 10 pounds. This is like eating only an extra third of a bagel a day. There are many published ranges of recommended serving sizes for different foods. The food guide on pages 186–192 lists some common serving sizes for a variety of foods, along with information on selected nutrients.

■ **Clock yourself.** Make it a habit to wait about 15 minutes before either taking another portion or starting to eat dessert or a snack. You'll often find that this is enough time for the urge to eat or to continue eating goes away.

Common Challenges of Losing Weight

"I need to lose 10 pounds in the next 2 weeks. I want to look good for a special event."

Sound familiar? Almost everyone who has tried to lose weight wants it off fast. There are hundreds of weight loss diets promising fast and easy ways to lose weight. However, these promises are false. There is no "magic bullet." If it sounds too good to be true, it probably is.

During the first few days of almost any weight loss plan, your body loses mostly water, along with some muscle. This can amount to 5 or even 10 pounds. Because of this, fad, and fast-weight-loss diets can say they are successful. But the pounds come right back on just as soon as you return to your old ways. Also, when you use fad diets, you may experience light-headedness, headaches, constipation, fatigue, and poor sleep, as such diets are often badly imbalanced in the kinds and amounts of foods allowed. Fat loss, what you really want to lose, typically comes about after a few weeks of eating fewer calories than your body needs.

Rather than wasting time with fad diets, do it right. Set small, realistic goals; do action planning; and use positive thinking and self-talk. (These activities are discussed in greater detail in Chapters 2 and 5.) The weight didn't go on overnight. It won't go away overnight.

"I just can't seem to lose those last few pounds."

Almost everyone reaches a time where weight loss stops (a plateau) despite continued hard work. This is frustrating and often makes us want to give up. Plateaus are often temporary. They can mean that your body now needs fewer calories and has adapted to its lower calorie intake and higher activity level. While your first impulse may be to cut your calories even further, this could actually make your body burn fewer calories, making more weight loss even harder.

This is a good time to ask yourself how much of a difference those last 1, 2, or even 5 pounds really makes. If you are feeling good and doing well with your blood sugar or cholesterol or other health issues, chances are you may not need to lose more weight. If you are relatively healthy, staying active, and eating a healthy diet, it is usually not bad to carry a few extra pounds. Also, you may have replaced some of your body fat with muscle, which will weigh more than fat—a type of weight gain that is good. However, if you decide that those pounds must go, try the following tactics:

- Instead of focusing on weight loss, focus on staying at the same weight and not gaining any weight for at least few weeks; then go back to your weight loss plan.

- Increase your physical activity. Your body may have adjusted to your lower weight and therefore needs fewer calories, so you may need to exercise more to burn more calories. Adding more exercise could help kick-start your body into burning more calories. (You can find tips for safely increasing your exercise in Chapter 6.)

- Keep thinking positive. Remind yourself of how much you have achieved. (Here's a tip: write that on sticky notes and post them where you will see them.)

"I always feel so deprived of the foods I love when I try to lose weight."

You are a special person. This means that the changes you decide to make have to meet your special likes, dislikes, and needs. Unfortunately, our brains can get channeled into what we don't want to do or should not be doing instead of being supportive or encouraging, especially when it comes to losing weight.

You think using both pictures and words. This calls for teaching yourself how to see things in a better light and telling your brain to stop thinking about certain things, and to replace those thoughts with positive ones that work for you (more on positive thinking can be found in Chapter 5). Here are a couple of examples:

- Replace thoughts that include the words *never, always,* and *avoid.* Instead, tell yourself that you can enjoy things occasionally, "but a healthier choice is better for me most of the time."

- Tell yourself that you are retraining your taste buds and that making healthier choices can help you manage your weight and feel better.

"I eat too fast or I finish eating before everyone else and find myself reaching for seconds."

If you are finishing meals in just a few minutes or before everyone else at the table, you are most likely eating too fast. You may be doing this for a number of reasons. You may be letting yourself get too hungry because too much time passes between meals or snacks and then you wolf food down when you finally do get to eat. You may be hurried, anxious, or stressed when you sit down to eat. Slowing down your eating pace can help you eat less and enjoy your food more. Here are some tips for cutting down your eating speed:

- Do not skip meals; you will avoid becoming overly hungry.

- Make it a game not to be the first person at the table to be finished eating.

- After eating something, if you find yourself saying "I think that was good—I better have more to make sure," that usually means you aren't paying attention to what you eat. Work on thinking about what you are eating and how you are enjoying it. Practice this without things that take your attention away, such as friends, video games, or television.

- Take small bites, chew slowly, and be sure to swallow each bite before taking another. Chewing your food well also helps you

enjoy your food more and feel better after the meal by lessening heartburn or other digestive upsets.

- Try a relaxation method about a half hour before you eat. Several methods are discussed in Chapter 5.

"I can't do it on my own."

Losing weight is challenging, and sometimes you just need some outside support and guidance. For help, you can contact any of the following resources:

- A registered dietitian through your health plan, local hospital, or the Academy of Nutrition and Dietetics website, http://www.eatright.org

- A support group such as Weight Watchers or Take Off Pounds Sensibly (TOPS), where you can meet other people who are trying to lose or maintain a healthy weight

- A weight loss program offered by your local health department, hospital, health plan, community school, or employer

Common Challenges of Keeping the Weight Off

"I've been on a lot of diets before and lost a lot of weight. But I've always gained it back, and then some. It's so frustrating, and I just don't understand why this happens!"

This happens to many people. In fact, it is the downside of quick-weight-loss diets, because they typically involve drastic changes. They do not focus on lifelong changes in eating habits,

exercise, and lifestyle. Typically, after you have gotten tired of the diet or have reached your goal weight, you return to your old ways, and the weight comes back on. Sometimes you even gain back more weight than you lost.

The key to maintaining a healthy weight is to develop healthy eating and exercise habits that you enjoy, that fit into your lifestyle, and that are part of a lifestyle that you can stick with. We have already given you many tips earlier in this chapter. Here are a few more:

- Set a personal weight gain "alarm"—say, a specific number of pounds gained (perhaps 3 pounds). If you hit this mark, go back on your regular program. The sooner you start, the faster the newly added pounds will come off.

- Monitor your activity level. Once you have lost some weight, exercise three to five times a week to improve your chances of keeping the weight off. Research suggests that to maintain weight loss, some people should be exercising nearly an hour a day—but no need to fear, this includes normal activities during the day as well as planned physical exercise. Also remember that increasing activity does not just mean exercising longer. It can mean going faster or doing something that is harder to do, such as walking uphill or swimming with paddles.

"I do OK keeping weight off for a short time. Then something happens beyond my control, and I stop caring about what I eat. Before I know it, I've slipped back into my old eating habits."

Everyone is going to slip at one time or another; no one is perfect. If it was only a little slip, don't worry about it. Just continue as if nothing happened and get back on your plan. If the slip is bigger, try to figure out why. Is there something that is taking a lot of your attention now? If so, weight management may need to take a back seat for a while. That's OK. The sooner you realize this, the better; just try to set a date when you will restart your weight management program. You may even want to join a support group and stay with it for at least 4 to 6 months. If so, look for a weight loss support group that does the following:

- It emphasizes healthy eating.

- It emphasizes lifelong changes in eating habits and lifestyle patterns.

- It gives support in the form of ongoing meetings or long-term follow-up.

- It does not make miraculous claims or guarantees. (Remember, if something sounds too good to be true, it probably is.)

- It does not rely on special meals or supplements.

Common Challenges of Gaining Weight

Sometimes long-term health problems make it difficult to gain weight or keep it on. This could be because your condition or its treatment makes it hard for you to eat because you aren't hungry, you are sad or depressed, your body is unable to use the food it gets, or it burns up calories faster than you can replace them.

When you aren't hungry or have trouble eating, few foods sound appealing. This is when it is more important to eat anything rather than worry about whether the foods you choose are "healthful." You need to eat for energy and strength and to support the body's nutrition needs, and that overrides being sure that what you eat is "healthy." During those times, feel comfortable about eating whatever you can; it will probably only be temporary and then you can return to healthy eating.

Here, too, slow and steady wins the race. Try the 200 Plan (see pages 207–208) by making sure to eat an extra 100 calories a day every day. This alone can result in a 10-pound weight gain over a year. Be sure to choose foods that you really enjoy, focusing on your favorites. Keep easy-to-fix or already-prepared foods handy so that you don't need to spend much time cooking.

If you experience a continual or extreme weight loss or have trouble keeping weight on, you're not alone. Let's look at some common challenges and some ideas for dealing with them.

"I don't know how to add calories to my current diet."

Here are some ways to increase the calories and nutrients you eat without increasing the amount of food you need to eat:

- Because fat gives us many more calories than carbohydrate or protein, choose foods that are higher in fat, but try to stick with foods that contain good fats (see page 191). For example, snack on calorie-rich foods such as avocados, nuts, seeds, or nut butter.

- Eat dried fruit or nectars instead fresh fruit or regular juice.

- Choose sweet potatoes instead of white potatoes.

- Use whole milk instead of lower-fat dairy products, and instead of broth or water in soups and sauces.

- Try a liquid supplement drink with or between meals.

- Drink high-calorie beverages such as shakes, malts, fruit whips, and eggnogs.

- Top salads, soups, and casseroles with shredded cheese, nuts, dried fruits, or seeds.

"I just don't have much of an appetite."

Check with your doctor or a registered dietitian to see if the following tips are appropriate for you.

- Eat tiny meals or smaller meals several times a day.

- Keep some nuts or dried fruit handy, and eat a few pieces each time you walk past the bowl.

- Eat the highest-calorie foods first, saving lower-calorie foods for later (for example, eat buttered bread before cooked spinach).

- Add extra whole milk or milk powder to sauces, gravies, cereals, soups, and casseroles.

- Add melted cheese to vegetables and other dishes.

- Use butter, margarine, or sour cream as toppings.

- Consider keeping a snack at your bedside so that you can eat something if you wake in the middle of the night.

Other common problems related to making changes in your eating habits are also discussed in Chapter 11. More information on body weight can also be found in the resources listed at the end of this chapter.

People come in many shapes and sizes—some of which can affect their health and their symptoms, whether they carry too much weight or not enough. There is no such thing as a perfect or "ideal" weight, but rather there is a range of pounds that is good for us. Being in a healthy weight range helps us achieve overall health and well-being, both for our body and our mind. The smartest and best approach to achieving a healthy weight range involves both healthy eating and being active. Once you get to your healthy weight, keeping it in a good range for you is most important. Tailoring how to meet your needs and how to match your lifestyle is the best way. Choose realistic lifelong strategies that you can stick to instead of trying quick fixes, which most often do not work. Set your sights on success by building on small changes over time.

Suggested Further Reading

Ferguson, James M., and Cassandra Ferguson. *Habits, Not Diets*, 4th ed. Boulder, Colo.: Bull, 2003.

Hensrud, Donald D., ed. *Mayo Clinic Healthy Weight for Everybody*. Rochester, Minn.: Mayo Clinic Health Foundation, 2005.

Nash, Joyce D. *Maximize Your Body Potential*, 3rd ed. Boulder, Colo.: Bull, 2003.

Schoonen, Josephine Connolly. *Losing Weight Permanently with the Bull's-Eye Food Guide*. Boulder, Colo.: Bull, 2004.

Other Resources

☐   Healthy Weight Network: http://www.healthyweight.net/

☐   National Weight Control Registry: http://www.nwcr.ws/

☐   Shape Up America: http://www.shapeup.org/

☐   Weight-control Information Network (WIN): http://win.niddk.nih.gov/index.htm

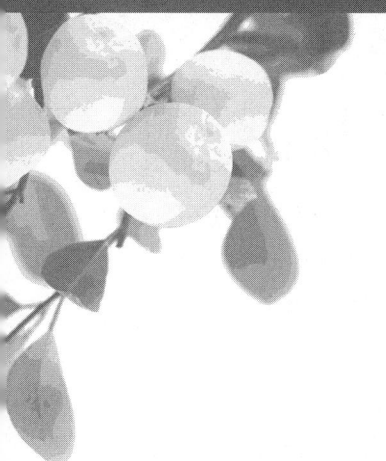

CHAPTER 13

Managing
Your Medicines

HAVING A CHRONIC ILLNESS usually means taking one or more medications. It is therefore a very important management task to understand your medications and to use them appropriately. This chapter will help you do just that.

A Few General Words About Medications

Few products are more heavily advertised than medications. If we read a magazine, listen to the radio, or watch TV, we see a constant stream of ads. These are aimed at convincing us that if we just use this pill, our symptoms will be cured. "Recommended by 90% of the doctors asked," they say. But be aware that they may have asked doctors working for the company or only a handful of doctors. And have you noticed that on TV, the ads present the benefits in a slow, upbeat voice, while the side effects are recited very rapidly? Almost as a backlash to this advertising, we have been taught to avoid excess medications. We have all heard about or experienced some of the bad effects of medications. It can be very confusing.

Your body is often its own healer, and given time, many common symptoms and disorders will improve. The prescriptions filled by the body's own "internal pharmacy" are frequently the safest and most effective treatment. So patience, careful self-observation, and monitoring with your doctor are often excellent choices.

It is also true that medications can be a very important part of managing a chronic illness. These medications do not cure the disease. They generally have one or more of the following purposes:

- **To relieve symptoms.** For example, an inhaler delivers medications that help expand the bronchial tubes and make it easier to breathe. A nitroglycerin tablet expands the blood vessels, allowing more blood to reach the heart, thus quieting angina. Acetaminophen (Tylenol) can relieve pain.

- **To prevent further problems.** For example, medications that thin the blood help prevent blood clots, which cause strokes and heart and lung problems.

- **To improve or slow the progress of the disease.** For example, nonsteroidal anti-inflammatory drugs can help arthritis by quieting the inflammatory process. Likewise, antihypertensive medications can lower blood pressure.

- **To replace substances that the body is no longer producing adequately.** This is how insulin is used to manage diabetes and thyroid medication for underactive thyroid.

Thus the purpose of medication is to lessen the consequences of disease or to slow its course. You may not be aware that the medication is doing anything, such as slowing the course of your disease—keeping you from getting worse or helping you get worse more slowly. You may not feel anything, and this may make you think that the drug isn't working. It is important to continue taking your medications, even if you cannot see how they are helping. If this concerns you, ask your doctor.

We pay a price for having such powerful tools. Besides being helpful, all medications have undesirable side effects. Some of these effects are predictable and minor, and some are unexpected and life-threatening. Some 5% to 10% of all hospital admissions are due to drug reactions. At the same time, not taking medications as prescribed is also a major cause of hospitalization.

Mind Power: Expect the Best

Medication affects your body in two ways. The first is determined by the chemical nature of the medication. The second is triggered by your beliefs and expectations. Your beliefs and confidence can change your body chemistry and your symptoms. This reaction is called the placebo effect. It is an example of how closely the mind and body are connected.

Many studies have shown the power of the placebo—the power of mind over body. When people are given a placebo (pill containing no medication), some of them improve anyway. Placebos can relieve back pain and chronic pain, fatigue, arthritis, headache, allergies, hypertension, insomnia, asthma, irritable bowel syndrome and chronic digestive disorders, depression, anxiety, and pain after surgery. The placebo effect clearly demonstrates that our positive beliefs and expectations can turn on our self-healing mechanisms. You can learn to take advantage of your powerful internal pharmacy.

Every time you take a medication, you are swallowing your expectations and beliefs as well as the pill. So expect the best!

Let's look at some ways to do that.

- **Examine your beliefs about the treatment.** If you tell yourself, "I'm not a pill taker" or "Medications always give me bad side effects," how do you think your body is likely to respond? If you don't think the prescribed treatment is likely to help your symptoms or condition, your negative beliefs will undermine the ability of the pill to help you. You can change these negative images into more positive ones. (Reviewing the discussion of positive thinking in Chapter 5 can help with this.)

- **Think of your medications the way you think of vitamins.** Many people associate healthful images with vitamins—more so than with medications. Taking a vitamin

makes you think that you are doing something positive to prevent disease and promote health. So if you regard your medications as health-restoring and health-promoting, like vitamins, you may obtain more powerful benefits.

- **Imagine how the medicine is helping you.** Develop a mental image of how the medication is helping your body. For example, if you are taking thyroid hormone replacement medication, tell yourself it is filling a missing link in your body's chemical chains to help balance and regulate your metabolism. For some people, forming a vivid mental image is helpful. An antibiotic, for example, might be seen as a broom sweeping germs out of the body. Don't worry if your image of what's happening chemically inside of you is not physiologically correct. It's your belief in a clear, positive image that counts.

- **Keep in mind why you are taking the medication.** You are not taking your medication just because your doctor told you to. You are taking your medication to help you live your life. It is therefore important to understand how the medicine is helping you. You can use this information to help the medicine do its job. Suppose a woman with cancer is given chemotherapy. She has been told that it will make her feel like she has the flu, she will vomit, and her hair will fall out. So of course, that is what she thinks about and that is what happens. But suppose she is also told that the symptoms will last only a few days, that hair falling out is a good sign because it means that cells that grow fast (cancer and hair) are being destroyed, and that her hair will grow back after chemo. In that case, she may regard her hair loss, flu-like symptoms, and vomiting as signs the drugs are working. She can then take actions to counter these effects and often have an easier time tolerating them. The presence of side effects can sometimes be your proof that the medicine is working.

Taking Multiple Medications

People with multiple problems often take many medications: a medication to lower blood pressure, anti-inflammatory drugs for arthritis, a pill for angina, a bronchodilator for asthma, antacids for heartburn, a tranquilizer for anxiety, plus a handful of over-the-counter (OTC) remedies and herbs. The more medications (including vitamins and OTC remedies) you are taking, the greater the risk of unpleasant reactions. Also, not all drugs like each other, and when they get together, they sometimes cause problems. Fortunately, it is often possible to take fewer medications and lower the risks. However, you should not do this without the help of your doctor. Most people would not change the ingredients in a complicated cooking recipe or throw out a few parts when fixing something in the car or home. It is not that these things can't be done. It is just that if you want the best and safest results, you may need expert help.

How you respond to any one medication depends on age, metabolism, daily activity, the waxing and waning of symptoms, your chronic conditions, your genetics, and your frame of mind. To get the most from your medications, your doctor depends on you. Report what effect, if any, the drug has on your symptoms and any side effects. Based on this critical information, your medications may be continued, increased, discontinued, or otherwise changed. In a good doctor-patient partnership, there is a continuing flow of information in both directions.

Unfortunately, this vital interchange is often shortchanged. Studies indicate that fewer than 5% of patients getting new prescriptions asked any questions about them. Doctors tend to interpret patient silence as understanding and satisfaction. Problems often occur because patients do not receive enough information about medications or do not understand how to take them. In addition, all too often people do not follow instructions. Safe, effective drug use depends on your doctor's expertise and equally on your understanding of when and how to take the drug, and the necessary precautions. You must ask questions. (Our discussion of communication in Chapter 9 can help.)

Some people are afraid to ask their doctor questions. They are afraid that they will seem foolish or stupid or that they might be perceived as challenging the doctor's authority. But asking questions is a necessary part of a healthy doctor-patient relationship.

The goal of treatment is to maximize the benefits and minimize the risks. This means taking the fewest medications, in the lowest effective doses, for the shortest period of time. Whether the medications you take are helpful or harmful often depends on how much you know about your medications and how well you communicate with your doctor.

What You Need to Tell Your Doctor

Even if your doctor doesn't ask, there is certain vital information about medications you should mention during every consultation.

Are you taking any other medications?

Report to your physician and your dentist all the prescription and nonprescription medications you are taking, including birth control pills, vitamins, aspirin, antacids, laxatives, alcohol, and herbal remedies. An easy way to do this is to carry a list of all medications along with the amount you take (dosage). Or bring all your medications to the doctor visit. Saying that you are taking "the little green pills" isn't very helpful.

This is especially important if you are seeing more than one physician. Each one may not know what the others have prescribed. Knowing all your medications and supplements is essential for correct diagnosis and treatment. For example, if you have symptoms such as nausea or diarrhea, sleeplessness or drowsiness, dizziness or memory loss, impotence or fatigue, they may be caused by a drug side effect rather than a disease. If your doctor does not know all your medications, he or she cannot protect you from drug interactions.

Have you had allergic or unusual reactions to any medications?

Describe any symptoms or unusual reactions caused by medications. Be specific: which medication and exactly what type of reaction? A rash, fever, or wheezing that develops after taking a medication is often a true allergic reaction. If any of these develop, call your doctor at once. Nausea, diarrhea, ringing in the ears, light-headedness, sleeplessness, and frequent urination are likely to be side effects rather than true drug allergies.

What are your chronic diseases and other medical conditions?

Many diseases can interfere with the action of a drug or increase the risk of using certain medications. Diseases involving the kidneys or liver are especially important to mention because these diseases can slow the metabolism of many drugs and increase toxic effects. Your doctor may also avoid certain medications if you now or in the past have had such diseases as high blood pressure, peptic ulcer disease, asthma, heart disease, diabetes, or prostate problems. Be sure to let your doctor know if you are possibly pregnant or are breastfeeding. Many drugs cannot be safely used in those situations.

What medications were tried in the past to treat your disease?

It is a good idea to keep your own records. What medications were used in the past to manage your condition, and what were the effects? Knowing what has been tried and how you reacted will help guide the doctor's recommendation of any new medications. However, the fact that a medication did not work in the past does not necessarily mean that it can't be tried again. Diseases change, and the same medication may work the second time.

What to Ask Your Doctor or Pharmacist

There is also important information that you need to know about your medications. Be sure to ask the following questions.

Do I really need this medication?

Some doctors prescribe medications not because they are really necessary but because they think patients want and expect drugs. Doctors often feel pressure to do something for the patient, so they prescribe a new drug. Don't pressure your doctor for medications. Many new medications are heavily advertised and promoted by their manufacturers. Quite a few medications that were heavily marketed were later found to be so hazardous that they were withdrawn. So be cautious about requesting the newest medications. If your doctor doesn't prescribe a medication, consider that good news. Ask about nondrug alternatives. In some cases, lifestyle changes such as exercise, diet, and stress management should be considered. When any treatment is recommended, ask what is likely to happen if you postpone treatment. Sometimes the best medicine is none at all, and sometimes it is taking a powerful medication early to avoid permanent damage or complications.

What is the name of the medication, and what dosage do I take?

Keep a record of each medication you take, noting its brand name, if any; the generic (chemical) name; and the dosage your doctor has prescribed. If the medication you get from the pharmacy doesn't match this information, ask the pharmacist to explain the difference. This is your best protection against medication mix-ups.

What is the medication supposed to do?

Your doctor should tell you why the medication is being prescribed and how it might help you. Is the medication intended to prolong your life, completely or partially relieve your symptoms, or improve your ability to function? For example, if you are given a medicine for high blood pressure, the medication is given primarily to prevent later complications (such as stroke or heart disease) rather than to stop a headache. On the other hand, if you are given a pain reliever such as ibuprofen (Motrin), the purpose is to help ease the headache. You should also know how soon you should expect results from the medication. Drugs that treat infections or inflammation may take several days to a week to show improvement, and antidepressant medications and some arthritis drugs typically take several weeks to start providing relief.

How and when do I take the medication, and for how long?

If medications are going to work you must take them *when* you are supposed to take them, *in the amounts* you are supposed to take them, and *as long as* you are supposed to take them. This is crucial to their safe and effective use. Does "every 6 hours" mean every 6 hours while awake or every 6 hours around the clock? Should the medication be taken before meals, with meals, or between meals? What should you do if you accidentally miss a dose? Should you skip it, take a double dose next time, or take it as soon as you remember? Should you refill and continue taking the medication until you have fewer symptoms or until you finish the current medication? Some medications are prescribed on an as-needed ("PRN") basis, so you need to know when to begin and end treatment and how much medication to take. You need to work out a plan with your doctor to suit your individual needs.

Taking the medication properly is vital. Yet nearly 40% of people report that their doctors failed to tell them how to take the medication or how much to take. If you are not sure about your prescription, contact your doctor or pharmacist.

What foods, drinks, other medications, or activities should I avoid while taking this medication?

Food in the stomach may help protect the stomach from some medications but make other drugs ineffective. For example, milk products or antacids block the absorption of the antibiotic tetracycline. This drug is best taken on an empty stomach. Some medications may make you more sensitive to the sun, putting you at increased risk for sunburn. Ask whether the medication prescribed will interfere with driving safely. Other drugs you may be taking, even over-the-counter drugs and alcohol, can either amplify or lessen the effects of the prescribed medication. Taking aspirin along with an anticoagulant medication can result in possible bleeding. The more medications you are taking, the greater the chance of an undesirable drug interaction. So ask about possible drug-drug and drug-food interactions.

What are the most common side effects, and what should I do if they occur?

All medications have side effects. Your doctor may have to try several medications before hitting on the one that is best for you. You need to know what symptoms to be on the lookout for and what action to take if they develop. Should you seek immediate medical care, discontinue the medication, or call your doctor? While the doctor cannot be expected to tell you every possible adverse reaction, the most common and most important ones should be discussed. Unfortunately, a recent survey showed that 70% of people starting a new medication did not recall being told by their physicians or pharmacists about precautions and possible side effects. So it may be up to you to ask.

Are there any tests necessary to monitor the use of this medication?

Most medications are monitored by the improvement or worsening of symptoms. However, some medications can disrupt body chemistry before any symptoms develop. Sometimes these adverse reactions can be detected by laboratory tests such as blood counts or liver function tests. In addition, the levels of some medications in the blood need to be measured on a regular basis to make sure you are getting the right amounts. Ask your doctor if the medication being prescribed has any of these special requirements.

Can a less expensive alternative or generic medication be prescribed?

Every drug has at least two names, a generic name and a brand name. The generic name is the name used to refer to the medication in the scientific literature. The brand name is the unique name given to the drug by its developer. When a drug company develops a new drug in the United States, it is granted exclusive rights to produce that drug for 17 years. After this 17-year period, other companies may market chemical equivalents of that drug. These generic medications are generally considered as safe and effective as the original brand-name drug but often cost much less. In some cases, your physician may have a good reason for preferring a particular brand. Even so, if cost is a concern, ask your doctor if a less expensive but equally effective medication is available.

You may also be able to save money by knowing how to use your insurance advantageously. For example, your copayment may be less if you obtain your medications from a company designated by your insurer. Also, many national pharmacies have discount programs for seniors and individuals with low income. It pays to ask and then ask again. And it is wise to shop around. Even in the same town, different stores sell the same medication at different prices.

Is there any written information about the medication?

Your doctor may not have time to answer all of your questions. You many not remember everything you heard. Fortunately, there are many other good sources of information, including pharmacists, nurses, package inserts, pamphlets, books, and Web sites. Several useful sources are listed at the end of this chapter.

How to Read the Prescription Label

One great source of information is the prescription label. The following illustration will help you learn how to read the labels on your prescriptions.

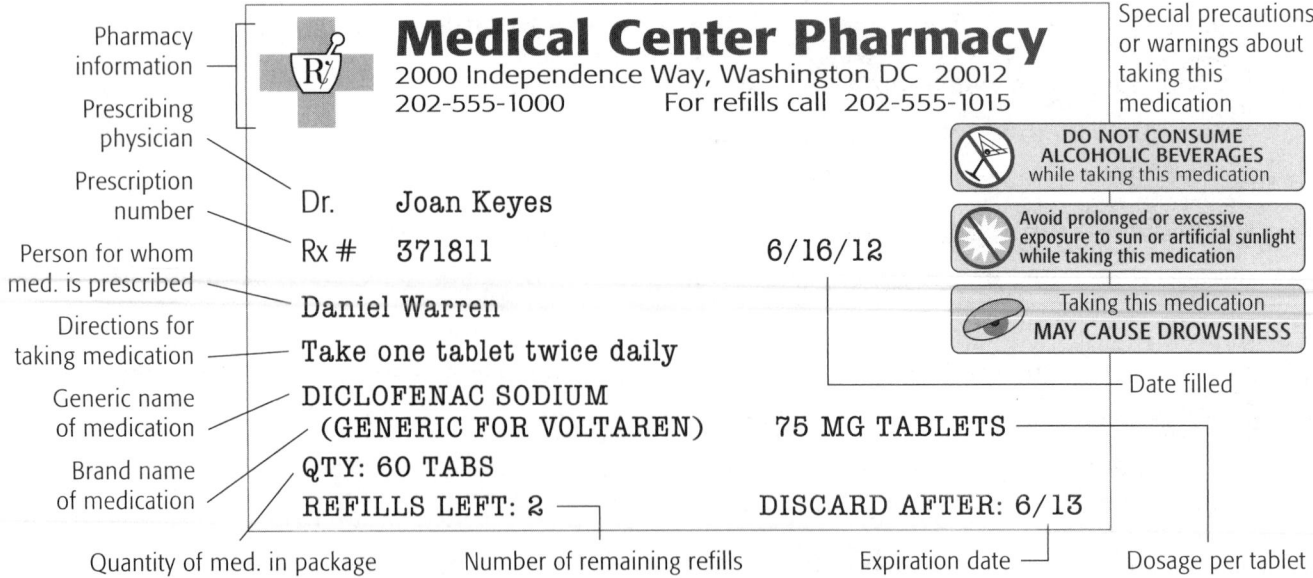

A Special Word About Pharmacists

Pharmacists are an underutilized resource. They have gone to school for many years to learn about medications, how they act in your body, and how they interact with each other. Your pharmacist is an expert on medications and can readily answer questions face to face, over the phone, or even via e-mail. In addition, many hospitals, medical schools, and schools of pharmacy have medication information services that you can call to ask questions. As a self-manager, don't forget pharmacists. They are important and helpful consultants.

Taking Your Medicine

No matter what the medication, it won't do you any good if you don't take it. Nearly half of all medicines are not taken as prescribed. This has been called "the other drug problem." There are many reasons why people don't take their prescribed medication: forgetfulness, lack of clear instructions, complicated dosing schedules, bothersome side effects, cost of the medications, and so on. Whatever the reason, if you are having trouble taking your medications as prescribed, discuss this with your doctor. Often simple adjustments can make it easier. For example, if you are taking many different medications, sometimes one or more can be eliminated. If you are taking one medication three times a day and another four times a day, your doctor may be able to simplify the regimen, perhaps even prescribing medications that you need to take only once or twice a day. Understanding more about your medications, including how they can help you, may also help motivate you to take them regularly.

If you are having trouble taking your medications, ask yourself the following questions and discuss the answers with your doctor or pharmacist.

- Do you tend to be forgetful?

- Are you confused about the instructions for how and when to use the medications?

- Is the schedule for taking your medications too complicated?

- Do your medications have bothersome side effects?

- Is your medicine too expensive?

- Do you feel that your disease is not serious or bothersome enough to need regular medications? (With some diseases such as high blood pressure, high cholesterol, or early diabetes, you may not have any symptoms.)

- Do you feel that the treatment is unlikely to help?

- Are you denying that you have a disease that needs treatment?

- Have you had a bad experience with the medicine you are supposed to be taking or another medication?

- Do you know someone who had a bad experience with the medication, and are you afraid that something similar will happen with you?

- Are you afraid of becoming addicted to the medication?

- Are you embarrassed about taking the medication, view it as a sign of weakness or failure, or fear you'll be judged negatively if people know about it?

- What are some of the benefits you might get if you take the medication as prescribed?

Remembering to Take Your Medicines

If forgetting to take your medications is a problem, here are some suggestions to help you remember:

- **Make it obvious.** Place the medication or a reminder next to your toothbrush, on the breakfast table, in your lunch box, or in some other place where you're likely to "stumble over" it. (But be careful where you put the medication if children are around.) Or you might put a reminder note on the bathroom mirror, the refrigerator door, the coffee maker, the television, or some other conspicuous place. If you link taking the medication with some well-established habit such as meal times or watching your favorite television program, you'll be more likely to remember.

- **Use a checklist or an organizer.** Make a medication chart listing each medication you are taking and the time when you take it, or check off each medication on a calendar as you take it. You might also buy a medication organizer at the drugstore. This container separates pills according to the time of day they should be taken. You can fill the organizer once a week so that all of your pills are ready to take at the proper time. A quick glance at the organizer lets you know if you have missed any doses and prevents double dosing. There are also Web sites that allow you to print out charts to help you track your medications; PictureRx (https://mypicturerx.com) is one, but it requires a subscription.

- **Use an electronic reminder.** Get a watch or mobile phone that can be set to beep at pill-taking time. There are also "high-tech" medication containers that beep at a preset time to remind you to take your medication. If you have a smartphone, you can also download apps that can track and remind you to take your medication.

- **Have others remind you.** Ask members of your household to remind you to take your medications at the appropriate times.

- **Don't run out.** Don't let yourself run out of your medicines. When you get a new prescription, mark on your calendar the date a week before your medications will run out. This will serve as a reminder to order and get your next refill. Don't wait until the last pill. Some mail-order pharmacies offer automatic refills, so your medications arrive when you need them.

- **Plan before you travel.** If you plan to travel, put a note on your luggage reminding you to pack your pills. Also, take along an extra prescription in your carry-on bag in case you lose your pills or your checked luggage.

Self-Medication

You may take nonprescription or over-the-counter (OTC) medications or herbs. In every two-week period, nearly 70% of people will take a nonprescription drug. Many OTC drugs are highly effective and may even be recommended by your doctor. But if you self-medicate, you should know what you are taking, why you are taking it, how it works, and how to use the medication wisely.

More than 200,000 nonprescription drug products are offered for sale to the American public, representing about 500 active ingredients. Nearly 75% of the public receives its education on OTC drugs solely from TV, radio, newspaper, and magazine advertising. This advertising is aimed at you.

The main message of drug advertising is that for every symptom, every ache and pain, and every problem, there is a pharmaceutical solution. While many of the OTC products are effective, many are simply a waste of your money. They may also keep you from using better ways to manage your illness or may interfere or interact badly with your prescription medications.

Whether you are taking prescribed medications or using over-the-counter medications or herbs, here are some helpful suggestions:

- **If you are pregnant or nursing, have a chronic disease, or are already taking multiple medications, consult your doctor before self-medicating.**

- **Always read drug labels and follow directions carefully.** Reading of the label, including review of the individual ingredients, may help prevent you from taking medications that have caused problems for you in the past. If you don't understand the information on the label, ask a pharmacist or doctor before buying it.

- **Do not exceed the recommended dosage or length of treatment** unless you have discussed the change with your doctor.

- **Use caution if you are taking other medications.** Over-the-counter and prescription drugs can interact, either canceling or exaggerating the effects of the medications. If you have questions about drug interactions, ask your doctor or pharmacist before mixing medicines.

- **Try to select medications with a single active ingredient rather than combination ("all-in-one") products.** In using a product with multiple ingredients, you are likely to get drugs for symptoms you don't even have, so why risk the side effects of medications you don't need? Single-ingredient products also allow you to adjust the dosage of each medication separately for optimal symptom relief with minimal side effects.

A Special Word About Alcohol and Recreational Drugs

The use of alcohol and recreational drugs (illegal or prescription medications used for nonmedicinal purposes) has been increasing in recent years, particularly among people over the age of 60. These drugs, whether legal or illegal, can cause problems. They can interact with prescription medications, making them less effective or even causing harm. They can fog judgment and cause problems with balance. This can in turn cause accidents and injure both you and others. In some cases, alcohol or recreational drugs can make existing long-term conditions worse. Alcohol use is associated with increased risk of hypertension, diabetes, gastrointestinal bleeding, sleep disorders, depression, erectile dysfunction, breast and other cancers, and injury. Limiting alcohol use to no more than two drinks per day is advised. "At risk" alcohol use for women is drinking more than seven drinks per week or more than three drinks per day and for men more than 14 drinks per week or more than four drinks in a day. This means that women of any age and anyone over age 65 should average no more than one drink per day and men under 65 should have no more than two drinks per day on average.

We are not here to judge but do have two pieces of advice:

- If you are at the "at risk" level for alcohol or are regularly using recreational drugs, seriously consider cutting down or stopping their use.

- Talk to your doctor about your use of these drugs. Doctors are often hesitant to raise the issue because they don't want to embarrass you. So it is up to you to bring up the subject. Doctors will be very willing to talk about it. They have heard it all, and they will not think less of you. An honest conversation may save your life.

- **When choosing medications, learn the ingredient names and try to buy generic products.** Generics contain the same active ingredient as the brand-name product, usually at a lower cost.

- **Never take or give a drug from an unlabeled container or a container whose label you cannot read.** Keep your medications in their original labeled containers or transfer them to a labeled medication organizer or pill dispenser. Do not make the mistake of mixing different medications in the same bottle.

- **Do not take medications that were prescribed for someone else,** even if you have similar symptoms.

- **Drink at least a half glass of liquid with your pills,** and remain standing or sitting upright for a short while after swallowing. This can prevent the pills from getting stuck in the esophagus.

- **Store your medications where children or young adults cannot find them.** Poisoning from medications is a common and preventable problem among the young, and the main sources of recreational drugs used by teens and young adults are the prescription medications of relatives or the relatives of friends. Despite its name, the bathroom medicine cabinet is not usually an appropriate place to store medications. A kitchen cabinet or tool box with a lock is far safer.

Medications can help or harm. What often makes the difference is the care you exercise and the partnership you develop with your doctor.

Suggested Further Reading

Castleman, Michael. *The New Healing Herbs: The Essential Guide to More Than 125 of Nature's Most Potent Herbal Remedies,* 3rd ed. New York: Rodale, 2010.

Graedon, Joe, and Teresa Graedon. *Best Choices from the People's Pharmacy.* New York: Rodale, 2006.

Griffith, H. Winter, and Stephen W. Moore. *Complete Guide to Prescription and Nonprescription Drugs, 2012.* New York: Perigee Books, 2011.

Physicians' Desk Reference. *The PDR Pocket Guide to Prescription Drugs,* 9th ed. New York: Pocket Books, 2010.

Rybacki, James J. *The Essential Guide to Prescription Drugs.* New York: HarperCollins, 2006.

Shane-McWhorter, Laura. *The American Diabetes Association Guide to Herbs and Nutritional Supplements.* Alexandria, Va.: American Diabetes Association, 2009.

Silverman, Harold M. *The Pill Book,* 14th ed. New York: Bantam Books, 2010.

Other Resources

☐ MedlinePlus: Drugs, Supplements, and Herbal Information, a service of the U.S. National Library of Medicine and National Institutes of Health: http://www.nlm.nih.gov/medlineplus/druginformation.html

☐ National Institutes of Health: Rethinking Drinking: Alcohol and Your Health: http://rethinkingdrinking.niaaa.nih.gov/

☐ Natural Medicines Comprehensive Database: http://naturaldatabaseconsumer.therapeuticresearch.com/home.aspx

☐ PictureRx: https://mypicturerx.com

☐ The National Center for Complementary and Alternative Medicine (NCCAM): http://nccam.nih.gov/

☐ WebMD: Drugs and Medications A–Z: http://www.webmd.com/drugs

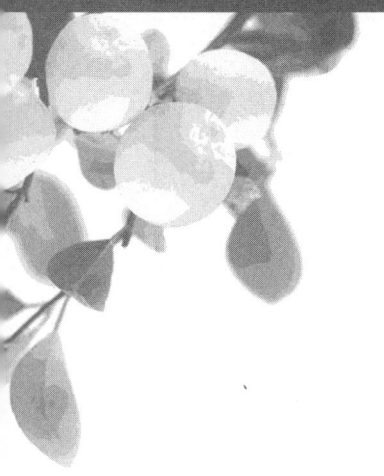

Making Treatment Decisions

W E HEAR ABOUT NEW TREATMENTS, new drugs, nutritional supplements, and alternative treatments all the time. Hardly a week goes by without a new treatment of some kind being reported in the news. Drug companies and nutritional supplement companies run commercials during the television news and place large ads in newspapers and magazines. Our e-mail boxes are filled with promises of new treatments or cures from spammers. We are bombarded in the market or pharmacy with signs and packaging for over-the-counter alternative treatments. Not only that, our health care providers may recommend new procedures, medications, or other treatments that we don't know much about.

What can we believe? How can we decide what might be worth a try?

An important part of managing our own care is being able to evaluate these claims or recommendations so that we can make an informed decision about trying something new. There are some important questions that you should ask yourself in the process of making a decision about any treatment, whether it is a mainstream medical treatment or a complementary or alternative treatment.

Where did I learn about this?

Was it reported in a scientific journal, a supermarket tabloid, a print or TV ad, a Web site, or a flyer you picked up somewhere? Did your doctor suggest it?

The source of the information is important. Results that are reported in a respected scientific journal are more believable than those you might see in a supermarket tabloid or in advertising. Results reported in scientific journals, such as the *New England Journal of Medicine, Lancet,* or *Science,* are usually from research studies. These studies are carefully reviewed for scientific integrity by other scientists, who are very careful about what they approve for publication. Many alternative treatments and nutritional supplements, however, have not been studied scientifically, so they are not as well represented in the scientific literature as medical treatments are. If this is the case, you need to be extra careful and critical about analyzing what you read or hear.

Were the people who got better like me?

In the past, many studies were done with easy-to-get people, so older studies were often done on college students, nurses, or white men. This has changed, but it is still important to find out if the people that got better were like you. Were they from the same age group? Did they have similar lifestyles? Did they have the same health problems as you do? Were they the same sex and race? If the people aren't like you, the results may not be the same for you.

Could anything else have caused these positive changes?

A woman returns from a two-week stay at a spa in the tropics and reports that her arthritis improved dramatically thanks to the special diet and supplements she received. But is it appropriate to attribute her improvement to the treatment when the warm weather, relaxation, and pampering may have had even more to do with her improvement?

It is important to look at everything that has changed since starting a particular treatment. It is common to take up a generally healthier lifestyle when starting a new treatment—could that be playing a part in the improvement? Did you start another medication or treatment at the same time? Has the weather improved? Are you under less stress than before you started the treatment? Can you think of anything else that could have affected your health?

Does treatment suggest stopping other medications or treatments?

Does it require that you stop taking another basic medication because of dangerous interactions? If the other medication is important, this will require a discussion with your health care provider before making a change.

Does treatment suggest not eating a well-balanced diet?

Does it eliminate any important nutrients or stress only a few nutrients that could be harmful to you? Maintaining a balanced diet is important for your overall health. Be sure that you're not sacrificing important vitamins or make certain that you're getting them from another source if you change your eating habits. Also be sure to avoid putting excessive stress on your organs by concentrating on only a few nutrients to the exclusion of others.

Can I think of any possible dangers or harm?

Some treatments take a toll on your body. All treatments have side effects and possible risks. Discuss these matters thoroughly with your health care provider. Only you can decide if the potential problems are worth the possible benefit, but you must have all the information in order to make that decision.

Many people think that if something is natural, it must be good for you. This may not be true. "Natural" isn't necessarily better just because it comes from a plant or animal. In the case of the powerful heart medication digitalis, which comes from the foxglove plant, it is "natural,"

but the dosage must be exact or it could be dangerous. Hemlock comes from a plant, but it is a deadly poison. Some treatments may be safe in small doses but dangerous in larger doses. Be careful.

Except in Germany, no regulatory agency is responsible for determining if what is listed on the label of a nutritional supplement is actually what's in the bottle. Supplements don't have the same safeguards as medications. Do some research about the company selling the product before you try it.

Can I afford it?

Do you have the money to give this treatment the time it needs to produce an improvement? Is your health strong enough to maintain this new regimen? Will you be able to handle it emotionally? Will this put a strain on your relationships at home or at work?

Am I willing to go to the trouble or expense?

Do you have the necessary support in place?

If you ask yourself all of these questions and decide to try a new treatment on your own, it is very important to inform your health care professional about it. After all, you are partners, and you will need to keep your partner informed on your progress during the time you are taking the treatment.

The Internet can provide information about new treatments very quickly and is therefore a resource for up-to-date information about these treatments. But be cautious. Not every piece of information on the Internet is correct

or even safe. Seek out the most reliable sources by noting the author or sponsor of the site and the URL (Internet address). Addresses ending in .edu, .org, and .gov are generally more objective and reliable; they originate from universities, nonprofit organizations, and governmental agencies, respectively. Some .com sites can also be good, but because they are maintained by commercial or for-profit organizations, their information may be biased in favor of their own products. One source of useful information about questionable treatments is

Quackwatch, a nonprofit corporation whose purpose is to combat health-related frauds, myths, fads, and fallacies (http://www.quack-watch.org). Other sites are accessible from the Quackwatch site. Sometimes it is wise to say no to conventional medical treatments as well. For example, various medical speciality organizations after reviewing the medical evidence have recommended that nearly 50 common treatments and procedures should NOT be done (see www.choosingwisely.org). (For more information on finding resources on the Internet and elsewhere, see Chapter 3.)

Making decisions about new treatments can be difficult, but a good self-manager uses the questions presented in this chapter and the decision-making steps in Chapter 2 to achieve the best personal results.

Other Resources

☐ American Board of Internal Medicine Foundation's Choosing Wisely: http://www.choosingwisely.org

☐ ConsumerLab: http://www.consumerlab.com

☐ National Center for Complementary and Alternative Medicine: http://nccam.nih.gov

☐ Quackwatch: http://www.quackwatch.org

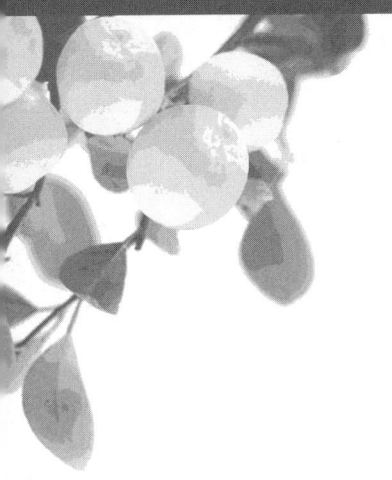

CHAPTER 15

Managing Chronic Lung Disease

SHORTNESS OF BREATH, TIGHTNESS IN THE CHEST, wheezing, persistent coughing, and thick mucus: if you have chronic lung disease, these symptoms may be all too familiar. When your lungs aren't working well, you may have trouble getting enough oxygen to your organs, and you may not be able to get rid of unhealthy waste air containing carbon dioxide. There are many types of lung disease; the most common are asthma, chronic bronchitis, and emphysema. In each of these diseases there is something getting in the way (an obstruction) of the airflow in and out of the lungs. Chronic bronchitis and emphysema are often referred to as chronic obstructive pulmonary disease (COPD). Although asthma, chronic bronchitis, and emphysema can be described separately, many people have a mixture of these diseases. Self-management and treatment of these conditions are similar and often overlap.

Special thanks to Cheryl Owen, RN, Karen Freimark, and Roberto Benzo, MD, for help with this chapter.

Understanding Asthma

Asthma is caused in two ways: by a tightening of the muscles in the walls of the airways known as *bronchospasm* and by inflammation and swelling of the airways (see Figure 15.1). The airways (bronchioles) are very sensitive, and when exposed to irritants such as smoke, pollens, dust, or cold air, the muscle contracts, and the airway narrows (see Figure 15.2). As the airway narrows, the flow of air is obstructed or blocked. This causes an "asthma attack" or flare-up characterized by shortness of breath, coughing, chest tightness, and wheezing (a high-pitched whistling sound as air pushes through narrowed airways). Treatment is aimed at relaxing the temporarily tightened airway muscles.

The irritants (sometimes called *triggers*) also cause inflammation of the airways. When this happens, the airways swell and produce mucus.

To make things worse, chemicals are released from the lining of the airways that make them even more sensitive to irritants. This sets up a vicious cycle leading to more bronchospasm and more inflammation.

An acute flare-up of asthma can be treated with medications that relax the muscles in the airways (bronchodilators), but that may not be enough. Effective treatment also includes avoiding irritants and the use of anti-inflammatory medications such as corticosteroids or cromolyn. These medications reduce the swelling, inflammation; and excessive sensitivity of the airways. To prevent attacks, you should avoid irritants, not smoke, and avoid secondhand smoke. If cold brings on symptoms, you should cover your nose with a scarf in cold weather and not exercise outside. In addition,

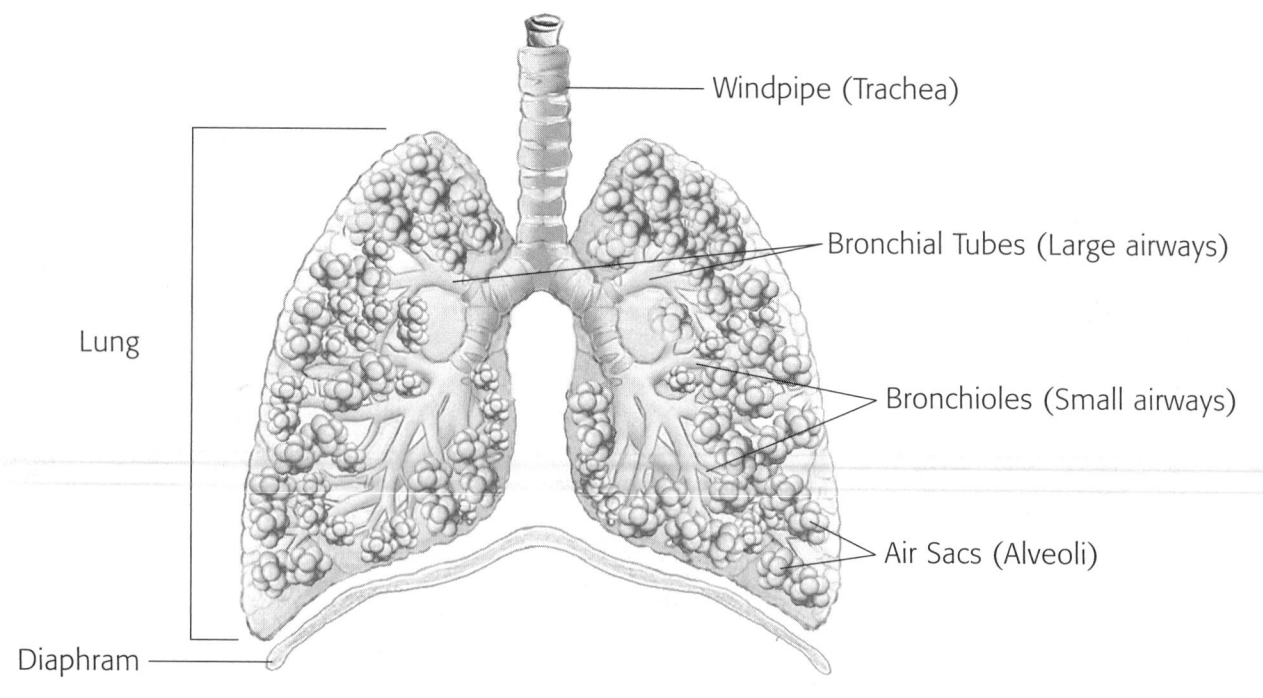

Figure 15.1 **Normal Lungs**

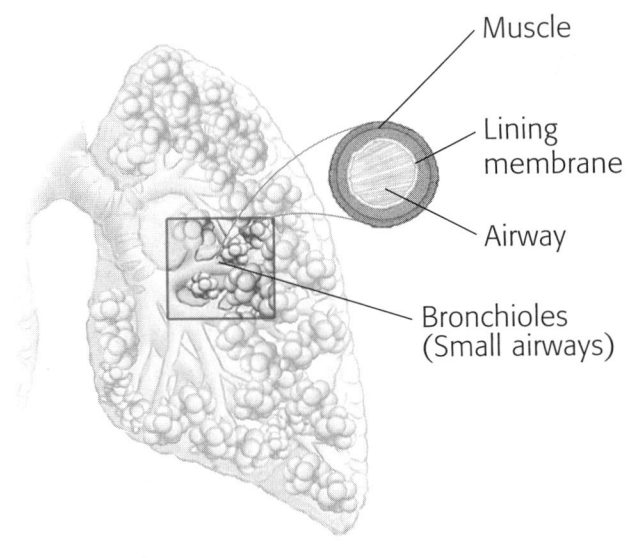

Figure 15.2 **The Bronchiole or Small Airway**

you may need to take anti-inflammatory medications *even when you have no symptoms.*

Asthma varies greatly from person to person. Symptoms may consist of mild wheezing or shortness of breath at night (asthma symptoms tend to be worse during sleep). The attacks may be mild and infrequent or severe and life-threatening. Asthma can usually be managed, but you must be an active partner. Learn your triggers and avoid them. Take action to prevent symptoms and acute attacks. Your health care provider may also teach you to monitor your lung function. Develop a plan with your doctor to recognize and treat symptoms. Learn how to breathe effectively and exercise properly. Although these measures cannot completely cure or reverse the disease, they can help you reduce symptoms and live a full, active life. By taking an active self-management role, you should be able to participate fully in work and leisure activities, sleep through the night without coughing or wheezing, and avoid urgent visits to the doctor or emergency department.

Understanding Chronic Bronchitis

In chronic bronchitis, the walls inside your airways become swollen and thick. This inflammation narrows the airways and interferes with breathing. The inflammation also causes the glands that line the airways to produce large amounts of thick mucus. The results are often a chronic cough that produces mucus (sputum) and shortness of breath.

Chronic bronchitis is primarily caused by smoking or inhaling secondhand smoke. Air pollutants, dust, and toxic fumes can also be causes. These keep the airways inflamed and swollen. The key to management is to stop smoking, stay away from smokers, and avoid other irritants. If this is done, especially early in the disease, you can often prevent it from becoming worse. If you have chronic bronchitis, you should get an influenza (flu) vaccine shot once a year and a onetime pneumococcal pneumonia vaccine as well. If you have a respiratory condition or are above age 65, you may need a second pneumonia vaccination. You should also avoid exposure to anyone with a cold or flu; these infections can make bronchitis much worse. Your doctor may also recommend the use of medications to thin and liquefy mucus as well as occasional treatment with antibiotics if symptoms get worse (increased cough with yellow-brown sputum, increased shortness of breath, fever).

Understanding Emphysema

In emphysema, the tiny air sacs (alveoli) at the very ends of the airways are damaged (see Figure 15.1). The air sacs lose their natural elasticity, become overstretched, and often break. If the air sacs are damaged, it is harder for your blood to get oxygen and to get rid of carbon dioxide. The tiniest airways also narrow, lose their elasticity, and tend to collapse when you breathe out. This traps the stale air in the air sacs and prevents fresh air from coming in.

A large amount of lung tissue can be destroyed before there are any symptoms. This is because most of us have more lung capacity than we need. However, eventually the lung capacity is lessened to the point where you begin to notice shortness of breath with activity or exercise. As the disease progresses, the shortness of breath becomes worse with less activity. It may be present even at rest. You may also have a cough that produces mucus.

Smoking and secondhand smoke are the major causes of emphysema. Cigarette smoking is the most common and most dangerous cause, but cigar and pipe smoking are also damaging. Even if you do not smoke, daily exposure to secondhand smoke is almost as bad. It is important that your home, car, and workplace be smoke-free. There is also a rare hereditary type of emphysema caused by not having enough of an enzyme that protects the elastic tissue in the lungs.

Emphysema tends to get worse over time, especially if smoking continues. The key to prevention and treatment is avoiding all smoking. Although quitting smoking sooner rather than later is better, quitting at any stage of the disease can help preserve remaining lung function. People with emphysema can learn a variety of self-management skills, from proper breathing to exercise. These will help them lead an active life. Medications and oxygen can sometimes be helpful in emphysema. We describe these later in this chapter.

Asthma, chronic bronchitis, and emphysema most often overlap, so you may have one or more of them. You may have pulmonary function tests (PFTs or spirometry tests) to evaluate your lung problem and the types of treatment that might help you. Although the treatment varies somewhat depending on the specific symptoms and disease, some of the principles and strategies of management are similar. Let's take a look at some self-management tools that are specific for chronic lung disease.

Avoiding Irritants and Triggers

The best way to manage chronic lung disease is to avoid the things that make it worse. Several irritants can trigger the symptoms of asthma and worsen the symptoms of other chronic lung disease. Fortunately, you can get rid of or avoid most of these.

Smoking

Smoking is the main cause of chronic bronchitis and emphysema and a major trigger of asthma. Whether you smoke yourself or are around people who smoke, smoking irritates and damages the lungs. The hot smoke dries, inflames, and narrows the airways. The poisonous gases paralyze the cilia, the tiny hairlike "sweepers" in your airways that help clean out dirt and mucus. The carbon monoxide in cigarette smoke robs your blood of oxygen and makes you feel tired and short of breath. The irritation from smoking makes infections more likely. This same irritation can irreversibly damage the air sacs in your lungs. Unfortunately, once air sacs are destroyed, they cannot be repaired. The good news is that most of these harmful effects can be eliminated by quitting smoking and by avoiding secondhand smoke.

If you have tried to quit and failed, do not give up. This is a common experience. Get help. Ask your health care professional or insurance plan about what can be done to help you quit smoking. This is not something you have to do on your own.

Air Pollution

Car exhaust, industrial wastes, household products, aerosol sprays, and wood smoke can irritate sensitive airways. On particularly smoggy days, check your radio and TV for air pollution alerts, and stay indoors as much as possible.

Cold Weather or Steam

For some people, very cold air can irritate the airways. If you can't avoid the cold air, try breathing through a cold-weather mask (available at most drugstores) or a scarf. For some people, steam, as from the shower, can also be a trigger.

Allergens

An allergen is anything that triggers an allergic reaction. If you have asthma, an attack may be triggered by almost anything, indoors and out. Avoiding your allergens completely can become a full-time job. Still, a few sensible measures significantly reduce exposure.

To avoid outdoor allergens, close the windows and use an air conditioner when pollen and mold spore counts are high. For some people the major allergic triggers are found indoors, in the form of house dust mites, animal dander, and molds. Often pets (dogs, cats, and birds) must be banished from the house or at least from bedrooms. Bathe dogs and cats weekly to reduce allergens. House dust mites tend to live in mattresses, pillows, carpets, upholstered furniture, and clothing. If this is a problem, vacuum your mattress and pillows and then cover them with an airtight cover. Wash bedding, including blankets and bedspread, weekly in hot water; avoid sleeping or lying on upholstered furniture; remove carpets from the bedroom; and if possible, avoid dusting and vacuuming and use a damp mop instead. Change heating and air-conditioning filters each month. Avoid air cleaners that produce ozone; these can make asthma worse. All of this takes time, but in the long run the effort will pay off.

Asthma symptoms can be triggered by perfumes, room deodorizers, fresh paint, and some cleaning products. Sometimes indoor air cleaners can be helpful in reducing allergens in the air.

Foods can be triggers for some people. The worst offenders are peanuts, beans, nuts, eggs, shellfish, and milk products. Food additives (such as sulfites in wine and dried apricots) can also sometimes trigger asthma symptoms.

If you cannot identify your triggers, allergy testing may be helpful. Immunotherapy ("allergy shots") may also help desensitize some people to certain allergens.

In addition to breathing problems, some people with respiratory conditions also have gastric reflux. This happens when acid from the stomach backs up and irritates the esophagus and airways. This may or may not cause heartburn symptoms. The irritation of the airways may cause coughing or trouble breathing. Treatment of reflux includes keeping your head and chest elevated when sleeping; avoiding smoking, caffeine, and foods that irritate the stomach; and when necessary, taking antacids and acid-blocking medications.

Medications

Some medications, including anti-inflammatory medications such as aspirin, ibuprofen (*Advil*), and naproxen (*Naprosyn, Aleve*) and beta-blockers such as propranolol (*Inderol*), can cause wheezing, shortness of breath, and coughing. ACE-inhibitor medications (lisinopril, benazepril) often used to treat hypertension and congestive heart failure and protect the kidneys in diabetes can also cause a dry, tickling chronic cough. If you suspect that you have symptoms related to a medication, do not stop your medication, but do talk to your health professional about it soon.

Infections

For individuals with lung problems, colds, flu, sinus infections, and infections of the airways and lungs can make breathing more difficult. Though you can't prevent all infections, you can reduce your risks. Be sure to get your flu and pneumonia shots. Try to avoid people with colds, wash your hands frequently, and don't rub your nose and eyes. Talk with your doctor about how to adjust your medications if you get an infection. Early treatment can often prevent serious illness and hospitalization.

Exercise

Exercise can be a problem or a benefit for people with chronic lung disease. On one hand, physical activity can improve strength and enhance the capacity of the heart and lungs. On the other hand, vigorous physical exercise can trigger asthma symptoms and cause uncomfortable shortness of breath in people with chronic lung disease. There are ways to choose exercise routines (see pages 254–256) and to adjust your medications before exercising to prevent exercise-induced asthma. If being able to exercise comfortably is a problem, discuss this with your physician.

Emotional Stress

Stress does not cause chronic lung disease. However, it can make the symptoms worse by causing the airways to tighten and breathing to become rapid and shallow. Many of the breathing and relaxation exercises in this book can help prevent the worsening of symptoms. Also, learning how to manage your disease helps you feel more in control and less stressed.

Note that triggers can add up. For example, your cat may not trigger an attack, but if you add a cold, cleaning chemicals, or stress, an attack may occur.

Monitoring Lung Disease

Lung disease changes over time. Sometimes it will be under better control than at other times. By monitoring your symptoms, you can often predict when a flare-up is coming and do something to keep from getting worse.

There are two ways to monitor lung disease. It is important to use at least one of them. For best results, use both symptom monitoring (for asthma, COPD, bronchitis, and emphysema) and peak flow monitoring (for asthma).

Symptom Monitoring (for Asthma, COPD, Bronchitis, Emphysema)

This monitoring requires that you pay attention to your symptoms and how they change. Here's how you can tell that a flare-up is coming:

- Symptoms (coughing, wheezing, shortness of breath, chest tightness, fatigue, increased or thickened sputum, or new fever) are worse, occur more often, or are greater in number than usual.

- More puffs than usual are needed of quick-relief medicine (such as an albuterol inhaler), or the medicine is required more often than twice a week (other than for physical activity).

- Symptoms cause you to wake up more frequently or are interfering with work, school, or home activities.

If you are having any of these changes in symptoms, discuss them with your doctor or other health professional.

Peak Flow Monitoring (for Asthma)

This uses a tool called a peak flow meter to measure if the breathing tubes are open enough for normal breathing. Peak flow measurements can let you know when a flare-up is starting (even before symptoms increase) and can help you figure out how bad the flare-up will be.

If you have moderate or severe asthma, the peak flow meter can become a best friend. It can alert you to problems before they become severe. It can help you and your doctor know when medications need to be increased and when they can be safely tapered. It can help you distinguish between worsening asthma and breathlessness caused by anxiety or hyperventilation. Most of all, it can help you manage your asthma better.

When the peak flow reading is closer to your personal best benchmark (to be described shortly), the breathing tubes are more open, and the asthma is under better control. When the peak flow reading is farther from your personal best, the breathing tubes are more closed. Even if you feel OK, a lower peak flow reading can warn you that a flare-up is starting and you need to take action and adjust your medications (see the Asthma Self-Management Plan on pages 242–243).

Asthma Self-Management Plan

Work out a plan with your doctor about what specific actions you should take and when. The following guide may be a place to start.

Managing Your Asthma: A Day-to-Day Self-Management Plan

GREEN ZONE: GO AHEAD

Your asthma is in good control.

No Symptoms

- You can sleep without waking.

- You have no cough, wheezing, chest tightness, or shortness of breath.

- "Quick-relief" medicines are needed no more than 2 days per week (except for exercise).

- You are able to participate in most activities without asthma symptoms.

- Work or school is not missed.

- You rarely, if ever, need emergency care.

- Your peak flow is 80%–100% of your personal best.

GO AHEAD

Take your medicine daily as prescribed, and avoid triggers.

YELLOW ZONE: BE AWARE

You are having a mild asthma attack.

Possible Symptoms

- You are experiencing some coughing.

- Wheezing is mild.

- You have slight chest congestion or tightness.

- Breathing when resting may be slightly faster than normal.

- You need to use quick-relief medications more than 2 days per week (except before exercise).

- Your peak flow is 50%–80% of your personal best.

If you do not have a peak flow meter or are not sure how to use it, ask your health professional. You will need to measure your personal best peak flow when you are feeling well and in good control so that you can then take quick action when your peak flow begins to drop. Because different meters can give different readings, use the same meter all the time.

You can keep track of your symptoms and peak flow measurements by writing them in an asthma diary. (Your medical professional can give you one, or you can make your own.) Keeping an asthma diary can help you figure out what triggers the asthma, whether the medicines are working, and when flare-ups are about to begin.

You'll need to work out an individual plan of action with your doctor (see the asthma self-management plan above). If you wait until your symptoms get worse, they will be more difficult to treat. Early action and adjustment of your medications can make a critical difference.

BE AWARE

1. Take quick-relief medicine every 4 hours as needed to relieve symptoms.

2. Increase the dose of your inhaled "controller" or "preventer" medicine until you no longer need quick-relief medicine and are back in the Green Zone. Do not take extra *Advair, Serevent,* or *Foradil.*

3. If symptoms continue more than 2 days or if quick-relief medicine is needed more than every 4 hours, see **Red Zone.** Call for advice if needed.

RED ZONE: STOP AND TAKE ACTION
You are having a severe asthma attack.

Possible Symptoms

- You are experiencing persistent coughing or wheezing.

- You have difficulty breathing when at rest.

- Coughing, wheezing, or shortness of breath wakes you up.

- Your breathing is faster than usual.

- Your symptoms are not getting better after 2 days in the Yellow Zone.

- Your peak flow is less than 50% of your personal best.

TAKE ACTION

If you need quick-relief medicine every 2 to 4 hours and you still have Red Zone symptoms, take the following steps:

1. Take quick-relief medications immediately. If symptoms do not improve after 20 minutes, take the medications again. If symptoms do not improve after another 20 minutes, take the medications for a third time and **contact your doctor.**

2. Start "burst" medicine, if prescribed. Keep in mind that it may take 4 to 6 hours for burst medicine to work.

3. *If you have taken steps 1 and 2 and there is no relief, you are having a severe asthma attack. Go to the nearest emergency department or call 911 now, and continue to take quick-relief medicine as needed.*

Medications

Medications cannot cure chronic lung diseases, but they can help you breathe easier. Effective management often involves more than one medication. Do not worry if you are prescribed several medications. A wide range of current medications are described in Table 15.1.*

Bronchodilators relax the muscles surrounding the airways, open the airways, and relieve wheezing and shortness of breath. Most inhaled bronchodilators can be used frequently and work within minutes. The exception is *Serevent* (salmeterol), which should be used no more often than every 12 hours.

---

*Because research on medications is changing rapidly, we recommend that you consult your physician, pharmacist, or a recent drug reference book for the latest information.

Table 15.1 **Medications Useful for Managing Chronic Lung Disease**

Medication	How It Can Help You	Comments
Bronchodilator Medications		
Beta-2 agonists *Examples:* Fast-acting beta agonists: albuterol (*Proventil, Ventolin*), pirbuterol (*Maxair*), metaproterenol (*Alupent, Metaprel*), terbutaline (*Brethine, Bricanyl*) **Long-acting beta agonists:** Salmeterol (*Serevent*), formoterol (*Foradil*) **Combinations:** *Advair* (long-acting beta agonist + inhaled corticosteroid), *Combivent* (ipratropium bromide + albuterol)	Relax and open airways Help prevent exercise-induced wheezing (These medications do not treat the underlying inflammation. For this you need an additional anti-inflammatory medication.)	These medications are usually inhaled, but some can also be taken by mouth either as pills or liquids. These medications are usually used as needed to treat suddenly worsening symptoms. Always carry these with you so you will have them at the first sign of increasing symptoms. If you tend to wheeze during exercise, bronchodilators can also be used 5 to 15 minutes before exercising. *Serevent* (salmeterol) and *Foradil* (formoterol) should not be used more frequently than every 12 hours and should always be taken in combination with an inhaled corticosteroid.
Anticholinergic medications *Examples:* ipratropium bromide (*Atrovent*), tiotropium (*Spiriva*)	Relax and open airways Inhibit mucus secretion	These medications are more commonly used to treat emphysema and chronic bronchitis than to treat asthma. They take longer than the beta agonists to open the airways, and to be effective, they need to be used regularly.
Methylxanthines and theophylline *Example:* aminophylline (*Slophyllin, Somophyllin, Slo-Bid, TheoDur, Resbid, Theolair-SR,* etc.)	Relax and open airways Long-acting; may help control nighttime wheezing	Theophylline is prescribed less frequently today for asthma because of the more widespread use of the beta-adrenergic bronchodilators and corticosteroid medications. Blood tests are used to measure the levels of theophylline. If it is too low, it may not be effective. If it is too high, it may be toxic.

Table 15.1 **Medications Useful for Managing Chronic Lung Disease (*continued*)**

Medication	How It Can Help You	Comments
Anti-Inflammatory Medications (Symptom Preventers or Controllers)		
Inhaled corticosteroids *Examples:* beclomethasone (*QVAR, Vanceril*), triamcinolone (*Azmacort*), flunisolide (*AeroBid*), fluticasone propionate (*Flovent*)	Gradually reduce inflammation, swelling, and spasm of the airways Reduce mucus production Decrease sensitivity of airways to irritants and allergens (These medications are *not* rapid-acting and are therefore not helpful for the immediate treatment of a severe asthma attack.)	You may need to take the inhaled steroid medication for 1 to 4 weeks to see its full benefit. Irritation and infection of the mouth can be greatly reduced by using a spacer (see page 248). Rinse excess medication out of your mouth after inhaling. If you are taking an inhaled bronchodilator as well as an inhaled steroid, use the bronchodilator first and wait 5 minutes before using the inhaled steroid. This increases the amount of steroid medication reaching the smaller airways.
Cromolyn sodium *Example: Intal*	Prevents asthma attacks by inhibiting the release of chemicals that cause airway inflammation, allergic reactions, and narrowing of the airways Helps prevent exercise-induced wheezing Should be used regularly, not just when symptoms worsen; this keeps inflammation down and prevents attacks Can also be used to prevent symptoms that occur from exercise or allergens (such as pets or pollens) if used 5 to 60 minutes before contact	This medication needs to be used regularly to reduce inflammation and may take 4 to 6 weeks for full benefit. If you are taking an inhaled bronchodilator as well as inhaled cromolyn, use the bronchodilator first and wait 5 minutes before using the cromolyn. This increases the amount of cromolyn reaching the smaller airways.

Continues on next page ▶

Table 15.1 **Medications Useful for Managing Chronic Lung Disease (*continued*)**

Medication	How It Can Help You	Comments
Anti-Inflammatory Medications (Symptom Preventers or Controllers)		
Systemic corticosteroids ("burst" medicines) *Examples:* prednisone, dexamethasone (*Decadron*), methylprednisolone (*Medrol*), triamcinolone (*Aristocort*)	Reduce inflammation, swelling, and spasm of the airways Reduce mucus production Decrease sensitivity of airways to irritants and allergens	These are often prescribed as "burst" medicines to be used during a severe asthma attack. If you are taking oral steroid medications, *do not suddenly stop taking them.* They need to be tapered over days or weeks on a schedule worked out with your doctor. Most of the serious side effects occur with long-term use of the medication. Stomach upset can be reduced by taking the oral steroid medication along with food. Although these medications are called "steroids," they are *completely different* from the anabolic steroids used illegally by some athletes, which can have devastating effects.
Leukotriene inhibitors *Examples:* montelukast (*Singulair*), zarfirlukast (*Accolate*)	Control allergen-induced asthma Improve nighttime symptoms Reduce the number of acute asthma attacks	These medications are used daily to prevent asthma. They should not be used to relieve an acute asthma attack.
Expectorants and mucolytics *Examples:* water, guaifenesin, potassium iodide, acetylcysteine, iodinated glycerol (*Organidin*)	May help make mucus thinner and easier to cough up	Be sure to drink 6 to 8 glasses of water a day to liquefy and thin mucus unless advised by your physician to limit how much you drink.

Anti-inflammatory medications may also be prescribed to reduce the inflammation, swelling, and reactivity of the airways. Medications to loosen mucus (mucolytics and expectorants) as well as antibiotics may be helpful if you have chronic bronchitis or emphysema.

Some of the medications may be used to relieve symptoms such as wheezing, while others may be used to prevent symptoms. Some medications may be used to both treat and prevent. When the medications are being used to prevent symptoms, they must be taken regularly, *even when symptoms are not present.* Too often people stop their medications because they feel better. Discuss with your doctor which medications to continue and which may be stopped as symptoms improve.

Some people worry that they will become addicted to the medications or that they may become "immune" and no longer respond to the medication. None of the medications used to treat lung disease are addictive. Nor do patients become "immune" to the medications. If your medications are not working well to control your symptoms, discuss this with your doctor so that adjustments can be made.

Metered-Dose Inhalers

Some lung medications, including bronchodilators, corticosteroids, and cromolyn, can be taken by inhalation. They come in a special canister called a metered-dose inhaler (MDI). When used properly, inhalers are a highly effective way of quickly delivering medication to your lungs. By breathing medicine directly into the lungs instead of swallowing it in pill form, you take less medication into the bloodstream, causing fewer side effects. Inhaling medication also allows more to reach the lungs. The key to using a metered-dose inhaler is to first exhale gently to empty your lungs and then inhale slowly through your mouth at the same time as you press down on the MDI canister to release the medication. Hold your breath for 10 seconds and then wait a minute before taking any additional puffs to let the previous puff work.

Learning to use an inhaler properly is more difficult than swallowing a pill. It takes proper instruction and some practice. One study revealed that whereas 98% of patients said they knew how to use their inhalers properly, fully 94% made errors in using them. So even if you think you are an expert, it is a good idea to have a health professional check out your technique every so often. Pharmacists can often help you learn the most effective and safe technique. If you

> ### Common Errors to Avoid When Using an Inhaler
>
> Forgetting to shake the canister
>
> Holding the inhaler upside down (mouthpiece should be on the bottom)
>
> Forgetting to exhale before inhaling with the inhaler
>
> Breathing through your nose
>
> Inhaling too fast
>
> Not holding your breath for 10 seconds
>
> Using an empty inhaler (see page 248)

have never been taught how to use an inhaler, ask your health professional for instructions. *Improper use of inhalers is one of the most important reasons for difficulty in controlling symptoms.* So if you are prescribed an inhaler, be sure to get help in using it properly. You can also watch videos on using an inhaler at http://www.kp.org/asthma or search for videos on the Internet.

Using the medications

Use the quick-acting symptom-relieving (bronchodilator) medication *first*. Wait several minutes for it to open up the breathing tubes so that the preventive controller (inhaled anti-inflammatory) medication can get into your lungs better.

Spacers or holding chambers

To make using an inhaler easier, safer, and more effective, many doctors strongly recommend using a spacer device or holding chamber. This is a chamber (usually a specially designed tube or bag) into which you spray the medication from the inhaler. You then inhale the medication from the spacer. The spacer makes it more likely that you can inhale the smaller, lighter droplets of medication farther into your airways. The spacer also collects on its walls some of the larger, heavier droplets of medication that would otherwise settle in your mouth or throat. This can reduce side effects such as yeast infections in the case of inhaled steroids. Some spacer devices have a whistle that sounds if you are inhaling too rapidly. This also reminds you not to take a fast breath. A fast breath deposits more of the medication in your mouth and less in your lungs.

Inhalers with spacers are easier to use than metered-dose inhalers without spacers. You don't have to worry about pointing the spray in the right direction, and your inhalation doesn't have to be as carefully timed and coordinated with the spray. Because more of the medication reaches your lungs and less is left in your mouth with a spacer, the medication tends to be safer and more effective. This is especially important if you are using a steroid inhaler.

If you are using a corticosteroid inhaler, rinse your mouth out with water after use. Do not swallow the water. Swallowing the water will increase the chance that the medication will get into your bloodstream. This may increase the side effects of the medication. Some powder may build up on the inhaler, but it is not necessary to clean the inhaler every day. Occasionally rinse the spacer or mouthpiece, cap, and case.

How to determine how many puffs are left in the metered-dose inhaler

An inhaler may still seem to release puffs of medicine even when there is no medicine left. The best way to tell how many puffs of medicine are left is to keep track of how many puffs

have been used already. There are two ways you can do this:

- Read the label on a new canister to find out how many puffs it contains. Write down one number for each puff on a sheet of paper. For example, if your canister has 100 puffs in it, you would write each number from 1 to 100 on a sheet of paper. Each time you take a puff of the medicine, cross off a number. When all the numbers are crossed off, the canister doesn't have any more medicine in it.

- Divide the number of puffs of medicine in the inhaler by the number of puffs you use each day. This gives you the number of days the medicine will last and lets you know when you will need to start using a new canister. For example, if the inhaler has 100 puffs and you take 2 puffs a day, the inhaler will last 50 days (100 puffs divided by 2 puffs a day = 50 days). Count off the days on a calendar, and mark the day when the inhaler will be empty. Ask your medical professional for a refill before you run out of medicine.

Note: If you cannot find the number of puffs on the label of the inhaler, ask your medical professional or your pharmacist.

Caution: In the past some people tried to float their MDI canister in water to figure out how many puffs were left. *This method does not work.* We recommend that you use one of the two methods we've just described.

Dry Powder Inhalers

Dry powder inhalers (DPIs) deliver the medicine as a powder. They are used without a spacer. When using a dry powder inhaler, you need to exhale first and then inhale *rapidly and deeply*. Note that unlike the *slow* inhalation described for metered-dose inhalers, with dry powder inhalers the inhalation needs to be *rapid*.

Nebulizers

Nebulizers are machines that deliver quick-relief medicine as a fine mist. They are often used in the clinic or the emergency room to give a 5- to 10-minute "breathing treatment" or at home for people who cannot use an inhaler with a spacer. Nebulizers are bulky and are less convenient than inhalers. Taking four to six puffs of quick-relief medicine from an inhaler with a spacer, when done correctly, works just as well as a breathing treatment with a nebulizer.

Oxygen Therapy

Some people with chronic lung disease cannot get enough oxygen from ordinary air because the lungs are damaged. If you are tired and short of breath because there is too little oxygen in your blood, your doctor may order oxygen.

Oxygen is a medicine. It is not addictive. Yet some people try not to use it for fear of becoming dependent on it. Other people do not like to be seen with oxygen equipment. Supplemental oxygen can provide the extra boost your body needs to remain comfortable and enable you do the things you want and need to do without extreme shortness of breath. Most important, it may slow down your disease and make your brain function better. Some people may require continuous use of oxygen, while others may need oxygen only to help them with certain activities such as exercise or sleep.

Oxygen comes in large tanks of compressed gas or small portable tanks of oxygen either as a gas or a liquid. If you are using oxygen, be sure to know the proper dose (flow rates and when to use it and for how long), how to use the equipment, and how to know when to order more. Do not worry. Your oxygen tank will not explode or burn. However, oxygen can help other things burn, so keep the tank at least 10 feet away from any open flame, including cigarettes.

How to Breathe Better

In addition to medications, there are other things you can do to improve your breathing.

Breathing Exercise

We breathe in and out nearly 18,000 times a day. It is not surprising that breathing is a central concern of people with lung disease. Yet many people find it surprising that proper breathing is a skill that has to be learned. This is especially important for people with lung disease. You can learn some ways to breathe that will enhance the functioning of your respiratory system.

Diaphragmatic or *abdominal breathing* helps strengthen respiratory muscles (especially the diaphragm) and helps rid the lungs of stale, trapped air. One of the primary reasons why people with lung disease feel short of breath and can't seem to get enough air in is that they don't get the old air out. These breathing exercises can help you empty your lungs more completely and take advantage of your full lung capacity.

(See pages 44–45 for instructions on how to do the breathing exercises.)

Posture

If you are slouched over, it may be very difficult to breathe in and out. Certain body postures make it easier to fill and empty your lungs. For example, if you are sitting, try leaning forward from the hips with a straight back. You can then rest your forearms on your thighs or rest your head, shoulders, and arms on a pillow placed on a table. Or use several pillows at night to make breathing easier. See page 47.

Clearing Your Lungs

Sometimes excess mucus blocks the airways, making it difficult to breathe. Your doctor or respiratory therapist may recommend certain positions for "postural drainage." For example, by lying on your left side on a slant with your feet higher than your head, you may be able to help the mucus from certain areas of the lung drain more effectively. Ask your doctor, nurse, or respiratory therapist which, if any, postures would be helpful for you. Also remember that drinking at least six glasses of water a day (unless you have ankle swelling or are told to limit fluid intake by your doctor) may help liquefy and loosen the mucus. See page 44.

Controlled Coughing

A deep cough, one that produces a strong jet of air, is a good way of clearing mucus from the airways. By contrast, a weak, hacking, tickle-in-the-throat type of cough can be exhausting, irritating, and frustrating. You can learn to cough from deep in your lungs and put air power into a cough to clear the mucus. Start by sitting in a chair or on the edge of the bed with your feet planted on the floor. Grasp a pillow firmly against your abdomen with your forearms. Take in several slow, deep belly breaths through your nose, and as you exhale fully with pursed lips, bend forward slightly and press the pillow into your stomach. On the fourth or fifth breath, slowly bend forward while producing two or three strong coughs without taking any quick breaths between coughs. Repeat the whole sequence several times to clear the mucus. See page 46.

Exercising with Chronic Lung Conditions

Exercise is among the simplest and best ways to improve your ability to live a full life with chronic lung disease. Physical activity strengthens the muscles, improves mood, increases energy level, and enhances the efficiency of the heart and lungs. Although exercise does not reverse the damage to the lungs, it can improve your ability to function within whatever limits you have due to your lung disease.

One of the most important things to remember when you start to exercise is to begin at a low intensity (for example, a slow rather than a brisk walk) and for short periods of time. You can gradually increase what you do as you find that you can do more with less shortness of breath. Good communication with your health care providers to manage your symptoms and adjust medications will let you get the most benefit and enjoyment from an exercise program.

Here are a few tips for exercising with a chronic lung condition:

- Use your medicine, particularly your inhaler, before you exercise. It will help you

Exercising with Asthma

Some people with asthma may cough or wheeze when they exercise. If you do, you may wish to discuss with your doctor using two puffs of albuterol (*Ventolin, Proventil*) or cromolyn (*Intal*) 15 to 30 minutes before starting exercise. Wearing a scarf or a mask over your face in cold weather may help prevent the cold air from triggering asthma. Swimming usually does not trigger asthma.

exercise longer and with less shortness of breath.

- If you become severely short of breath with only a little effort, your doctor may want to change your medicines or even have you use supplemental oxygen before you begin your conditioning activities. Mild shortness of breath is normal during exercise, but it may take you some time to find the right combination of exertion and time to stay in your comfort zone.

- Take plenty of time to warm up and cool down during conditioning activities. This should include exercises such as pursed-lip breathing and diaphragmatic or abdominal breathing (see page 45).

- Everyone experiences a normal "anticipatory" increase in heart rate and breathing rate even before exercise begins. This can be worrisome if you are afraid of getting too short of breath. Pursed-lip and diaphragmatic breathing will help you relax and stay calm.

- Pay attention to your breathing to make sure you breathe in deeply and slowly and use pursed-lip breathing when you breathe out (see pages 44–45). Learn to take two or three times longer breathing out as you do breathing in. For example, if you are walking briskly and notice that you can take two steps while you're breathing in, you should breathe out through pursed lips over four to six steps. Breathing out slowly will help you exchange air in your lungs better and will probably increase your endurance.

- Remember that arm exercises may cause shortness of breath and a faster heart rate sooner than leg exercises.

- Cold and dry air can make breathing and exercise more difficult. This is why swimming is an especially good activity for people with chronic lung disease.

- Strengthening exercises such as calisthenics, light weightlifting, and rowing may be helpful, particularly for people who have become weakened or deconditioned it is helpful whether due to medications or other causes

Exercising with Severe Lung Disease

If you can get out of bed, you can exercise 10 minutes a day. Here is how you do it. Every hour, get up and walk slowly across the room or around your chair for 1 minute. Doing this 10 times a day gives you 10 minutes of exercise. Then you can increase gradually to a daily exercise routine

Sleep Apnea

If you snore and you tend to feel sleepy during the day, you may have a special type of breathing problem called sleep apnea. If you have sleep apnea, your throat becomes blocked during sleep. Then for short periods of time (10 seconds or more), you may stop breathing (this is called apnea). If you have sleep apnea, you probably don't know it until someone says something to you about your snoring. This condition is one of the most common undiagnosed serious health problems today.

Sleep apnea may cause you to wake up feeling tired or with a headache or to feel sleepy or have trouble with concentration throughout the day. Sleep apnea can also lead to more serious problems such as high blood pressure, heart disease, and stroke.

It can even mimic the memory problems seen in dementia and Alzheimer's disease. Sleep apnea is diagnosed by doing a sleep study in a laboratory or wearing a small monitor at home.

You can treat sleep apnea at home by making lifestyle changes. These include losing weight, if appropriate; sleeping on your side; avoiding alcohol; not smoking; and using medication to relieve nasal congestion and allergies. You also can use a breathing device that uses gentle air pressure to keep tissues in the throat from blocking your airway. This is known as continuous positive air pressure (CPAP). Or your doctor may recommend using a dental device (oral breathing device) to help keep your airway open.

that will help you feel stronger and more comfortable moving. Here are some things to remember as you start to get more active:

- Don't hurry. Many people with lung disease hurry up to get there before their breath runs out. It is much better to slow down. Move slowly, breathing as you go. At first, this will take a real effort. With practice, you will find that you can go farther more comfortably. If you are afraid to try this alone, have someone walk with you, carrying a chair (a folding "cane chair" might be useful), or use a walker with a seat so that you can sit down if necessary.

- As you begin to feel stronger and more confident, walk 2 minutes every hour. You have

just doubled your exercise and are now up to 20 minutes a day. When this feels comfortable, change your pattern to walking 3 to 4 minutes every other hour. Wait another week or two, and then try 5 minutes three or four times a day. Next, try 6 to 7 minutes two or three times a day. You now have the basic idea. Most people with severe lung disease can build up to walking 10 to 20 minutes, once or twice a day, within a couple of months.

- If being up on your feet is a problem, try using a restorator (portable bicycle crank and pedals). This is especially helpful if you have a low level of endurance, do not have standby help, or are afraid of exertion. The restorator lets you sit where you are and use your legs to pedal. It's a good device to build confidence and get accustomed to exertion in a secure atmosphere.

Asthma, chronic bronchitis, and emphysema are not curable. But you can, in partnership with your health care team, work to reduce the symptoms and improve your ability to live a rich, rewarding life. The goal is to control your symptoms so that you can do daily activities, exercise, sleep comfortably, and prevent having to go to the hospital or emergency department.

Suggested Further Reading

Haas, François, and Sheila Spencer Haas. *The Chronic Bronchitis and Emphysema Handbook.* New York: Wiley, 2000.

Marcus, Bess, Jeffrey S. Hampl, and Edwin B. Fisher. *How to Quit Smoking Without Gaining Weight.* New York: Pocket Books, 2004.

Plaut, Thomas F., and Teresa B. Jones. *Asthma Guide for People of All Ages.* Amherst, Mass.: Pedipress, 1999.

Shimberg, Elaine Fantle. *Coping with COPD: Understanding, Treating, and Living with Chronic Obstructive Pulmonary Disease.* New York: St. Martin's Griffin, 2003.

Snowdrift Pulmonary Foundation. *Frontline Advice for COPD Patients.* Denver: Snowdrift Pulmonary Foundation, 2002; free download at http://www.copd-alert .com/Frontlin.pdf

Other Resources

☐ American Lung Association, (800) 586-4872: http://www.lung.org

☐ Asthma and Allergy Foundation of America, (800) 7-ASTHMA or (202) 466-7643, http://www.aafa.org

☐ COPD Foundation, (866) 316-COPD: http://www.copdfoundation.org

☐ Kaiser Permanente: http://www.kp.org/asthma

☐ National Asthma Education and Prevention Program: (301) 951-3260: http://www.nhlbi.nih.gov/about/naepp/

☐ National Heart, Lung, and Blood Institute, (301) 592-8573: http://www.nhlbi.nih.gov

☐ National Jewish Health: (800) 222-5864 (Lungline): http://www.nationaljewish.org

☐ Pulmonary Paper: (800) 950-3698: http://www.pulmonarypaper.org

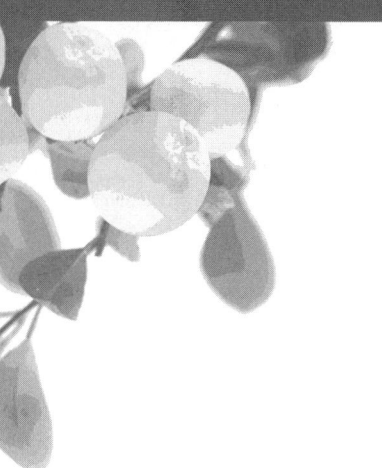

CHAPTER 16

Managing Heart Disease, High Blood Pressure, and Stroke

WE NOW KNOW A LOT ABOUT the treatment of heart disease, high blood pressure, and stroke and have many ways to prevent and treat these life-threatening diseases. We can save lives and keep people out of hospitals. People with heart disease and even those who have had strokes can look forward to long, healthy, and enjoyable lives.

There are many forms of heart disease. The arteries that supply the heart muscle can be blocked, as in atherosclerosis. When a person has heart failure, the heart muscle is damaged and unable to push blood effectively to the lungs and the rest of the body. If the valves inside the heart are damaged, the result is valvular heart disease. Again, blood may not reach the rest of the body. The electrical system that controls the beating of the heart can also be disrupted. This causes the heart to beat too fast, too slow, or irregularly (this is called arrhythmia). We will talk about all of these as well as other problems with the circulatory system, including strokes and high blood pressure.

Coronary Artery Disease

Coronary artery disease, the most common form of heart disease, causes most heart attacks and heart failure. Coronary arteries are blood vessel "pipelines" that wrap around the heart. The coronary arteries deliver the oxygen and nutrients the heart needs to perform its job. Healthy arteries are elastic, flexible, and strong. The inside lining of a healthy artery is smooth, so blood flows easily. Arteries narrow as they become clogged with cholesterol and other substances. This is called atherosclerosis, also known as coronary artery disease (CAD). The blocked or narrowed area is called a stenosis.

Atherosclerosis is a gradual process that occurs over many years. The first step is damage to the wall of the artery. This damage can be caused by high cholesterol, high triglycerides, diabetes, smoking, or high blood pressure. This damage allows the low-density lipoprotein cholesterol (LDL cholesterol, the "bad" cholesterol) to enter the artery wall and cause inflammation. Some people have this damage as early as their teens.

Over time, more cholesterol is deposited and the fatty areas grow larger and larger. These fatty areas are called plaques. They can completely block off blood flow in an artery. Plaques can also crack open, causing a blood clot to form at the injured site. In both cases, blood flow to the heart is blocked, and the person may experience angina (temporary chest pain) or a heart attack. A heart attack is also known as a myocardial infarction (MI) and, if not treated immediately, can cause permanent damage to the heart muscle. When a part of the heart muscle has been damaged, that part can no longer help the heart pump blood.

The pain of angina or a heart attack may be on the left side of the chest over the heart but may also radiate to the shoulders, arms, neck, and jaw. Some people with angina or a heart

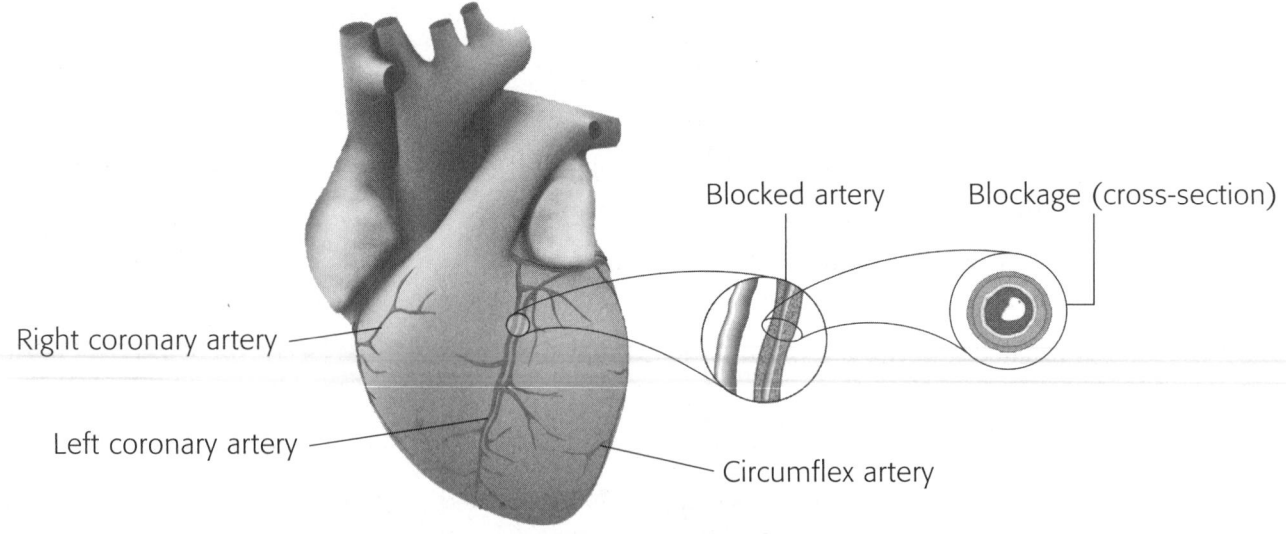

Figure 16.1 **The Arteries of the Heart**

attack may also experience nausea, sweating, shortness of breath, and fatigue.

Symptoms of heart disease in women may be different from those just described, which are typical for men. Women may be unusually tired and experience sleep disturbances, shortness of breath, nausea, cold sweats, dizziness, and anxiety. These symptoms are more subtle than the crushing chest pain often associated with heart attacks. This may be because women tend to have blockages not only in their main arteries but also in the smaller arteries that supply blood to the heart—a condition called small vessel heart disease. Many women show up in emergency rooms after heart damage has already occurred. This is because their symptoms are not the ones that most people think of as symptoms of a heart attack. (See "Seek Emergency Care Immediately" on page 259.)

Arrhythmias

People with heart disease may notice irregular heartbeats (palpitations). This is caused by irregularities in the conduction system or electrical wiring of the heart. Damage to this system can result in irregular heartbeats, skipped beats, or racing beats. Physicians refer to these as arrhythmias or dysrhythmias.

Most irregular heartbeats are minor and not dangerous. However, some types of arrhythmias can cause problems. Dangerous arrhythmias are sometimes accompanied by episodes of fainting, dizziness, shortness of breath, or irregular heartbeats lasting minutes. Such arrhythmias may be more dangerous for people with severely weakened hearts and those with heart failure.

Sometimes the heart can beat irregularly and you may not notice the difference. If you notice irregular heartbeats, take note of how frequently they occur, how long they last, how fast your heart is beating (check your pulse), and how you feel during the episode. This information will help your doctor decide whether or not your arrhythmias are dangerous. Remember that infrequent, short bouts of irregular beats are common for people both with and without heart disease. They are generally not cause for concern and should not require any change in activity or treatment.

Peripheral Vascular Disease

Peripheral vascular disease (PVD), also called peripheral arterial disease (PAD) or peripheral artery occlusive disease (PAOD), occurs when the arteries in the legs harden, form plaque deposits, and narrow (atherosclerosis). Atherosclerosis in the legs is usually the result of the same disease process that happens with atherosclerosis in heart disease.

The main symptom of PVD is leg pain when walking (claudication). Some people may experience leg sores that don't heal or heal slowly. Some of the treatments and medication are similar to those for heart disease: stopping smoking (most important), exercise, medications, and sometimes surgery to help restore blood flow to the legs.

Heart Failure

"Heart failure" does not mean that your heart has stopped working or is going to stop. It means that your heart's pumping ability is weaker than normal; your heart still beats, but with less force. This condition is sometimes called congestive heart failure because fluid tends to collect in the lungs and legs.

Heart failure can be treated and its symptoms managed, even when the heart cannot be returned to normal. What are the signs and symptoms of heart failure?

- **Excessive tiredness, fatigue, and weakness.** When your heart is not pumping with enough force, your muscles do not get enough oxygen. You may be more tired than usual and not have enough energy for normal activities.

- **Shortness of breath.** Sometimes breathing becomes more difficult due to excess fluid in your lungs. You may have trouble catching your breath, a frequent or hacking cough, difficulty breathing when lying flat, or wake up at night due to difficulty breathing. If you need to prop yourself up with many pillows or sleep in a recliner, this may be a sign of heart failure.

- **Weight gain and swelling.** These are common signs of heart failure. The weight gain is due to fluid retention. When your body is holding on to extra fluid, your weight will go up. Sometimes weight gain happens rapidly (in days), and sometimes it happens more slowly. You may have swelling (edema) in your feet and ankles, your shoes and socks may be too tight, rings on your fingers may become too tight, your stomach may feel bloated, and there may be a tightness at your waistline.

- **Changes in how often you urinate.** When you urinate (pass water), your kidneys are helping your body get rid of extra fluid. At night more blood is pumped to your kidneys because your brain and muscles are resting and need less blood. This allows your kidneys to "catch up." You may have more frequent urination at night or at all times.

Although heart failure is a serious condition, keeping daily track of your weight and eating a low-sodium diet can relieve symptoms and prevent unnecessary trips to the hospital.

Track Your Weight

It is important that you weigh yourself properly and frequently if you are to catch trends that may be indicative of health problems. Here's how to do it:

Seek Emergency Care Immediately

If you are having symptoms that might mean a heart attack or stroke, *you must seek medical care immediately.* New treatments are available that can dissolve blood clots in the blood vessels of the heart and brain. These restore blood flow and prevent heart or brain damage. However, these treatments *must be given within hours of the heart attack or stroke*—the sooner, the better. In the United States, call 911 or emergency services if you have any of the following symptoms: *Do not wait!*

Heart Attack Warning Signs

- Severe, crushing, or squeezing chest pain

- Pain or discomfort in one or both arms, the back, neck, jaw, or stomach

- Chest pain lasting longer than 5 minutes when there is no apparent cause and is not relieved by rest or heart medications (nitroglycerin)

- Chest pain occurring with any of the following: rapid or irregular heartbeat, sweating, nausea or vomiting, shortness of breath, light-headedness or passing out, or unusual weakness. For women, chest pain may not be present with these symptoms.

If you think you are having a heart attack:

1. Stop what you are doing

2. Sit down.

3. Call 911. (Do not try to drive yourself.)

4. If you are not allergic to aspirin, take one adult (325 mg) or four baby (81 mg) aspirin tablets.

Stroke Warning Signs

- Sudden numbness or weakness of the face, arm, or leg, especially on one side of the body

- Sudden confusion, trouble speaking, or trouble understanding

- Sudden trouble seeing in one or both eyes that does not clear with blinking

- Sudden trouble walking, dizziness, loss of balance or coordination

- Sudden severe headache with no known cause

Minutes matter! Fast action can save lives—maybe your own. Don't wait more than 5 minutes to call 911 (in the United States) or your local emergency response number.

- Weigh yourself at about the same time every day. We suggest weighing every morning, just after waking up (after urinating and before eating).

- Weigh yourself with the same amount of clothing on or without clothing.

- Use the same scale. Check to be sure the scale is set to zero before weighing yourself. Make sure the scale is on a hard surface.

- Write your weight on a daily weight log or other record (a calendar works well).

- Repeat weighing if you have doubts about the scale or your weight.

- Bring your daily weight log to all your medical appointments.

- Call your health care professional if you have a weight gain of 2 to 3 pounds (or more) in a day, a gain of 5 pounds (or more) in 5 days, shortness of breath, or increased swelling of feet or ankles.

Eat Healthy, Low-Sodium Foods

Sodium is an important mineral that helps regulate fluid levels in your body. Too much sodium makes your body hold on to too much fluid. People with heart failure need to eat less sodium to avoid retaining excess fluid that can back up in their lungs and cause shortness of breath. To learn more about healthy eating and how to keep you sodium low, see page 182.

Stroke

Strokes happen when a blood vessel in the brain is blocked or bursts. Without blood and the oxygen it carries, part of the brain starts to die. The part of the body controlled by the damaged area of the brain can't work properly.

There are two types of stroke:

- An **ischemic stroke** (the most common stroke) happens when a blood clot blocks a blood vessel in the brain. The clot may form in the blood vessel or travel from somewhere else in the blood system, such as the heart valves or arteries in the neck.

- A **hemorrhagic stroke** happens when an artery in the brain leaks or bursts. This causes bleeding inside the brain.

The symptoms of a stroke depend on the area of the brain that is damaged. You may experience any of the following:

- Sudden numbness, tingling, weakness, or paralysis in your face, arm, or leg, especially on only one side of your body

- Sudden vision changes (like a curtain coming down)

- Sudden trouble speaking

- Sudden confusion or trouble understanding simple statements

- Sudden problems with walking or balance

Brain damage from a stroke can begin within minutes. It is important to know the symptoms of stroke and act fast (see "Seek Emergency Care Immediately" on page 259). Quick treatment (within 90 minutes) can help limit damage to the brain and increase the chance of a full recovery. If you are with someone who has these symptoms, call 911 even if the person says no. You may prevent brain damage and save a life.

Sometimes the symptoms of a stroke develop and then go away within minutes. This is called a transient ischemic attack (TIA) or ministroke. Do not ignore these symptoms. They may be a warning sign that a stroke may soon happen. See your doctor if you have symptoms that seem like a stroke, even if they go away quickly. Getting early treatment for a TIA can help prevent a stroke.

If you have had a stroke, you may notice improvements for several months. Stroke rehabilitation ("rehab") programs can be especially helpful in recovery as well as in preventing future strokes. They are most helpful if started as soon after a stroke as your doctor says is safe. This is usually days, not weeks, later.

Not smoking; getting regular exercise; keeping your blood pressure, cholesterol, and diabetes under control; and taking certain medications can also improve recovery and help prevent future strokes.

High Blood Pressure

High blood pressure (hypertension) increases the risk of heart disease, stroke, and kidney and eye damage. Blood pressure is a measurement of the amount of pressure in an artery, expressed as two numbers. The *systolic* pressure (the higher first number) is the pressure in the artery when the heart contracts and pushes out a wave of blood. The *diastolic* pressure (the lower second number) is the pressure when the heart relaxes between contractions.

The two pressures are recorded in millimeters of mercury (mm Hg). So a blood pressure of 120/80 ("120 over 80") means that the systolic pressure is 120 mmHg and the diastolic pressure is 80 mm Hg. Both numbers are important because a high reading for either type of pressure can cause damage.

High blood pressure is often called the silent disease because most people who have it have no symptoms and cannot really tell if their blood pressure is high. The only way to find out is to measure it. But because people whose blood pressure is high feel perfectly well, they find it hard to believe that anything is wrong and so may not want treatment. However, the silent disease may not stay silent. Over years, untreated high blood pressure can damage blood vessels throughout the body. In some people this damage to blood vessels can cause

strokes, heart attacks, heart failure, or damage to the eyes or kidneys. The reason for treating high blood pressure is to prevent these serious complications. That's why it is extremely important to control your blood pressure even if you feel perfectly well.

Why do you have hypertension? Over 90% of hypertension is called "primary" or "essential," which really means that the cause is not known.

What is normal blood pressure? A healthy blood pressure is below 120 systolic and 80 diastolic (120/80). "Prehypertension" is below 140/90. Hypertension is considered 140/90 or higher. For most people, lower blood pressure usually means less risk of complications. And for some people—for example, those with diabetes or chronic kidney disease—it may be important to keep their blood pressure in a lower range.

Your blood pressure varies, however, from minute to minute. Hypertension is diagnosed when blood pressure measurements are high at two or more separate times. Except in severe cases, the diagnosis is never based on a single measurement. That's one reason it is important to have repeated measurements of your blood pressure.

Some people's blood pressure tends to go up only in the doctor's office. This is a stress reaction called "white-coat hypertension." So it is very helpful to have additional measurements for both diagnosing hypertension and monitoring blood pressure treatment. There are many ways to get your blood pressure checked. Ask at the pharmacy, fire station, or senior center. You can even get a machine and take your blood pressure at home. Collect three or four blood pressure readings, and see how these change, depending on what you are doing. Take these with you to the doctor.

Blood pressure can often be lowered by a combination of a low-sodium diet, exercise, maintaining a healthy weight, limiting alcohol, and using prescribed medications. While some people are reluctant to use these medications due to fear of side effects, the surprising news is that many people with high blood pressure actually feel better (less fatigue, fewer headaches, and so on) when they take the medications.

Diagnosing Heart Disease

Sometimes the symptoms of heart disease are clear and "classic," such as chest pain with physical activity. Fortunately, there are now many tests available to determine if heart disease is present and how severe it is. The following are the most common tests and treatments.

- **Blood tests.** Blood tests to measure fat-like substances (cholesterol and triglycerides) estimate your risk of heart disease. They are also used to monitor the effects of cholesterol-lowering medications. If you are having chest pains, your physician may order tests of cardiac enzymes such as troponin to confirm the diagnosis of a heart attack. With heart failure, blood levels of a hormone called BNP may rise.

- **Electrocardiogram.** An electrocardiogram (EKG or ECG) measures your heart's electrical activity. It can show a lack of oxygen to the heart, a heart attack, heart enlargement, and irregular heart rhythm. It is a "snapshot" of your heart's activity. Sometimes EKGs need to be repeated to see if a heart attack is occurring. An EKG cannot

predict your risk for a future heart attack. Sometimes a portable Holter monitor is worn for several hours or days to detect abnormal heart rhythms that come and go.

- **Echocardiogram.** Painless ultrasound waves are bounced off the heart. This produces detailed images of the heart. A computer converts echoes and displays them on a TV screen. The pictures are recorded and can show heart size, heart motion, valve function, and certain types of heart damage. This test may also be done with exercise (stress testing) to see how the heart responds to stress.

- **Stress test.** Sometimes problems appear only when the heart is under increased stress. (In this case stress refers to something that makes the heart work harder, not emotional stress.) This test is done while exercising on a treadmill or stationary bicycle or after the injection of a chemical to stimulate the heart without exercising. An EKG is attached to the chest. The EKG, blood pressure, and symptoms are monitored during the test and for a few minutes after the test. A stress test is done for the following reasons:

To evaluate symptoms associated with exercise or exertion

To confirm suspicion of heart disease

To evaluate treatment

To assess progress after a heart attack

To determine irregularities in heart rhythm

A positive test result suggests the presence of coronary artery disease.

■ **Nuclear scan.** A weak radioactive substance such as thallium is injected into a vein. A scanner or special camera is used to take two sets of pictures, with and without stress (induced by exercise or medication), which are compared. This test shows blood distribution to the heart muscle and how well the heart is pumping.

■ **Cardiac catheterization and coronary angiography.** A long plastic tube called a catheter is inserted through a major blood vessel (usually in the groin) and gently guided into the heart. A dye is then injected into the catheter. This allows the coronary arteries to show up on X-rays. This test helps your physician decide the best treatment if the arteries are clogged. It can also give information about the function of the heart muscle and the valves.

Prevention and Treatment of Heart Disease, High Blood Pressure, and Stroke

There are three general approaches to help prevent and treat heart disease: lifestyle changes, medications, and procedures and surgery. Most people will benefit from one or more of these.

Lifestyle Changes and Nondrug Treatments

Heart attacks, strokes, and high blood pressure can often be prevented or controlled by taking the following actions:

■ **Not smoking.** Smoking damages the inner lining of the blood vessels and raises blood pressure. Quitting is the best thing you can do for your health. Fortunately, there are now a variety of support programs (from telephone counseling to online and group programs) and medications (from nicotine gum and patches to calming medications) that can help you quit and stay quit.

■ **Exercising.** Exercise strengthens your heart. It can also lower your cholesterol and blood pressure and help you control your weight. Inactive people double their risk for heart disease. Even small amounts of daily physical activity can lower your risk of heart disease and help you feel better and have more energy (see Chapters 6, 7, and 8).

■ **Healthy eating.** Cholesterol is a fatlike substance in the blood. It can cause fatty deposits called plaque to build up and narrow your blood vessels. The higher your cholesterol level, the greater your risk for heart disease. See page xxx for ways to lower cholesterol. Unfortunately, not all cholesterol can be controlled by what you eat. The body also makes cholesterol, and medications may be necessary. No matter how it is done, through lifestyle changes or medications (or both), lowering cholesterol considerably reduces the risk of heart attacks and strokes.

- **Maintaining a healthy weight.** Being overweight makes your heart work harder and can raise your LDL ("bad") cholesterol and blood pressure and increase your chances of developing diabetes. The highest risk is excess weight around the midsection. Regular exercise and healthy eating are the most important steps to help prevent weight gain, maintain weight, or lose weight. See Chapters 11–12.

- **Managing emotional stress.** Stress increases your blood pressure and heart rate, which can damage the lining of the blood vessels. This can lead to heart disease. (See Chapter 5.)

- **Limiting alcohol.** Whereas drinking a little (one drink per day for women, two drinks per day for men) may *reduce* the risk of heart disease, drinking more or binge drinking (more than five drinks at one time) can *increase* the risk of both heart disease and high blood pressure. So if you do use alcohol, limit the use.

- **Controlling diabetes.** If you have diabetes, your risk for heart disease more than doubles because high blood sugar damages the blood vessels. By controlling your blood sugar and taking certain heart-protective medications, you can greatly lower the risk of heart attack and stroke. See page 285.

- **Controlling high blood pressure.** See Chapter 11 for ways to recognize foods high in cholesterol.

Medications for a Healthy Heart

A variety of medications are available to treat heart disease and high blood pressure. Some of these are also very useful in preventing future heart attacks, stroke, and kidney damage. We used to think that medication should only be used if lifestyle changes such as healthy eating and exercise failed. Newer research suggests that the way to get the greatest benefit is to combine certain medications with lifestyle changes.

In Table 16.1 we briefly discuss some of the most common and most effective medications. If you have heart disease, diabetes, stroke, peripheral arterial disease, chronic kidney disease, or an abdominal aortic aneurysm, be sure to consult your doctor to find out if some or all of these heart-protective medications are right for you. If one medication is not working for you or is causing side effects, discuss this with your doctor. Usually an alternative medication can be found that will work. Most heart medications are taken for a lifetime and continue to work to reduce the risk of heart disease, heart failure, and stroke. These are not addicting and usually can be used safely over many years. Do not start or stop these medications without discussing with your doctors.

Heart Procedures and Surgery

With certain heart problems or when using medications alone is not sufficient, several types of heart procedures and surgery may be helpful.

- **Coronary or "balloon" angioplasty.** Coronary angioplasty relieves the symptoms of coronary artery disease by improving blood flow to the heart by opening the blockages. A catheter (long narrow tube) with a balloon at the tip is inserted into the artery to widen a narrow passage in the vessel. Your physician may choose to insert a tiny mesh tube called a stent to help keep the narrowed vessel open. Many stents ("drug-eluting stents") contain medications that may help prevent the artery from clogging up again.

- **Coronary artery bypass surgery.** Bypass surgery creates a new route for blood flow to your heart. A blood vessel from your leg or chest wall is used to create a detour around the blockage in the coronary artery. One or more blocked arteries may be bypassed. The surgery usually requires several days in the hospital, and the recovery time can be weeks to months.

- **Valve replacement.** Sometimes it may be necessary to have heart surgery to repair or replace a damaged heart valve.

- **Surgery and devices for rhythm problems.** The nerves of the heart can be interrupted by surgery to control or prevent certain types of irregular rhythms. Also, devices such as pacemakers and implantable defibrillators may be permanently attached to the heart to treat abnormal heart rhythms.

Exercising with Heart Disease

Exercise can be both safe and helpful for many people with heart disease, with and without surgery. To make the most of your exercise, work closely with your health providers to find the best exercise program for your needs. Remember that regular, well-chosen exercise is an important part of treatment and rehabilitation. Exercise can lower your risk for future problems, reduce the need for hospitalization, and improve your quality of life.

When Not to Exercise

Some heart conditions limit the kinds and amount of exercise you do. You should follow your doctor's advice about exercise and exercise if you have poor circulation to the heart (ischemia), if you experience irregular heartbeats (arrhythmia), or if your heart is unable to pump enough blood to the rest of your body. If your heart disease is severe, your doctor may want to change your treatment before giving you clearance to exercise. For example, if you have an arrhythmia, your doctor may want to treat you with a medicine that controls your heartbeat. If you have poor circulation to the heart muscle, the physician may recommend medications, bypass surgery, or "balloon" angioplasty to improve blood flow to the heart muscle before clearing you for conditioning activities.

Table 16.1 Medications Useful for Managing Heart Disease, High Blood Pressure, and Stroke

Medication	How It Can Help You	Comments
Blood thinners or anticoagulants *Examples:* coated "baby" aspirin (81 mg), warfarin (*Coumadin*), clopidogrel (*Plavix*)	Blood thinners lower the risk of a blood clot. This decreases the risk of a heart attack and stroke, especially if you have already had a heart attack or a stroke or have diabetes.	Aspirin can cause stomach irritation and may even cause small ulcers and bleeding. Usually, taking the low-dose (81 mg) aspirin with a special coating and taking it with food can protect the stomach. Although aspirin can reduce the overall risk of strokes caused by blood clots, it can slightly increase the risk of having a certain type of stroke from bleeding. Sometimes clopidogrel is used to help prevent blood clots.
Cholesterol-lowering statins (HMG-CoA reductase inhibitors) *Examples:* lovastatin (*Mevacor*), simvastatin (*Zocor*), atorvastatin (*Lipitor*), pravastatin (*Pravachol*)	Statins work to lower your LDL (bad) cholesterol by blocking the production of cholesterol in the liver. They also increase your HDL (good) cholesterol and may help prevent blood clots and inflammation inside your arteries. The latest evidence suggests that even if your cholesterol levels are normal, if you have heart disease or diabetes, taking a statin medication can lower your risk of future heart disease or stroke.	People who take statins daily are much less likely to have a heart attack or to die from a heart attack or stroke. If you have severe muscle pain, severe weakness, or brown urine while taking one of these drugs, contact your health care professional immediately. Statins may be combined with other drugs to lower cholesterol and reduce triglycerides.
Calcium channel blockers *Examples:* amlodipine (*Norvasc*), felodipine (*Plendil*), nifedipine (*Adalat, Procardia*), verapamil (*Calan, Isoptin SR*), diltiazem (*Cardizem, Dilacor*)	These medications relax the muscles around the arteries, lowering blood pressure. This makes it easier for your heart to pump blood.	Verapamil and diltiazem may make heart failure worse but can be used safely if you do not have heart failure.

*Because research on medications is changing rapidly, we suggest that you consult your physician, a pharmacist, or a recent drug reference book for the latest information.

Table 16.1 Medications Useful for Managing Heart Disease, High Blood Pressure, and Stroke (*continued*)

Medication	How It Can Help You	Comments
Beta-blockers *Examples:* atenolol (*Tenormin*), metoprolol (*Lopressor, Toprol XL*), propranolol (*Inderal*), acetabutol (*Sectral*), nadolol (*Corgard*), carvedilol (*Coreg*)	Beta-blockers reduce the workload of the heart by relaxing the heart muscle and slowing the heart rate. This allows your heart to pump blood more easily. Beta-blockers are used to treat high blood pressure, heart failure, irregular heart beats, blocked arteries, and angina (chest pain). This medication reduces sudden death (without symptoms or warning) from heart attack in people with coronary heart disease. If you monitor the intensity of your exercise by heart rate, be aware that because beta-blockers slow your heart rate, they may change your target heart rate range and maximal heart rate. Ask your doctor about this.	Early side effects usually go away over time. You may need to take a beta-blocker for 2 to 3 months before you feel better. But throughout this time, it can protect your heart from getting weaker. People with poorly controlled asthma and diabetes need to discuss whether they can use beta-blockers.
Angiotensin-converting enzyme (ACE) inhibitors *Examples:* lisinipril (*Prinivil, Zestril*), captopril (*Capoten*), enalopril (*Vasotec*) and **Angiotensin receptor blockers (ARBs)** *Example:* losartan (*Cozaar*)	ACE inhibitors and ARBs relax blood vessels so that blood flows more easily to the heart. This allows oxygen-rich blood to reach the heart. They also lower blood pressure and can help reduce symptoms and improve survival in heart failure. They are also used to treat and prevent kidney problems, especially in people who also have diabetes	Some people taking these drugs develop a mild cough or tickle in the back of the throat. If the cough is not very bothersome, it is not necessary to stop the medication. But if the cough is annoying, an ARB can sometimes be substituted.
Antiarrhythmics *Examples:* amiodarone (*Cordarone*), flecainide (*Tambocor*), various beta-blockers and calcium channel blockers	These drugs help the heart beat more slowly or more steadily.	

Continues on next page ▼

Table 16.1 Medications Useful for Managing Heart Disease, High Blood Pressure, and Stroke (*continued*)

Medication	How It Can Help You	Comments
Diuretics *Examples:* hydrochlorothiazide (*HCTZ, Esidrix*), furosemide (*Lasix*), chlorthalidone (*Hygroton*), bumetanide (*Bumex*), triamterene + hydrochlorothiazide (*Dyazide, Maxzide*)	Diuretics ("water pills") reduce the amount of fluid in the body, including the buildup of fluid in the lungs that can occur in heart failure. Your body gets rid of this excess fluid when you urinate. Getting rid of excess fluid decreases the amount of work your heart needs to do and can help reduce blood pressure, swelling, and the buildup of fluids in the lungs. Certain diuretics have been shown to reduce the risk of heart attack and stroke.	If you take your last dose of diuretic medication no later than 6:00 P.M. you may not need to get up as often at night to urinate. Depending on the medication, you may need to take extra potassium.
Digoxin *Example: Lanoxin*	Digoxin is used in heart failure to help your heart pump with more strength. It helps control heart rate.	
Nitrates *Examples:* nitroglycerin (*Nitrostat, Nitro-Bid, Nitro-Dur*), isosorbide dinitrate (*Isordil*)	Nitrates relax the walls of blood vessels and increase the supply of blood and oxygen to the heart. These can help relieve chest pain (angina).	Nitroglycerin, in the form of sublingual (under-the-tongue) tablets or as a spray, is taken at the first sign of chest discomfort or tightness. Do not swallow or chew the tablet. ***If the discomfort is not gone in 5 minutes, call 911 immediately.*** Continue taking the nitroglycerin approximately every 5 minutes until the discomfort is gone or help arrives. Keep a fresh supply on hand by refilling your prescription every 6 months, once you open the bottle.

*Because research on medications is changing rapidly, we suggest that you consult your physician, a pharmacist, or a recent drug reference book for the latest information.

Tips for Safe Exercise

If you do not have any restricting conditions or a doctor's advisory, it is safe for you to begin the conditioning program outlined in this book. The following are exercise considerations for people with different kinds of heart disease.

- Strengthening activities, such as isometrics, weightlifting, or rowing, can increase blood pressure and stress your heart needlessly. This can be dangerous if you have high blood pressure or your heart has trouble pumping. If you and your doctor think strengthening is important for you, you will need to pay special attention to not holding your breath while you exercise. Remember to breathe out as you exert. One way to be sure to breathe is to count out loud or breathe out through pursed lips.

- If you have not exercised since your heart disease began, you and your doctor may decide that supervision by experienced professionals is a good way to start. Most communities have cardiac rehabilitation programs or professionally staffed gyms at a local hospital or community center.

- Once you are cleared for activity by your physician, keep the intensity well below the level that causes symptoms such as chest pain or severe shortness of breath. For example, if you get chest pain during an exercise treadmill test when your heart is beating at 130 beats per minute, you should not let your heart get above 115 beats per minute when you exercise. If you cannot easily judge your intensity to stay below your "symptom zone," you can wear a pulse rate monitor (available at medical supply and sporting good stores) and check your heart rate at any time. Other ways to monitor the intensity of your exercise are the talk test and your perceived exertion (see page 126).

- If your heart has decreased pumping strength, avoid activities that cause you to strain. Try safer and more helpful conditioning activities such as light calisthenics, walking, swimming, and stationary bicycling.

- Exercise while lying down—as when you swim or pedal a special "recumbent" stationary bicycle—can help improve the efficiency of the heart's pumping action and is less tiring than exercise while standing up.

- Always remember that if you develop new or different symptoms, such as chest pain, shortness of breath, dizziness, or rapid or irregular heartbeat while at rest or while exercising, you should stop what you are doing and contact your physician.

Exercising with Stroke

If you have had a stroke that affected your arm or leg, you may have had physical and occupational therapy. You may recognize many of the exercises in this book as the ones you did in therapy. If you are still seeing a therapist or doing a home exercise program, talk with the therapist about adding new activities. If you are making your own exercise decisions now, you can use the exercises in this book to continue to improve flexibility, strength, and endurance. If you have weakness in your arm or leg or have trouble with balance, it is important that you think of safety when you choose which exercises to do. Having another person with you, sitting instead of standing, and using a counter, sturdy chair, or wall rail for support are some ideas for adapting exercises to meet your needs. You can also think of ways for your stronger side to help your weaker side exercise. A stationary bicycle with toe clips on the pedals will let your stronger leg help both legs exercise. Doing arm exercise holding a cane, walking stick, or towel in both hands will let both arms move. Remember, even if the arm and leg weakness is permanent, you can still increase your physical activity and general health with exercise.

Exercising with Peripheral Vascular Disease (Claudication)

Exercise for people with leg claudication is generally limited by the leg pain that develops during exercise. The good news is that conditioning exercises can help improve endurance and reduce leg pain for most people. Start with short walks or bicycling, and continue to the point when you start to have leg pain. Stop and rest or slow down until the discomfort eases and then start again. At the beginning, repeat this cycle for 5 to 10 minutes, increasing gradually as you get more comfortable. Many people find that they can gradually increase the length of time they can walk comfortably or exercise with this method. A good goal is to be able to keep going for 30 to 60 minutes, which is long enough to get noticeable fitness benefits too. If leg pain continues to keep you from being physically active, talk to your doctor about your options. Remember, arm exercises won't usually cause leg pain, so be sure to include them as an important part of your overall conditioning program.

The Outlook

We can do a lot to prevent heart disease and stroke and to help people with these conditions live long, full lives. The combination of healthy lifestyle, selective use of medications, and cardiac procedures when needed has dramatically lowered the risk of heart attack, stroke, and early death. You also have an important job to do. It is up to you to eat well and exercise, manage stress, and take your medications as prescribed. If you do not do your part, your health care team will be much less effective. Part of good care and self-management for people with serious heart conditions involves planning for the future and making their wishes known regarding end-of-life issues and medical care (see Chapter 19).

Suggested Further Reading

American Heart Association. *To Your Health: A Guide to Heart-Smart Living.* New York: Clarkson Potter, 2001.

American Medical Association. *Guide to Preventing and Treating Heart Disease: Essential Information You and Your Family Need to Know about Having a Healthy Heart.* Hoboken, N.J.: Wiley, 2008.

Casey, Aggie, Herbert Benson, and Ann MacDonald. *Mind Your Heart: A Mind/Body*

Approach to Stress Management, Exercise, and Nutrition for Heart Health. New York: Free Press, 2004.

Casey, Aggie, Herbert Benson, and Brian O'Neill. *Harvard Medical School Guide to Lowering Your Blood Pressure.* New York: McGraw-Hill, 2005.

Granato, Jerome. *Living with Coronary Heart Disease: A Guide for Patients and Families.* Baltimore: Johns Hopkins University Press, 2008.

Heller, Maria. *The DASH Diet Action Plan: Proven to Lower Blood Pressure and Cholesterol Without Medication.* New York: Grand Central Life & Style, 2011.

Ornish, Dean. *Eat More, Weigh Less: Dr. Dean Ornish's Advantage Ten Program for Losing Weight Safely While Eating Abundantly.* New York: Quill, 2001.

Ornish, Dean. *The Spectrum: A Scientifically Proven Program to Feel Better, Live Longer, Lose Weight, and Gain Health.* New York: Ballantine, 2008.

Rippe, James M. *Heart Disease for Dummies.* Hoboken, N.J.: Wiley, 2004.

Taylor, Jill Bolte. *My Stroke of Insight: A Brain Scientist's Personal Journey.* New York: Viking, 2009.

Other Resources

- [ ] American Heart Association (AHA), (800) 242-8721: http://www.americanheart.org/

- [ ] American Stroke Association, (888) 478-7653: http://www.strokeassociation.org/

- [ ] HeartHub: http://www.hearthub.org/

- [ ] National Heart, Lung, and Blood Institute (NHLBI), (301) 592-8573: http://www.nhlbi.nih.gov/

- [ ] National Institute of Neurological Disorders and Stroke, (800) 352-9424: http://www.ninds.nih.gov/

- [ ] National Institutes of Health: http://health.nih.gov/

- [ ] National Stroke Association, (800) STROKES (787-6537): http://www.stroke.org/

- [ ] National Women's Health Information Center: http://www.womenshealth.gov/

- [ ] The DASH Diet, http://www.nhlbi.nih.gov/hbp/prevent/h_eating/h_eating.htm

- [ ] WomenHeart: The National Coalition for Women with Heart Disease, (202) 728-7199: http://www.womenheart.org/

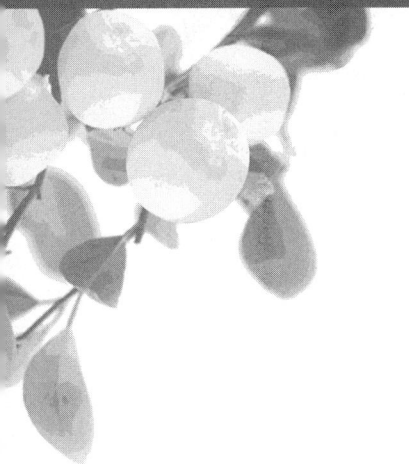

CHAPTER 17

Managing Chronic Arthritis and Osteoporosis

*L*ITERALLY, THE WORD *ARTHRITIS* MEANS "inflammation of a joint." However, as the word has come to be used, *arthritis* commonly refers to virtually any kind of damage to a joint. Although most forms of arthritis cannot be cured, you can learn to reduce pain, maintain mobility, and use medications to manage symptoms or slow the progression of the disease.

The most common form of chronic arthritis is osteoarthritis. It is the arthritis that generally affects us as we age, causing knobby fingers, swollen knees, or back pain. Osteoarthritis is not caused by inflammation, although sometimes it may result in inflammation of a joint. The cause of osteoarthritis is not precisely known but involves deterioration or a wearing away of the cartilage that cushions the ends of bone together with degeneration of bones, ligaments, and tendons associated with the joint.

Many other kinds of chronic arthritis are due to inflammation. The most common forms are those caused by rheumatic diseases such as rheumatoid arthritis, metabolic

273

diseases such as gout, and psoriasis. With these diseases, the lining of the joint becomes inflamed and swollen and also secretes extra fluid. As a result, the joint becomes swollen, warm, red, tender, and painful to move. If present for a time, inflammatory arthritis can also result in destruction of cartilage and bone. Such destruction can ultimately lead to deformity. The cause of the inflammation associated with these diseases is not precisely known, but with respect to gout, it is clearly related to the formation of uric acid crystals in the joint fluid, and in the case of rheumatic diseases, it is thought to be due to a form of autoimmunity (an immune or allergic reaction of the body against itself).

Most arthritic diseases do not affect only the joints. Joints are crossed by tendons from nearby muscles that move the joints and by ligaments that stabilize the joints. When the joint lining is inflamed or the joint is swollen or deformed, those tendons, ligaments, and muscles can be affected. They may become inflamed, swollen, stretched, displaced, thinned out, or even broken. Also, in many places where tendons or muscles move over each other or over bones, there are lubricated surfaces to make the movement easy. These surfaces are called bursas. With arthritis, they too may become inflamed or swollen, causing bursitis. Thus arthritis of any kind does not simply affect the joint. It can affect all of the structures in the area around the joint.

Consequences of Arthritis

The irritation, inflammation, swelling, or joint deformity of arthritis can cause pain. The pain may be present all the time or only sometimes, as when moving the joint. Of all the symptoms of arthritis, pain is the most common.

Arthritis can also limit movement. The limitation may be due to pain, to swelling that prevents normal bending, to deformity of the joint or tendons, or to weakness in nearby muscles.

In addition, arthritis can cause problems in areas distant from the joint. For example, if arthritis affects the joints of one leg, that leg may be favored during walking or other motion. The person's posture is altered, and an extra burden is placed on other muscles and joints. Abnormal posture or extra burdens can create pain on the other side of the body or in areas distant from the site of the arthritis.

Stiffness of joints and muscles may also occur, particularly after periods of rest such as sleeping and sitting. The stiffness makes it difficult to move. However, if you are able to get going, or if you can get heat to the affected joint and muscles (hot pad or hot shower), the stiffness may lessen or disappear. For most people, the stiffness lasts only a short while; for others it can last all day.

Another common consequence of arthritis is fatigue. Here again, the precise cause is not known. Inflammation itself causes fatigue. So does chronic pain, and so does the effort of movement when joints and muscles don't work right. In addition, fatigue can be caused by the worries and fears that often accompany arthritis. Whatever its cause or combination of causes, fatigue is an issue most arthritis patients must confront.

Depression may also accompany chronic arthritis. People with chronic arthritis often have trouble doing what they need or want to do. This can make them feel helpless, angry, and withdrawn, which may lead to depression. Depression can make other symptoms such as pain, fatigue, and disability seem worse. It can reduce an individual's work or social functioning. It can damage family relationships, as well as the capacity for independent living. Usually the depression is the situational type, meaning that it comes from the difficulties caused by the arthritis and is not a mental illness. Often it improves when the arthritis improves, but it can also be helped through self-management practices (see Chapter 2), managing pain and depression (see Chapter 4), and by the use of antidepressant medication.

Fibromyalgia is a condition that sometimes accompanies chronic arthritis but usually exists alone. Though not inflammatory, it creates muscle tenderness and joint pain similar to that of chronic inflammatory arthritis. The cause is not yet known. Anti-inflammatory treatment does not usually help. However, much of the self-management therapy used by patients with chronic arthritis is beneficial for people with fibromyalgia.

Although arthritis can have very damaging effects, much can be done to offset or eliminate these effects. The remainder of this chapter will describe aspects of appropriate management and lead you to helpful self-management techniques described in detail elsewhere in this book.

Prognosis: What Does the Future Hold?

Most chronic arthritic diseases, if left untreated, would have different outcomes for different people. Some people would progress more or less steadily, with increasing disability. Others would experience disease that waxed and waned over many years, possibly getting slowly worse but maybe not. Some individuals might even have the disease or symptoms disappear spontaneously. With modern treatment, most patients can be helped to reduce the limitations from their arthritis, and in some the progression can be slowed or stopped.

There is no real cure for any of the forms of chronic arthritis. As just noted, for some fortunate people, the arthritis will subside partly or completely on its own. Medical treatment can usually suppress the inflammation and the symptoms but must often be continued for long time periods. Proper self-management can greatly enhance improvement and the prevention of disability. This depends largely on the participation of the person with arthritis and sometimes the person's family. Therefore, a prognosis—what the future holds—cannot be predicted accurately for any individual. It depends partly on medical treatment, partly on the individual's own self-management efforts, and partly on good fortune.

Because there is no cure for chronic arthritis, medical treatment is aimed at preventing or controlling inflammation, swelling, and pain and improving physical function. The medications commonly used either help pain or reduce inflammation and swelling, or do both. When inflammation is reduced, pain usually declines and function increases.

It is important to realize that most people with chronic arthritis can lead normal or nearly normal lives. Proper use of medications and self-management practices make this possible. Thus one should not abandon major life plans.

Rather, one should adjust them to accommodate treatment needs and remember that treatment plans can often be modified to meet the particular needs or wishes of the person with chronic arthritis.

Common Types of Arthritis and Their Treatment

As noted earlier, arthritis can be the result of either loss of cartilage or bone in a joint or inflammation of a joint. Treatment depends on the type.

Osteoarthritis

Osteoarthritis is a result of degenerative changes in the cartilage and bones in joints. Cartilage cushions the ends of bones and allows them to move smoothly over one another. Because of this degeneration, the bone surfaces become rough and painful when in motion. The roughness may also irritate the joint lining (the synovium), causing it to produce more than normal amounts of joint fluid. The extra fluid results in swelling. Occasionally, small pieces of damaged cartilage will break off, float in the fluid, catch on a moving surface, and increase pain. Also, bone ends may grow small spurs (called osteophytes) that create, for instance, knobs on fingers and heel spurs. Although osteoarthritis can affect any joint, it most commonly affects the hands, knees, hips, shoulders, and spine. In general, its presence increases as we age.

The cause of osteoarthritis is not known, and there is no specific medical treatment to prevent or arrest the degenerative changes. Treatment is therefore aimed at maintaining joint function and reducing pain.

With osteoarthritis, the saying "use it or lose it" is particularly true. Unless the affected joints are used, they will slowly lose mobility, and the surrounding muscles and tendons will weaken. Fortunately, exercise will not make the osteoarthritis worse, and as movement improves with exercise and surrounding tissues strengthen, pain often declines. Thus exercise is the centerpiece of treatment. Use of exercise is discussed later in this chapter and Chapters 7 and 8 of this book.

Because osteoarthritis damages joint cartilage, an exercise program also protects cartilage. Cartilage needs joint motion and some weight bearing to stay healthy. In much the same way that a sponge soaks up and squeezes out water, joint cartilage soaks up nutrients and fluid and gets rid of waste products by being squeezed when you move the joint. If the joint is not moved regularly, cartilage deteriorates.

To help with osteoarthritic pain, the best medications are acetaminophen (Tylenol) and aspirin. Drugs such as ibuprofen (Motrin) and naproxen (Aleve), along with aspirin, are known as nonsteroidal anti-inflammatory drugs, or NSAIDs. When there is no inflammation involved in the arthritis, as is commonly the case with osteoarthritis, the anti-inflammatory activity of these drugs is not important. The benefit from these anti-inflammatory medications comes from their pain-reducing effect, which is similar to that of aspirin. Therefore, aspirin or acetaminophen (Tylenol) is usually as effective as the NSAIDs.

Heat to the joint and pain-controlling measures such as relaxation and cognitive distraction can be very helpful (see Chapter 5). Heat before exercise often makes the exercise easier. For pain at night in hands, feet, or knees, gloves, socks, and a sleeve over the knees can greatly improve sleep.

When swelling from irritation or mild inflammation is present, draining and injection of the joint with a corticosteroid medication often corrects the problem, sometimes with lasting benefit.

If the disease progresses to deformity, discomfort, and weakness that make normal living impossible, surgical joint replacement is available. Artificial joints commonly function like normal joints and permit recovery of lost strength in muscles and tendons.

Two additional therapies for osteoarthritis have been introduced. Both are intended to improve damaged cartilage or substitute for it. One is glucosamine, taken daily in pill form. The other is hyaluronan, injected into the joint as a lubricant. Studies suggest that glucosamine diminishes symptoms from osteoarthritis in the short term with potency similar to low doses of aspirin. However, the studies are not definitive, and long-term outcomes have not been established. Fortunately, glucosamine appears to have no significant adverse effects. Use of hyaluronan is more complicated because it requires injections into the joint and is also expensive. But as of this writing, both methods of treatment appear not to be of certain benefit to people

with osteoarthritis, and they have no theoretical or practical value in other forms of arthritis.

Chronic Inflammatory Arthritis

The rheumatic diseases (rheumatoid arthritis, lupus erythematosus, and others), psoriasis, and gout are the commonest forms of chronic inflammatory arthritis. Inflammatory arthritis can also occur in association with inflammatory diseases of the intestines or liver. It may appear with infections such as Lyme disease or streptococcal and virus illnesses. In those settings, it will sometimes clear with antibiotic treatment or with time, but sometimes it will become chronic.

The most commonly used medications for chronic inflammatory arthritis, with the exception of gout, fall into the following categories:

■ **Nonsteroidal anti-inflammatory drugs (NSAIDs).** As noted earlier, these drugs have both pain-reducing and anti-inflammatory effects. They are usually the first drugs used to treat arthritis because they are often helpful and tend to have the least severe side effects. Representatives of this group include aspirin, ibuprofen (*Motrin*), naproxen (*Naprosin, Aleve*), sulindac (*Clinoril*), and diclofenac (*Voltaren*). Acetaminophen (*Tylenol*), though not an NSAID, is also used to reduce pain, but it has no anti-inflammatory effect. Most of the NSAIDs can damage the stomach and intestines, but this can be minimized by always taking the medications in the middle of a meal. This sounds simple, but many people don't follow this advice all the time.

A few years ago, three new NSAIDs became available: celecoxib (*Celebrex*), rofecoxib (*Vioxx*), and valdecoxib (*Bextra*). They were designed to have anti-arthritic abilities similar to other NSAIDs but to be less damaging to the stomach and intestines. However, *Vioxx* and *Bextra* have been withdrawn from sale or restricted in use because over time they can cause heart and blood vessel disease. *Celebrex* remains available.

- **"Disease-modifying" drugs.** The drugs in this category are all anti-inflammatory drugs, more powerful than the NSAIDs but also potentially more toxic. The term "disease-modifying" implies slower progression or reversal of inflammatory arthritis, but healing from these drugs usually does not occur. Members of this group are gold (*Myochrysine*), methotrexate (*Rheumatrex*), sulfasalazine (*Azulfidine*), hydroxychloroquine (*Plaquenil*), and leflunomide (*Arava*). They are usually used in inflammatory arthritis if NSAIDs fail. They are not used for osteoarthritis.

  In recent years, evidence has emerged indicating that earlier use of "disease-modifying" agents slows the progression of the disease. Because the NSAIDs do not achieve such slowing, most patients with rheumatoid arthritis now receive treatment with second-line agents early in the course of their disease. Such an early benefit from "disease-modifying" drugs may also be true for other forms of chronic inflammatory arthritis. Use of these medications should be discussed with a rheumatologist, a physician with special training in treating arthritis and associated diseases.

- **Corticosteroids.** Corticosteroids are powerful anti-inflammatory drugs that also suppress immune function. Both effects are helpful with inflammatory arthritis, especially for rheumatic diseases in which the body's immune system appears to play a role in causing the disease (autoimmune disease). Most corticosteroids in use are synthetic versions of a normal human hormone, cortisol, which is present in everybody. Corticosteroids are the most rapid-acting and effective of the anti-arthritic drugs but may cause serious adverse effects when used for long periods of time. Prednisone (*Deltazone*) is the most commonly used corticosteroid and is often given with another anti-inflammatory drug to get a faster response.

- **Cytotoxic drugs.** These drugs, developed to treat cancer, also have anti-inflammatory and immunosuppressive effects. Examples include cyclophosphamide (*Cytoxan*), azathioprine (*Imuran*), cyclosporine (*Neoral*), mycophenolate (*CellCept*), and rituximab (*Rituxan*). These drugs can be quite toxic but also very effective. They are usually used only after other drugs have failed to control the problem. They are never used for osteoarthritis.

- **New biological agents.** A biological material called tumor necrosis factor (TNF) plays an important role in the inflammation of rheumatoid arthritis. TNF is a product of cells involved in the inflammatory and immune responses and is a member of the cytokine family. Two methods of counteracting TNF have been developed. One treatment uses an antibody to TNF called infliximab (*Remicade*) or adalimumab (*Humira*). The other treatment method uses a soluble receptor obtained from cells to neutralize the TNF. This material is called etanercept (*Enbrel*). *Remicade* is given intravenously, whereas *Humira* and *Enbrel* are injected subcutaneously (under the skin). Antibodies to other cytokines have been developed and can sometimes be effective. The new biological therapies can be very helpful when other treatments fail. However, their effects may not last, they can occasionally cause serious infections, and they are expensive.

For gout, the main treatment goal is reducing the blood uric acid level with drugs such as allopurinol (*Zyloprim*), colchicine (*Colcrys*), probenecid (*Benuryl*), and the newer febuxostat (*Uloric*). For chronic gout arthritis, most of the drugs and other methods of management for chronic inflammatory arthritis are also used.

For inflammatory arthritis, drugs are frequently used in combination. The combinations are usually based on the individual's response to particular drugs. Thus many combinations are used, sometimes including the biological agents. Although a certain combination may work best for a particular person, recent evidence indicates that no one combination is clearly superior to the others.

Some years ago, each type of inflammatory arthritis was treated with a particular group of drugs. Today, almost all of the drugs discussed here are used for any type of inflammatory arthritis. The choice of drugs depends on the person's condition and responses; commonly, milder drugs are used first, and more powerful ones are used when milder ones fail. However, as mentioned earlier, stronger drugs are now often used earlier in rheumatoid arthritis in an effort to prevent joint destruction.

It is almost impossible to predict beforehand whether any of the drugs will be helpful. Therefore, the treatment of chronic arthritis with drugs is a trial-and-error process. For chronic inflammatory arthritis, only occasionally do drugs other than corticosteroids provide an immediate benefit. Usually many days or even weeks are necessary before the full effects of the drug are felt.

Problems can be caused by the toxic effects of the drugs. All drugs can cause harm as well as benefit. Sometimes a particular drug can be very helpful for the arthritis but also cause so much harm that it cannot be used. Again, it is impossible to predict which drugs will be harmful in an individual patient. With some of the drugs, toxic effects cannot be recognized by the individual, and so the individual must be monitored with blood counts, liver function studies, analyses of urine, or other tests. People starting on any drug treatment for chronic arthritis should make sure they understand the signs and symptoms of potential harm, including rash, upset stomach, or unusual thoughts, and notify the physician if such symptoms appear. Also, discuss with your doctor whether you need to have regular blood or urine tests to monitor for toxic effects of the medications.

The unpredictability of benefits and harms from drug therapy creates uncertainty for both the patient and the physician. The best way to deal with this uncertainty is to ensure that you understand the treatment plan and the alternatives and that you have a clear way to communicate with the physician if the plan is not succeeding.

Sometimes, despite drug treatment, joints are damaged to the point where they no longer work effectively. Fortunately, modern surgical techniques allow for replacement of many types of joints, and replacement joints often function almost as well as natural joints. This is especially true for hips and knees. Modern surgery is efficient, and recovery is usually rapid.

Other Ways to Manage Chronic Arthritis

In addition to treatment with drugs or surgery, there are many other management approaches to achieve good results with chronic arthritis.

The goal of proper management is not just to avoid pain and reduce inflammation; it is to maintain the maximum possible use of affected joints. This involves maintaining the greatest motion of the joint and the greatest strength in muscles, tendons, and ligaments surrounding the joint. The key to this goal is exercise, which is an essential part of any good management program. The exercise should be regular, consistent, and as vigorous as possible. Exercise will not make the arthritis worse. In fact, failing to exercise can increase arthritis symptoms because of loss of joint mobility and physical deconditioning. Although exercise may increase pain temporarily, this is normal during joint and muscle reconditioning.

Maintaining good posture and normal motion of joints helps protect joints from deterioration, sustains mobility, and eases pain. The inactivity that results from long time periods spent sitting or lying down can worsen posture, reduce joint flexibility, and cause weakness even in the joints not affected by arthritis. Also after inactivity, especially sleeping, stiffness is common. It can be reduced by mild exercise in bed before arising or by a hot bath or shower. For some people, mild exercise before going to bed will reduce stiffness the next morning.

Appropriate exercise programs are described in Chapters 6, 7, and 8, and more specific recommendations for people with arthritis are found later in this chapter. It is wise to exercise as many joints as possible, including those without arthritis, in order to maintain general physical condition. However, chronic arthritis can affect the bones of the neck. Therefore, to prevent nerve damage, it is best to avoid extreme neck movements and strong pressure on the back of the neck or head. Because heat makes exercise easier, it is helpful to exercise when warm. Examples are exercise during or after a bath and, for hands and wrists, after washing dishes.

In addition to improving mobility, heat is also useful to reduce pain in joints and muscles, at least temporarily. When combined with rest, it can be very soothing. Alternatively, some people find cooling a warm joint with ice to be helpful. Cooling, however, does not increase mobility.

Control of fatigue is important. Rest periods between activities and restful sleep at night are essential for control (see Chapter 8 on sleeping better). When pain disturbs sleep at night, different types of beds (firm beds, foam beds, air beds) and the use of mild sleep medications can be of significant help. For some people with arthritis, low doses of antidepressive medication at bedtime will effectively control night pain and improve sleep.

Sometimes when joint function remains limited, use of assistive devices can be of benefit. Many types of devices are available (braces, canes, special shoes, grippers, reachers, walkers).

What you eat has little effect on most types of chronic arthritis, particularly osteoarthritis and rheumatoid arthritis. What you eat, however, is important for gout, where use of alcohol and eating certain meats can provoke attacks. People with gout should discuss this with their physicians. In rare cases, food allergies can cause attacks of arthritis. There is some evidence that eating oils from cold-water fish can help people with rheumatoid arthritis; however, the benefit is small. Of course, if you are overweight, losing weight can reduce the extra burden on joints, especially those that bear weight (hips, knees, feet). People with chronic arthritis should eat balanced, pleasurable meals and maintain a normal weight. Ways to do this are discussed in Chapters 11 and 12.

It is not surprising that sometimes in the struggle against arthritis, an individual becomes depressed. Usually this is a situational depression resulting from the consequences of chronic arthritis and not a mental illness. It is important to recognize the depression and to seek advice from health professionals. There are many ways to combat depression; the important thing is to know it is present and take steps to control it. (see Chapter 4).

Most people with chronic arthritis are able to lead productive, satisfying, and independent lives. The most important step in achieving this is to take an active part in managing your own arthritis. All of the components of management mentioned here either are the responsibility of the individual or are best done with the individual's participation.

Osteoporosis

Osteoporosis is not arthritis but rather a condition that is usually a result of aging and affects the bones. In osteoporosis, bones lose calcium and become more brittle. Then they are more susceptible to fracture than normal.

Normal bone structure is maintained primarily by calcium and vitamin D intake and physical activity. In women, it is also maintained by estrogen, so after menopause, when estrogen production declines, osteoporosis increases. As we age and are less physically active, bone weakening becomes more likely. In addition, the risk of osteoporosis is increased by smoking and heavy drinking, by some endocrine diseases, and by long-term use of corticosteroids as medications. This last is especially important for patients with inflammatory arthritis who must often use corticosteroids for treatment.

Although osteoporosis can cause bone pain, it usually does not cause specific symptoms. Therefore, the diagnosis is made by bone imaging. Because X-rays can detect only advanced osteoporosis, the imaging is done with a DXA scan, which measures bone mineral density.

Most physicians use the DXA scan for people who are at risk of osteoporosis; the result allows them to establish the diagnosis, determine its severity, and guide treatment.

The prevention and treatment of osteoporosis involve the dietary supplements and actions listed in the box on page 283. An appropriate intake of calcium and vitamin D is particularly important. If the osteoporosis does not respond to these steps or is severe, there are medications that strengthen bones, primarily estrogens and bisphosphonates, such as alendronate (Fosamax), ibandronate (Boniva), and risedronate (Actonel). If you cannot tolerate bisphosphonates or can't take them for another medical reason,

you may benefit from another class of medicines known as selective estrogen receptor modulators (SERMs) such as raloxifene (Evista). SERMs produce estrogen-like effects on bones and reduce the risk of vertebral fractures. They are less effective than bisphosphonates, but they can still be helpful. Use of these drugs should be discussed thoroughly with your physician; although they are generally safe, they can have adverse effects.

A mild form of osteoporosis called osteopenia can also be diagnosed by DXA scan. This can usually be managed by the supplements and actions in the box on page 283, and medications are unnecessary unless the osteopenia is progressing.

Exercising with Arthritis or Osteoporosis

Regular exercise is crucial to the management of all types of chronic arthritis and osteoporosis.

Osteoarthritis

Because osteoarthritis begins as primarily a problem with joint cartilage, an exercise program should include taking care of cartilage. Cartilage needs joint motion and some weight bearing to stay healthy. As noted earlier, in much the same way that a sponge soaks up and squeezes out water, joint cartilage soaks up nutrients and fluid and gets rid of waste products by being squeezed when you move the joint. If the joint is not moved regularly, cartilage deteriorates.

Any joint with osteoarthritis should be moved through its full range of motion several times daily to maintain flexibility and cartilage health. Judge your activity level so that pain is not increased. If hips and knees are involved, walking and standing should be limited to 2 to 4 hours at a time, followed

by at least an hour off your feet to give the cartilage time to decompress. Using a cane on the opposite side of the painful hip or knee will reduce joint stress and often get you over a rough time. Good posture, strong muscles, and good endurance, as well as shoes that absorb the shocks of walking, are important ways to protect cartilage and reduce joint pain. Knee-strengthening exercises (Exercises 15, 18, and 19 in Chapter 7) performed daily can help reduce knee pain and protect the joint. Being overweight makes knee pain worse, and losing weight can reduce pain. Regular exercise is an important part of losing weight and keeping it off.

Chronic Inflammatory Arthritis

Exercise will not damage joints in chronic arthritis and is important for all types of chronic inflammatory arthritis. Its purposes are to maintain joint mobility, strengthen ligaments and tendons around the joint, and maintain or

To Prevent or Slow Osteoporosis

- **Get enough calcium.** For adults under 50, 1,000 mg a day; for those over 50, 1,200 mg a day. Foods high in calcium include milk, yogurt, sardines, cheese, and fortified oatmeal. To check on calcium content read your food labels.

- **Get enough vitamin D.** Vitamin D is important for bone health. Although you can get vitamin D in some foods and from the sun, you will probably need to take a vitamin D supplement. Check with your doctor, as these recommendations may change. The recommendation of the U.S. Osteoporosis Association is 400 units a day for adults under 50 and 800 to 1,000 units a day for older adults.

- **Be physically active.** Get exercise by walking, bicycling, or dancing. It is also very important to do strengthening exercises for the shoulders, arms, and upper back.

- **Avoid lifting heavy objects and high-impact exercise,** especially if you have osteoporosis.

- **Sit up straight, and don't slouch.** Good sitting posture puts less pressure on the back.

- **Don't bend down to touch your toes when standing.** This puts unnecessary pressure on your back. If you want to stretch your legs or back, lie on your back and bring your knees up toward your chest.

- **Maintain a healthy weight.** If you are overweight, losing even just a little weight will help reduce pressure on bones.

- **Don't smoke,** or if you do, stop or reduce your smoking.

- **Limit alcohol** to no more than one or two drinks a day.

- **Prevent falls** to protect yourself from injury in the following ways:

  Remove throw rugs, electrical cords, and items left on the stairs that may cause you to trip and fall.

  Make sure that your home is well-lit, including stairwells and entryways.

  Do not walk on ice, polished floors, or other slippery surfaces.

  Avoid walking in unfamiliar places.

  Use a cane or walker regularly if your balance is poor, and install grab bars, especially in the bathroom, to keep you safe at home.

  Wear low-heeled shoes with good arch supports and rubber soles.

  Check your vision, and get new glasses if you do not see well.

  Regain and maintain your balance; check out the balance exercises in Chapter 7.

- Talk with your doctor about medications if these steps are not adequate.

increase the strength of muscles that move the joint. Gentle flexibility exercises can also help with morning stiffness. When the joint is inflamed, mild exercise in all joint motions is good within the limits created by pain. When the inflammation is suppressed or eliminated by medication, full regular exercise is desirable. It should be done daily. Specific types of exercise are described in Chapter 7. They involve all the movements normal to the involved joint and should be done against increasing resistance (weights, elastic bands, compressible balls, spring structures). The goal is to achieve maximum function for the affected joints, and that is possible for most people.

Osteoporosis

Regular exercise plays an important part in preventing osteoporosis and strengthening bones already showing signs of disease. Endurance and strengthening exercises are the most effective for strengthening bone. Flexibility and back- and abdomen-strengthening exercises are important for maintaining good posture. Look for the "VIP" exercises and the weight symbol for strengthening exercises in Chapter 7. You can help yourself with a regular exercise program that includes some walking and general flexibility and strengthening of your shoulders, hips, back, and stomach muscles.

Suggested Further Reading

Arthritis Foundation. *The Arthritis Foundation's Guide to Good Living with Osteoarthritis.* Atlanta: Arthritis Foundation, 2000.

Arthritis Foundation. *The Arthritis Foundation's Guide to Good Living with Rheumatoid Arthritis.* Atlanta: Arthritis Foundation, 2000.

Arthritis Foundation. *Change Your Life! Simple Strategies to Lose Weight, Get Fit, and Improve Your Outlook.* Atlanta: Arthritis Foundation, 2002.

Arthritis Foundation. *Living Better with Fibromyalgia.* Atlanta: Arthritis Foundation, 1996.

Arthritis Foundation. *Walk with Ease: Your Guide to Walking for Better Health, Improved Fitness, and Less Pain.* Atlanta: Arthritis Foundation, 1999.

Backstrom, Gayle, and Bernard Rubin. *When Muscle Pain Won't Go Away: The Relief Handbook for Fibromyalgia and Chronic Muscle Pain,* 3rd ed. Dallas, Tex.: Taylor, 1998.

Davidson, Paul. *Chronic Muscle Pain Syndrome: The 7-Step Plan to Recognize and Treat It— and Feel Better All Over.* New York: Berkley Books, 2001.

Foltz-Gray, Dorothy. *Alternative Treatments for Arthritis: An A-to-Z Guide.* Atlanta Arthritis Foundation, 2007.

Lorig, Kate, and James Fries. *The Arthritis Helpbook,* 6th ed. Reading, Mass.: Perseus, 2006.

Sayce, Valerie, and Ian Fraser. *Exercise Beats Arthritis: An Easy-to-Follow Program of Exercise,* 3rd ed. Boulder, Colo.: Bull, 1998.

Other Resources

☐   Arthritis Foundation, http://www.arthritis.org/

☐   National Institutes of Health, http://www.niams.nih.gov/

☐   Osteoporosis Foundation, http://www.osteofoundation.org/

☐   U.S. National Library of Medicine, http://www.ncbi.nlm.nih.gov/pubmedhealth/PMH0002223/

CHAPTER 18

Managing Diabetes

*L*IVING WELL WITH DIABETES requires both good medical care and effective self-management. In this chapter we will help you learn about the disease and what you do to manage it.

What Is Diabetes?

Diabetes is a disease that makes it difficult for the body to turn food into energy. To understand diabetes, it is helpful to know a little about the digestion process, the function of the pancreas and insulin, and how these relate to diabetes (see Figure 18.1.)

Some of the food we eat (sugar, starch, and other carbohydrates) is broken down in the digestion process into a simple sugar called glucose. Glucose is absorbed into the bloodstream from your stomach, causing the level of blood glucose (also known as

1) **The Mouth:** Starts the process of food intake. Chews and breaks up the food so it may be passed down to the stomach.

2) **The Stomach and Intestines:** Break down the food into nutrients, simpler substances the body can absorb. One is simple sugar or glucose.

3) **The Pancreas:** Produces hormones and substances that help with digestion. One of these hormones is insulin.

4) **Insulin:** Enters the bloodstream. It acts like the key that allows the glucose to enter the cell.

5) **Simple Sugar or Glucose:** Enters the bloodstream, and, with the help of insulin, gives nutrients to the cells, producing energy.

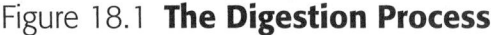

Figure 18.1 **The Digestion Process**

blood sugar) to rise. For the cells of your body to use the glucose as fuel, it needs the help of insulin. Insulin is a hormone produced by the pancreas, a small gland located below and behind your stomach. Insulin helps the blood glucose get from the bloodstream into the cells. Once inside the cells, the glucose is burned to give your body energy.

Glucose in the body can be compared to the gasoline in a car; each is a fuel and a source of energy. Gasoline alone, however, is not enough to make the car move. We also need a key to start the motor, which allows the gasoline to be converted into energy. Like the car, our bodies also need a key that enables us to use glucose as energy. Insulin is this key; it opens the door to allow the glucose to pass from the bloodstream into the cells, where it produces energy for the body.

For people with diabetes, insulin is not able to carry out this function for one of two reasons.

The pancreas may not produce enough insulin (this is called Type 1 diabetes), or the insulin that is produced cannot be used efficiently by the body (Type 2 diabetes). In either case the unabsorbed glucose remains in the bloodstream (see Table 18.1). The result is high blood glucose. When the kidneys filter the blood, excess glucose spills out in the urine. This causes two of the symptoms of diabetes: frequent urination and large amounts of sugar in the urine. This is how diabetes got its name, officially *diabetes mellitus*. The Greek word *diabetes* means "to pass through," and the Latin word *mellitus* means "sugar" or "honey."

The exact cause of diabetes is not known. Type 1 diabetes, which requires insulin as medication, usually starts in childhood; it is an autoimmune disease in which the body's immune system may damage the pancreatic cells that produce insulin.

Type 2 diabetes is sometimes called adult-onset diabetes. However, we are seeing more

Table 18.1 **Overview of Type 1 and Type 2 Diabetes**

Characteristics	Type 1 Diabetes (insulin dependent)	Type 2 Diabetes (may or may not need insulin and may need oral medications)
Age	Usually begins before age 20, but can occur in adults	Usually begins after age 40, but can occur earlier
Insulin	Little or no insulin is produced by the pancreas	The pancreas produces insulin, but it may not be enough or it cannot be used by the body
Onset	Sudden	Slow
Gender	Males and females equally affected	More females are affected
Heredity	Some hereditary tendency	Strong hereditary tendency
Weight	Majority experience weight loss and are thin	Majority are overweight
Ketones	Ketones found in the urine	Usually there are no ketones in the urine
Treatment	Insulin, diet, exercise, self-management	Diet, exercise, self-management, and when necessary, oral medication and/or insulin

and more teens and even children developing Type 2 diabetes. Type 2 diabetes does not seem to be an autoimmune disease. Rather, it tends to run in families and may start as a result of other factors. These include being overweight, lack of exercise, eating, and other lifestyle habits or some other illness. It is more common among people who are overweight. Excess body fat does not allow the body to make proper use of insulin. Insulin is produced, but the body is resistant to it. This resistance prevents the body from moving the glucose from the blood into the cells of the body efficiently. Glucose builds up in the blood because the body cannot use it. Fortunately, we know some ways to prevent this type of diabetes, as will be discussed shortly.

The important difference between the two types of diabetes is that Type 1 requires a daily supplement of insulin, whereas the majority of people with Type 2 may not initially need extra insulin to control the disease. However, if blood glucose levels cannot be well controlled with diet, exercise, and oral medications, supplementary insulin can be tremendously helpful in Type 2 diabetes.

Diagnosing Diabetes

Diabetes is usually diagnosed and monitored with blood tests. Monitoring is done by a combination of home testing of blood glucose (see page 289) and laboratory testing of hemoglobin A1C. The A1C measures your average blood glucose over the past 2 to 3 months. This

How Do I Know If I Have Diabetes?

Some people with diabetes have no symptoms, while others may have some or all of the following:

- Extreme tiredness
- Extreme thirst
- Frequent urination, especially at night
- Blurry vision or a change in vision
- Increased hunger

- Unintentional weight loss
- Sores or cuts that heal slowly
- Numbness or tingling in the feet
- Frequent infections of skin, gums, bladder, or vagina (yeast infections)

laboratory test helps you understand how well you are able to keep your diabetes under control. A1C results range from about 4 to about 16. It is also the test your doctor uses to monitor your diabetes and how well your treatment program is working to control your diabetes. For people with diabetes, the usual aim is to keep the A1C below 7 (though some doctors recommend a slightly higher goal for patients, especially those over 65 and with other health conditions).

Recently the results of the A1C are sometimes reported as a calculated eAG (estimated average glucose) blood test. The eAG is easier for some people to understand in that it is reported in the same units and ranges as your daily blood glucose monitoring. It is recommended that you have an A1C at least every year, and more often if you are adjusting your treatment plan.

Complications from Diabetes

High blood sugar over months and years can lead to serious complications. For most people, the higher the blood glucose level, the higher the chance of complications.

Although extremely high blood sugar levels can cause loss of consciousness and even death, most complications are related to damage done to blood vessels and nerves throughout the body. This can lead to heart disease and stroke, kidney damage, loss of vision, pain and loss of feeling in the feet, and slow healing of infections and wounds.

Fortunately, you can greatly reduce or delay such complications through healthy eating, exercise, weight control, controlling blood pressure and cholesterol, taking certain medications, and not smoking.

Prevention

Type 2 diabetes is a growing epidemic. Like most chronic disease, diabetes does not happen overnight. Instead it happens slowly over time. There are many people who have a condition known as *prediabetes*. This means that their blood sugar levels are higher than normal but not high enough to be diagnosed as diabetes. Prediabetes is an early warning sign. But the good news is that maintaining a healthy weight and being physically active can often reverse prediabetes and delay or prevent the development of Type 2 diabetes.

Some of the risks for diabetes, such as having a brother, sister, or parent with diabetes, cannot be changed. But most of the risks can be reduced by healthy eating, regular exercise, and weight control. Sometimes just losing 5 or 10 pounds can stop or slow the development of diabetes.

If you are at risk for diabetes, talk with your health professional. Knowing early about diabetes can help you prevent complications. It's worse to have diabetes and not know it.

Self-Management

Successful diabetes management includes maintaining blood sugar in a safe range, detecting early problems, and taking action to prevent complications. This involves working closely with your doctor and health care team and practicing effective self-management, which includes all of the following:

■ Monitoring your blood glucose

■ Observing symptoms and knowing what to do

■ Following a healthy eating plan

■ Engaging in regular physical activity

■ Managing stress and emotions

■ Dealing with sick days, infections, and other illnesses

■ Using prescribed medications in a safe and effective way

■ Getting necessary tests, exams, and immunizations

Blood Glucose Monitoring

Management of diabetes is aimed at keeping blood glucose in a safe range. The only way to tell if blood glucose is in a safe range is to monitor it. Monitoring is *not* a treatment. It is a tool you can use to find out how you are doing and make any needed day-to-day changes in diet and exercise, as well as changes in your medications, as recommended by your health care team.

There are two ways to monitor blood glucose levels:

■ **A1C and estimated average glucose (eAG) tests.** These are in fact the same blood test, but the results can be reported in two different ways. The test is ordered by your doctor and done in a laboratory; it shows your average blood glucose levels over approximately 3 months (see page 288).

■ **Home blood glucose monitoring.** This consists of a series of blood glucose tests you can do at home using a small drop of blood, glucose strips, and a home glucose meter. The meter is about the size of a cellphone and can be taken with you anywhere. The meter is easy to use. You can check your blood sugar at home, at work, or anywhere else. Be sure to get instructions on how to monitor your blood sugar and what equipment you will need. In this way you will ensure accurate results. It is especially helpful to have a doctor, nurse, pharmacist, or diabetes educator observe your technique and give you tips.

Because blood sugar levels change often throughout the day and night, you will want to learn how your eating, exercise, medications, stress, illness, and infections all affect your blood sugar. Monitoring can help with this. Checking your own blood sugars gives you and your doctor more flexibility in making decisions about how to control your blood sugar levels. Checking your blood glucose may also help you evaluate and take action if your blood sugar is too high or too low (see page 298).

How often should I monitor?

How often you check your blood glucose depends on how you and your health care team are going to use the information. Remember, monitoring is not a treatment. It is used to give you information so that you can make needed changes. You may want to monitor several times a day or perhaps once a week. If you are using insulin more than once a day or are using an insulin pump, you should monitor at least three times per day. You should monitor anytime you want to know how you are doing with your self-management plan. There are a few times when it is especially important to monitor, including these:

- When you start a new medication

- When you change the dose of a medication

- Anytime you think you might have low or high blood sugar

- Days when you are sick

The important thing about monitoring is that the information is *for you.*

Blood sugar targets

When you monitor your own blood sugar, it is important to know your blood sugar targets. Talk with your doctor about your personal targets. For many people, the blood sugar targets are as follows:

> Before a meal, including in the morning after fasting: 70 to 130 mg/dL
>
> 2 hours after a meal: less than 180 mg/dL

Remember that your doctor may recommend slightly different targets for you.

We suggest that you conduct an experiment. On two days, one a weekday and one a weekend day, monitor your blood glucose five times: first thing in the morning before eating, before a meal, 2 hours after a meal, before exercising, and again after exercising. We know that this is a lot of finger sticks, but you have to do this only once, and you will learn a lot. You can plot your blood sugars on the accompanying chart.

If there are things about these numbers you do not understand or if you want help to figure out what these numbers mean, talk with your health care provider or diabetes educator.

Points to keep in mind

Blood sugar naturally rises and falls during the course of the day. It is usually lowest in the morning when you wake up and highest an hour or two after you eat.

Your target range is likely from a low of about 70 first thing in the morning to a high of 180 after

Your Blood Glucose Profile

Use the following table to plot your blood glucose profile.
Then ask yourself the questions below it.

My Daily Glucose Results

Day 1

When Tested	Time of Day	Blood Glucose Level (mg/dL)
First thing in the morning (before eating or taking medicine)		
Before a meal		
2 hours after lunch or dinner		
Before exercising		
After exercising		

Day 2

When Tested	Time of Day	Blood Glucose Level (mg/dL)
First thing in the morning (before eating or taking medicine)		
Before a meal		
2 hours after lunch or dinner		
Before exercising		
After exercising		

Questions to Ask Yourself

- Was your blood sugar within the recommended range?
- Are any of your numbers under or over your recommended target?
- Do you notice any daily pattern?
- Are there times during the day that your glucose is lower than target range?
- Are there specific times during the day that your glucose is higher than target range?
- Can you think of any reasons why your blood glucose acted as it did?

meals. Do not be concerned if your blood sugar fluctuates within this target range.

What is important is that your blood sugars be about the same each day in relationship to the same activities (for example, an hour or two after meals or after exercising).

You may also be instructed by your doctor or diabetes educator on how to check your urine at home for ketones if your blood sugars tend to be high. Ketones in the urine is a sign that your body is using fat for energy instead of using glucose because not enough insulin is available to use glucose for energy.

If you have been managing your diabetes, (eating well, exercising, and taking your medication) and your early morning reading is almost always high, you should talk to your doctor. You may go to bed with your blood sugars in a target range, but then find that the levels jump up in the morning. This is known as the "dawn effect" or "dawn phenomenon." Blood sugars may rise a few hours before getting up in the morning in response to release of hormones and extra glucose from the liver. To prevent or correct high blood sugar levels in the morning, your doctor may, based on the results of blood testing throughout the night, recommend not eating carbohydrates close to bedtime, adjusting your dosage of medication or insulin, or switching to a different medication.

Observing Symptoms and Taking Action

Although it is important to know how you feel when your blood glucose is very low or high, this is not a reliable way to manage diabetes. First, many people do not have symptoms until their blood sugar is already very high or low. Some people

with diabetes are unaware of any symptoms they may have during periods of high or low blood sugars. This makes it very difficult to stay within their appropriate blood glucose range. Second, many of the symptoms are the same for both high and low blood sugar. Without knowing the actual blood glucose level, one does not know what to do. The only way for you to know about your blood glucose on a day-to-day basis is to monitor it.

Maintaining a Safe Blood Glucose Level

The goal of diabetes management is to keep blood sugars in a target range. Sometimes your blood glucose may get too high (hyperglycemia) or too low (hypoglycemia). The causes of hyperglycemia and hypoglycemia include the following:

- Too little or too much medication or insulin
- Eating at irregular hours or missing or skipping meals
- Having too little or too much food (especially carbohydrates)
- Increased or decreased physical activity
- Having an illnesses, infection, or surgery
- Emotional stress

It is critically important that you learn to recognize the symptoms, take self-care corrective action, and know when and how to seek medical assistance (see Table 18.2 on page 294–295).

We recommend that people with diabetes wear an emergency bracelet or carry an emergency card in their wallet (or both). The emergency card should also have information about the medications you are taking, your doctor's contact information, and an emergency contact person's name and number. We also recommend that you always carry a "remedy food" or fast-acting carbohydrate source with you to quickly manage a low blood sugar.

Adopting a Healthy Eating Plan

Healthy eating is the core of diabetes self-management. You are the only one who can manage your blood sugar. The good news is that this is not as hard as it might seem. Small changes in your eating can make important differences in your blood glucose levels and how you feel. Let's start with some reassurance. You do not have to go hungry. You do not need special foods. You can still eat the foods you like. Healthy eating for diabetes is healthy eating for your whole family. In Chapter 11 there is information about healthy eating. Here we will give the important basics for people with diabetes. If you have diabetes, you need to be more careful than other people about when, how much, and what types of foods you eat. This is because the type of food, the timing of when you eat, and the amount you eat all effect your blood sugar.

All food affects blood sugar. However, carbohydrates (carbs) are the nutrients that do the most to determine blood sugar levels. Your job is to monitor your carbs, especially refined carbohydrates like sugar. You can do this by learning about the carbohydrate content in different foods, eating healthy foods with fewer carbs, watching your portion size, and knowing the number of carbs in a portion. We discuss all of these in Chapter 11.

Choose vegetables, fruits, and whole grains. These foods give you good nutrients, energy, and fiber, fewer calories, and less fat. Limit high-carbohydrate snacks, such as candy, cakes, cookies, sodas, and ice cream. These raise your blood glucose and add fats and calories without giving you healthful nutrients. We are not saying you can't ever have the foods you love. You just need to limit these foods. Think about having 45 to 60 grams of carbs to spend at each meal If you spend 40 grams of these carbs on cake, consider limiting your other carbs for this meal. Remember, moderation is the key to successful management of blood glucose.

Planning meals when you have diabetes may sound complicated. To help you out, here's a simple tip for healthy eating. Try the plate method to plan your meals (see Figure 18.2). For each meal, half your plate should be non-starchy vegetables (spinach, broccoli) and fruit, a fourth of your plate should be some lean protein (fish, meat, beans, etc.), and the last fourth can be a starch such as potatoes, whole-grain bread, or rice. Note that this plate is a little different from the one in Figure 11.1 in Chapter 11 for people who do not have diabetes.

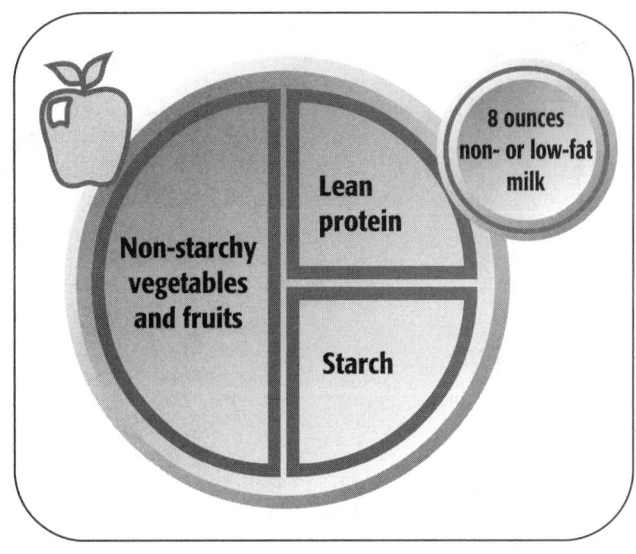

Figure 18.2 **The Diabetes Plate**

Table 18.2 **Hyperglycemia and Hypoglycemia***

	Hyperglycemia (blood glucose too high)	**Hypoglycemia (blood glucose too low)**
Symptoms	Extreme tiredness Extreme thirst Blurry vision or a change in vision Increased hunger Increased need to urinate	Feeling sweaty, shaky, or dizzy Hard, fast heartbeat Headache Confusion or irritability or sudden change in mood Tingling around your mouth or in your fingers
What to do if you suspect this condition	If possible, check your blood sugar. If it is above 250, take the actions indicated here. If you cannot check your blood sugar and think you have high blood sugar, take the following actions immediately: Drink water or other sugar-free liquids to prevent dehydration. If you take insulin, follow your instructions for taking extra insulin. Check you blood sugar every 4 hours. Seek immediate medical attention if you develop any of the symptoms described below.	If you feel symptoms of low blood sugar, check your blood sugar immediately. If your blood sugar is below 70 mg/dL† or if you are in a place where you cannot test your blood sugar, or still have symptoms of low blood sugar, take the following actions: Eat a 15 g "remedy food" or fast-acting carbohydrate source—for example, 3 glucose tablets, 3 packets of sugar, or ½ cup (4 ounces) of fruit juice or regular soda. Wait 15 minutes, note your symptoms, and, if possible, check your blood sugar again. After 15 minutes, if the symptoms are not better or your blood sugar level is still less than 70 mg/dL, eat another remedy food and wait 15 minutes. If your symptoms are still not better, call the doctor or nurse. Do not wait—it is critical to get immediate medical help. If your symptoms are better and your next meal is more than 1 hour away, eat a snack (for example, half a sandwich, some low-fat cheese, a few crackers, or a cup of milk).

Table 18.2 **Hyperglycemia and Hypoglycemia (*continued*)**

	Hyperglycemia (blood glucose too high)	Hypoglycemia (blood glucose too low)
When to call the doctor or seek immediate medical help	If you feel confused, disoriented, agitated, or weak If you have symptoms of dehydration, such as extreme thirst, dry mouth, and cracked lips, or have not urinated for 8 hours If you are running a fever, are vomiting, or have diarrhea If you have a strong, fruity breath odor (similar to nail polish or acetone) If your breathing is rapid and deep If your blood sugar level is over 300 mg/dL for 8 hours or much higher than usual	If you have slurred speech, poor coordination, or clumsy movements If you have seizures or loss of consciousness If your symptoms are not better after repeating the "what to do" steps If you have low blood sugar (less than 60 mg/dL) twice in one day If your blood sugar is repeatedly lower than usual without cause

*Depending upon your condition and history, your doctor may provide you with slightly different instructions for managing high or low blood sugars.

†Some people experience symptoms of hypoglycemia with blood sugars slightly higher than 70 mg/dL. This is another reason it is important for you to check your blood sugars, know your body, and learn how you feel at different levels.

Here is one final suggestion. Most people would benefit from smaller portions. A portion may be smaller than you think. For example, a portion of rice or pasta containing 15 grams of carbohydrate is $1/3$ cup. This does not mean you cannot have more than a portion. It means you need to keep your total grams of carbs per meal between 45 and 60. You can learn about portion sizes and the carbohydrate content of common foods in Chapter 11.

It is generally better to eat smaller meals every 4 to 5 hours during the day. Be sure not to skip breakfast. This is when your body most needs fuel as you have not eaten for a long time.

To learn more about managing your eating plan, we recommend that you spend some time with a certified diabetes educator. This is a person who has been specially trained to teach diabetes management. A registered dietitian (RD) can also help you tailor your eating plan to your lifestyle. Some additional resources are listed at the end of this chapter.

Managing Physical Activity

Regular exercise, along with healthy eating, is a core element of controlling blood glucose levels and improving health for everyone with diabetes. However, people who are taking medication to control diabetes should discuss any change in exercise habits with their doctor, dietitian, or health educator because changes in activity levels often require changes in medication and eating schedules.

Exercise is beneficial for people with diabetes in several ways. Mild to moderate aerobic exercise decreases the need for insulin and helps control blood glucose levels by increasing the sensitivity of body cells to insulin and lowering blood glucose levels both during and after exercise. This type of regular exercise is also essential for losing weight and reducing cardiovascular risk factors such as high levels of blood lipids (cholesterol and triglycerides) and high blood pressure.

The exercise program recommended for people with diabetes is generally the same as the conditioning program described in Chapter 7. Mild to moderate aerobic exercise for approximately 30 minutes at a time performed as part of a general conditioning program is a safe and effective way to help control diabetes and stay healthy. Most people with diabetes should aim for at least 150 minutes a week. If you would like to do more exercise—for example, if you wish to run a marathon—check with your health care team, as you may need to make adjustments to your eating or medications (or both).

Additional considerations for people with diabetes are to begin an exercise program only when your diabetes is well under control, keep in touch with your doctor to make changes in medication and diet if needed, and coordinate eating, medication, and exercise to avoid hypoglycemia (low blood sugar). It is often helpful to check your blood sugar levels before and after exercise so that you develop a sense of how your body responds to exercise. If you do not take insulin, plan to be active within an hour after eating your meals or snacks to prevent low blood sugar. If you have Type 1 diabetes and your blood sugar is less than 100 mg/dL before exercising, eat 15 to 30 grams of carbohydrate before you start exercising unless advised otherwise by your health care team. Stop exercising right away if you are dizzy, have shortness of breath, feel sick to your stomach, or are in pain. Drink extra fluids before, during, and after exercise. If you have problems with sensation in your feet or poor circulation, be sure to check your feet regularly and protect yourself from blisters and abrasions. It is especially important to inspect your feet and practice good skin and nail hygiene regularly. Shoe inserts can be tailored to help protect the soles of the feet.

For more information on how to develop and maintain an exercise program, see Chapter 7.

Managing Stress and Emotions

After learning that you have diabetes or if you develop diabetes-related complications, you may be feeling angry, scared, or depressed. These feelings are normal, understandable, and manageable. For people with diabetes, stress and emotions such as anger, fear, frustration, and depression can raise blood sugar levels. For this reason, it is important to learn effective ways to deal with these feelings. Hiding or ignoring your feelings is not healthy. You will find lots of tools for dealing with stress and negative emotions in Chapters 4 and 5.

Managing Sick Days, Infections, and Other Illnesses

People with diabetes, like all people, sometimes get sick. When you get an infection, a cold, or the flu, your blood sugar tends to go up. How your body uses food and diabetes medicines changes. For this reason, it is important to plan for sick days and to know what to do and when to seek help. The following points should be included in your plan.

Planning Ahead

- Have a family member or friend who is able to help you when needed. This person should know what to do, when to call the doctor, or when to take you to the emergency department.

- Have plenty of both sweetened and unsweetened or sugarless (or sugar-free) liquids on hand.

- Have a thermometer at home and know how to use it.

- Have your emergency medical information on hand (including doctor's number and list of medications and dosages).

- Be sure to ask your health care providers under what circumstances you should call them. (Some general guidelines are provided below.)

When You Get Sick

- Take your usual dose of insulin or pills unless you have a special "sick-day plan," you are vomiting, or your health care team tells you otherwise.

- Test your blood sugar two to four times a day. If your blood sugar is over 300 mg/dL, test every 3 to 4 hours. Write down the results and time.

- If you take insulin and your blood sugar is above 300 mg/dL, test your urine for ketones. Record whether you have small, moderate, or large amounts.

- Watch for symptoms of hypoglycemia or hyperglycemia (see pages 294–295).

- Track how much fluid you drink. To prevent dehydration, try to sip at least 8 ounces (1 cup) of fluids every hour while awake. If your blood sugar is over 240 mg/dL, use sugar-free drinks such as broth, tea, or water. If your blood sugar is low, eat or drink ½ to 1 cup of a sugared liquid (fruit juice or regular soft drink).

- Check your temperature twice a day and record it.

- Keep eating if possible. Small frequent meals or snacks can help.

- Keep in touch. Tell a family member or friend how you are feeling and have the person check in with you frequently.

When to Call Your Health Care Professional

- If your blood sugar is less than 60mg/dL two times in one day

- If your blood sugar is over 300 mg/dL for 8 hours or your blood sugars are much higher than they usually are

- If your temperature rises above 101°F (38.3°C) or if it stays above 100°F (37.8°C) for more than 2 days

- If you vomit or have diarrhea for more than 24 hours

- If you are not able to drink liquids or eat food or keep down medications for more than 8 hours

- If you have a small level of ketones in your urine as indicated on the test strips

- If you experience deep or troubled breathing, an extremely dry mouth, or a fruity odor to your breath

- If you have been sick longer than expected and are not getting better

- You are not feeling well and are unsure what you should do to care for yourself

When to Seek Immediate Emergency Care

- If your blood sugar is over 500 mg/dL

- If you find moderate to large amounts of ketones in your urine

When you call your health care professional, be prepared. Have the following information: your type of diabetes, your blood sugar level (if you know it), your temperature, if you have ketones in your urine, your symptoms, the medications you are taking, and what you have done to treat your symptoms.

Medications: Helping You Control Blood Glucose and Prevent Complications

In addition to healthy eating and exercising, most people with diabetes benefit from medications. These help keep blood sugar, blood pressure, and cholesterol levels in the target ranges. Although they can be helpful, many people do not like taking medications. For some of us, not taking medications is a point of pride. We might want to manage our conditions naturally. In some cases it is possible to manage without medications. However, most people with diabetes, if they are going to maintain blood glucose control and prevent complications, need to take one or more medications. Medications can help prevent such complications as heart attack, stroke, kidney disease, and early death. Unfortunately, you cannot wait to see what happens before you decide to take medications to reduce your risks. Once diabetes complications have appeared, they usually cannot be reversed.

Blood sugar medications

Your doctor will recommend medications based on your type of diabetes, how well your blood sugar is controlled, and your other medical conditions.

- **Insulin for Type 1 diabetes.** Insulin is required throughout your life because your body does not produce insulin.

- **Medications for Type 2 diabetes.** There are several types of pills that can be used separately or in combination to help control your blood sugar. Oral or injected insulin is also a safe and effective choice for many people with Type 2 diabetes.

Medications to prevent complications

In addition to using medications to control blood sugar, studies have shown that certain other medications can reduce the risk of developing diabetes complications. Because of their protective benefit, these medications are recommended even if your blood pressure and cholesterol are in the target ranges. Depending on your age and medical conditions, common types of preventive medications may include the following:

- **Aspirin.** Low-dose aspirin (81 mg) reduces risk for heart attack and stroke by decreasing the chance of a sudden blockage in an artery.

- **ACE inhibitors or ARBs.** These specialized medications to control blood pressure protect your kidneys and reduce the chance of having a heart attack or stroke.

- **Statins.** These decrease inflammation and lower cholesterol, reducing the chance of a heart attack or stroke.

Talk with your doctor if you are not taking these additional preventive medicines to find out whether you should be taking them.

Diabetes medications

Some people with Type 2 diabetes can manage their blood glucose without insulin or other diabetes medications by controlling their exercise, diet, and weight, sometimes losing only 10 to 15 pounds (4–6 kg). The rule of thumb is that a weight loss of 7% will help bring blood glucose into a healthy range. This means 14 pounds if you weight 200 pounds. However, along with diet and exercise, most patients with Type 2 diabetes will need the help of oral medications or insulin to safely control their blood sugar and help prevent complications. The medications do not take the place of healthy eating and regular physical activity. Table 18.3 lists the most common medications currently used to treat diabetes.

Insulin is used to treat everyone with Type 1 diabetes and for many people with Type 2 diabetes. It is used to replace the insulin that is not produced or is inadequately utilized by the body. Using insulin injections is now one of the safest and most effective ways to control blood glucose and prevent complications. Research now supports using insulin earlier in the treatment of Type 2 diabetes if blood sugar levels are quite high, if oral medications do not control blood sugar, or if you experience side effects from oral medications. Some patients are initially fearful of using insulin, but once started, they find that

Table 18.3 **Common Medications Used for Diabetes**

Medication	How It Can Help You Control Blood Glucose	Comments
Biguanides *Examples:* Metformin (*Glucophage, Fortimet, Glucophage XR, Glumetza, Riomet*)	Decrease the production and release of glucose from the liver. Decrease insulin resistance.	May cause some diarrhea and nausea. Take with food. These medications must be used with caution in people with heart failure, kidney failure, or liver problems.
Sulfonylureas and glinides		
Examples: **Sulfonylureas:** glipizide (*Glucotrol*), glyburide (*Micronase, DiaBeta*), tolazamide (*Tolinase*), tolbutamide (*Orinase*), chlorpropamide (*Diabinese*) **Glinides:** repaglinide (*Prandin*), nateglinide (*Starlix*)	Help pancreas produce and release more insulin	May cause some weight gain.
Alpha-glucosidase inhibitors *Examples:* acarbose (*Precose*), miglitol (*Glyset*)	Slow the digestion and absorption of carbohydrates, thereby reducing after-meal blood sugar peaks	May cause some bloating and gas. Take with first bite of meal.
Repaglinide (*Prandin*)	Stimulates pancreas to release more insulin right after meals	

the injections are rather easy and nearly painless (usually causing less discomfort than the finger stick required to check blood sugar). In addition, controlling blood sugar levels is often much easier with the use of insulin. Remember, using insulin is a good thing and a wise decision if recommended by your doctor.

There are several types of insulin, depending on how fast and how long they work. It is important that you know the type of insulin you are taking, the company that makes it, the dose (number of units you are taking), and when to take it (before a meal or snack or soon after taking the first bite of your food). Also make sure that the insulin you are taking has not passed its expiration date. If you feel that you could benefit from learning more about the use of insulin, talk with your doctor or diabetes educator. Your doctor may also work out with you a written plan for how to adjust your insulin

Table 18.3 **Common Medications Used for Diabetes (*continued*)**

Medication	How It Can Help You Control Blood Glucose	Comments
Thiazolidinediones *Examples:* Pioglitazone (*Actos*), rosiglitazone (*Avandia*)	Decrease insulin resistance by helping cells use insulin better to decrease blood sugar levels	May cause some weight gain and fluid buildup. These drugs are not recommended for people with heart failure or liver problems, and their effectiveness at reducing heart attacks, stroke, and death is uncertain.
Insulin	Helps the cells in the body get the blood sugar out of the bloodstream and into the cells where it can be used to provide energy for the body	Different types of insulin vary in how fast they work and how long they work. Quicker-acting insulin may be given around mealtimes to help lower blood sugar levels. Longer-acting insulin may provide a more constant blood glucose level throughout the day and overnight. Sometimes a combination of short-acting and long-acting insulin may be used.
Injectable hormones *Examples:* pramlintide (*Symlin*), exenatide (*Byetta*)	May help control your blood sugar level	

Note: Many new medications for managing blood glucose are being developed and evaluated each year. Be sure to discuss with your doctor which medications might be right for you.

dose ("sliding scale") based on your daily home blood glucose measurements. Some patients with diabetes may also benefit from the use of the newer insulin pumps. You will also find a list of resources at the end of this chapter.

If you do need medications, you should know when to take them and never skip a dose. Most of these drugs are taken once or twice a day, usually right before meals. Check with your doctor before stopping or changing your medicines, even if you

don't feel well. When traveling, always keep your medications with you, not in your luggage.

Other medications, including over-the-counter medications and some natural remedies and dietary supplements, can sometimes interact with diabetes medications. Therefore, it is important that your doctor and pharmacist know all the medications you are taking, including prescription and nonprescription drugs and any vitamins, minerals, supplements, herbals, and natural medicines used.

Here is one last piece of advice about medications. If you start a new drug and experience side effects, be sure to tell your health care team right away. A change in medicine or in the dosage of the current medicine may clear up some side effects.

Preventing Complications

Diabetes can cause other problems in the body. These can often be delayed and sometimes avoided by maintaining good blood glucose control. Remember that most complications are directly related to this control. The following are the most common complications of diabetes:

- **Heart disease and stroke.** It may surprise you that heart disease and stroke are the biggest killers of people with diabetes. High blood sugar levels can harden and block the arteries. The good news is that there are many things you can do to help reduce these potential problems.

- **Nerve damage.** Diabetes can cause damage to nerves (neuropathy), resulting in a burning or tingling sensation, numbness, or severe pain, especially in the feet and hands. Nerve damage can also lead to sexual problems such as erection problems in men and vaginal dryness in women. Nerve damage can also lead to problems with digestion and urination.

- **Kidney damage.** Diabetes can damage the blood vessels in the kidney, especially when the blood pressure is high, causing kidney failure. The first sign may be detected by a test for small amounts of protein in the urine.

- **Vision problems.** Blurred vision can occur when high blood sugar levels temporarily cause the lens in the eye to swell. More serious and permanent damage to the blood vessels in the retina in the back of the eye (retinopathy) can lead to poor vision or even blindness.

- **Infections.** Diabetes can decrease immune function and reduce blood flow, which can lead to slower healing and more frequent infections of the skin, feet, lungs, and other parts of the body.

- **Gum disease.** People with diabetes have a greater risk for gum (periodontal) disease and infection. That's why it is important to discuss your diabetes with your dentist and to get regular dental checkups.

Here's a handy checklist to make sure you are doing the things and getting the care that will help significantly prevent or delay these and other complications of diabetes. They may even save your life!

- **Maintain safe blood glucose levels.** A healthy diet, regular exercise, a healthy weight, and (if needed) medications are the keys to controlling blood sugar levels and preventing complications.

- Control your blood pressure. The target blood pressure reading for people with diabetes are usually 130/80 or less (or as recommended by your doctor). Lower blood pressure means less stress on your heart and blood vessels, eyes, and kidneys. To prevent complications of diabetes, controlling blood pressure can be as important as controlling blood glucose levels.

- **Control your blood cholesterol.** LDL ("bad") cholesterol, rather than total cholesterol, is the measure that is usually monitored for people with diabetes. The target level for people with diabetes is 100 or less (and some studies suggest an even lower target level of 70; check with your doctor). Remember that taking a statin medication may further reduce the risk of heart attack and stroke even if your cholesterol level is low without the statin.

- **Protect your kidneys.** Along with regular testing, taking an ACE inhibitor or ARB medication can help lower blood pressure as well as protect your kidneys.

- **Get regular checkups, exams, and immunizations.**

  - Have an A1C test at least once a year.

  - Have kidney function tests at least once a year.

  - Have cholesterol and lipid tests at least once a year.

  - Have eye exams (including inspection of the retina at the back of your eyeball) every 1 to 2 years (or as recommended by your doctor), and report any changes in vision to your doctor. This retinal exam is different from a test by an optometrist, who checks your vision to see if you need glasses or corrective lenses.

  - Remind your health care provider to check your feet at each visit or at least once a year. One way to do this is to always take off your shoes and socks in the examining room. (See below for other tips about foot care.)

  - Have your blood pressure checked at every visit (or as recommended by your provider) and keep track of the numbers.

  - Have a flu shot every year and a pneumonia vaccination at least once (may need to be repeated after age 65).

  - Have a dental exam once a year or as recommended by your provider; floss and brush your teeth at least once a day.

- **Check out your feet.** When you have diabetes, your feet need extra care and attention. Diabetes can damage the nerve endings and blood vessels in your feet, making you less likely to notice when your feet are injured. Diabetes also limits your body's ability to fight infection and get blood to areas that need it. If you get a minor foot injury, it could become an ulcer or a serious infection.

  - Examine your feet every day. You or someone else should look between the toes and on the tops and bottoms of the feet for cuts, cracks, sores, corns, calluses, blisters, ingrown toenails, extreme dryness, bruises, redness, swelling, or pus.

  - Wash your feet every day. Use warm (not hot) water. Check the water temperature with your wrist or another part of your body, not your feet, and dry thoroughly, especially between the toes. Do not soak your feet.

- Cut your toenails straight across. If you can't safely trim your toenails yourself, ask a family member to do it or get professional help. Also, do not clean under your toenails or remove skin with sharp objects. (Many senior centers have a day or two a month when a professional comes in to cut toenails.)

- If your feet are dry, rub on a mild lotion before bed. Do not put lotion between your toes. Avoid lotions that contain alcohol or other ingredients that end in *-ol*, as these tend to dry out the skin.

- Wear comfortable shoes and socks (never go barefoot except when bathing or in bed). Your shoes should support, protect, and cover your feet. If your feet sweat, use powder. Before putting on shoes, check inside for rough places or any sharp objects such as tacks or nails on the sole of the shoe. Break in new shoes gradually. Avoid socks with tight, elastic tops.

- To avoid "hot spots," do not wear the same shoes two days in a row. If you have any problems with your feet, change your shoes in the middle of the day.

- Have your doctor or other clinician check your feet at each office visit.

- Always get early treatment for foot problems. A minor irritation can lead to a major problem.

- **Take these additional precautions.**
  - Be sure to tell your health care provider if you are taking aspirin (81 mg tablet) to lessen your risk of heart attacks and stroke.

  - Do not smoke, or if you do smoke, take steps to quit.

  - In general, it is a good idea to avoid alcohol. For the person with diabetes, alcohol can cause a sudden and drastic drop in blood glucose, and it adds calories that can lead to weight gain. If you do drink, make sure you have some food with it to avoid a low blood sugar reaction, which can happen if you have alcohol on an empty stomach.

  - Protect your skin. Don't get sunburned, and keep your skin clean.

  - Wear a MedicAlert necklace or bracelet, and carry with you a list of all your medications.

  - At every visit and if you are hospitalized or go to the emergency department, remind the doctor and nurse that you have diabetes.

The Bottom Line: Your Role Is Important

Most complications of diabetes can be prevented, delayed, and treated. You have an important role. Let us quickly review what you must do:

- Maintain your blood glucose level within your normal range.

- Be aware of your body and symptoms.

- Report changes early. Time is important.

- Make sure you get regular checkups, exams, tests, and immunizations.

To become a good diabetes self-manager, there is lots to learn. Putting all of this into action is sometimes difficult. Set personal goals to control your diabetes, review them regularly, and revise them as needed. Be sure to talk to your doctor or diabetes educator about your questions, problems, and concerns. Find other information and resources in your community. Take a diabetes education program. Consider joining a diabetes support group either in your community or online. Some resources are listed at the end of this chapter.

Suggested Further Reading

American Diabetes Association. *A Field Guide to Type 2 Diabetes: The Essential Resource from the Diabetes Experts.* Alexandria, Va.: American Diabetes Association, 2004.

American Diabetes Association. *Complete Guide to Diabetes*, 5th ed. Alexandria, Va.: American Diabetes Association, 2011.

Arsham, Gary, and Ernest Lowe. *Diabetes: A Guide to Living Well*, 4th ed. Alexandria, Va.: American Diabetes Association, 2004.

Beaser, Richard S., and Amy P. Campbell. *The Joslin Guide to Diabetes: A Program for Managing Your Treatment.* New York: Simon & Schuster, 2005.

Bierman, June, Virginia Valentine, and Barbara Toohey. *Diabetes: The New Type 2: Your Complete Handbook to Living Healthfully with Diabetes Type 2.* New York: Tarcher, 2008.

Polonsky, William H. *Diabetes Burnout: What to Do When You Can't Take It Anymore.* Alexandria, Va.: American Diabetes Association, 1999.

Raymond, Mike. *The Human Side of Diabetes.* Chicago: Noble Press, 1992.

Schade, David S., Patrick J. Boyle, and Mark R. Burge. *101 Tips for Staying Healthy with Diabetes and Avoiding Complications.* Alexandria, Va.: American Diabetes Association, 1996.

Walker, Rosemary, and Jill Rodgers. *Diabetes: A Practical Guide to Managing Your Health.* New York: DK, 2005.

Other Resources

☐ American Diabetes Association (ADA), 1660 Duke Street, P.O. Box 25757, Alexandria, VA 22313; (888) DIABETES: http://www.diabetes.org/. The ADA publishes a bimonthly magazine called *Diabetes Forecast*. It is filled with practical tips on diabetes care and relates personal experiences of people with diabetes.

☐ International Diabetes Center, 4959 Excelsior Boulevard, Minneapolis, MN 55416: http://www.Idcdiabetes.org/. The center offers a variety of inexpensive pamphlets, booklets, and slide sets dealing with various facets of diabetes care.

☐ Joslin Diabetes Foundation, One Joslin Place, Boston, MA 02215; http://www.joslin.harvard .edu/. This world-famous facility has separate divisions for research, education, and youth. Its efforts involve all facets of diabetes management and research. It is one of eight Diabetes Research and Training Centers designated by the National Institutes of Health.

☐ National Diabetes Education Program, http://www.ndep.nih.gov/. On this site you will find a wide variety of materials to help you self-manage your diabetes.

☐ National Diabetes Information Clearinghouse, 7910 Woodmont Avenue, Suite 1811, Bethesda, MD 10014; http://diabetes.niddk.nih.gov/. This organization publishes a list of nutrition information related to diabetes management.

CHAPTER 19

Planning for the Future: Fears and Reality

PEOPLE WITH CHRONIC ILLNESSES often worry about what will happen to them if their disease becomes truly disabling. They fear that at some time in the future they may have problems managing their lives and their illness. One way people can deal with fears of the future is to take control and plan for it. They may never need to put their plans into effect, but there is reassurance in knowing that they will be in control if the events they fear come to pass. We'll examine the most common concerns and offer some suggestions that may be useful.

What If I Can't Take Care of Myself Anymore?

Regardless of our state of health, most of us fear becoming helpless and dependent. But this fear is even greater among people with potentially disabling health problems. And it usually has physical as well as financial, social, and emotional components.

Physical Concerns of Day-to-Day Living

As your health condition changes, you may need to consider changing your living situation. This may involve hiring someone to help you in your home or moving to a place where more help is provided. How you make this decision depends on your needs and how they can best be met. Keep in mind that we are talking about physical, social, and emotional needs. All must be considered.

Start by evaluating what you can do for yourself and what activities of daily living (ADLs) will require some kind of help. ADLs are the everyday things such as getting out of bed, bathing, dressing, preparing and eating meals, cleaning house, shopping, and paying bills. Most people can do all of these things, even though they may have to do them slowly, with some modification, or with some help from gadgets.

Some people, though, may eventually find one or more of these tasks no longer possible without help from somebody else. For example, you may still be able to fix meals but no longer able to do the shopping. Or if you have problems with fainting or sudden bouts of unconsciousness, you might need to have somebody around at all times. You may also find that some things that you enjoyed in the past, such as gardening, are no longer pleasurable. Using the problem-solving steps discussed in Chapter 2, analyze and make a list of what the potential problems might be. Once you have this list, solve the problems one at a time, first writing down every possible solution you can think of. For example:

Can't go shopping

- Get daughter to shop for me
- Find a volunteer shopping service
- Shop at a store that delivers
- Ask a neighbor to shop for me
- Use the Internet
- Get home-delivered meals

Can't be by myself

- Hire an around-the-clock attendant
- Move in with a relative
- Get a Lifeline Emergency Response system
- Move to a board-and-care home
- Move to a retirement community

When you have listed your problems and the possible solutions to the problems, select the solution that seems the most workable, acceptable, and within your financial means (step 3 of problem solving).

The selection will depend on your finances, the family or other resources you can call on, and how well the potential solutions will solve your problem. Sometimes one solution will be the answer for several problems. For instance, if you can't shop and can't be alone, and household chores are reaching the point of a need for help, you might consider a retirement community that will solve all of these problems, one that offers meals, regular house cleaning, and transportation for errands and medical appointments.

Even if you are not of retirement age, many facilities accept younger people, depending on the facility's particular policies. Some facilities for the retired take residents at age 50, or younger if one member of the household is the minimum age. If you are a young person, the local center for people with disabilities or "independent living center" should be able to direct you to an out-of-home care facility appropriate for you. When looking for a retirement community, consider the levels of care that are offered. These usually include *independent living,* where you have your own apartment or small house; *assisted living,* where you get some help with dressing, taking medications, and other tasks; and *skilled nursing,* which includes help with all ADLs and some medical care.

It may help to discuss your wishes, abilities, and limitations with a trusted friend, relative, or social worker. Sometimes another person can spot things we ourselves overlook or would like to ignore. A good self-manager often makes use of other resources, which is step 6 in the problem-solving steps in Chapter 2.

Make changes in your life slowly, one step at a time. You don't need to change your whole life to solve one problem. Remember that you can always change your mind. Don't burn your bridges behind you. If you think that moving out of your own place to another living arrangement (relatives, care home, or elsewhere) is the thing to do, don't give up your present home until you are settled in your new home and are sure you want to stay there.

If you think you need help, hiring help at home is less drastic than moving. If you can't be alone and you live with a family member who is away from home during the day, going to an adult or senior day care center may be enough to keep you safe and comfortable while your family is away. In fact, adult day care centers are ideal places to find new friends and activities geared to your abilities.

A social worker at your local senior center, center for people with disabilities, or hospital social services department can be very helpful in providing information about resources in your community. This person can also give you ideas about how to deal with your care needs. There are several kinds of professionals who can be of great help. As previously mentioned, social workers are good for helping you decide how to solve financial and living arrangement problems and locating appropriate community resources. Some social workers are also trained in counseling the disabled or the elderly in relation to emotional and relationship problems that may be associated with your health problem.

An occupational therapist can assess your daily living needs and suggest assistive devices or rearrangements in and around your home to make life easier. They can also help you figure out how to keep doing pleasurable activities that are limited because of disability.

Most hospitals have a discharge planner on staff. This person, usually a nurse, will see you before you go home and check that you know how to care for yourself and also that you have the help you need. It is very important that you be honest with this person. If you have concerns about your ability to care for yourself, say so. Solutions are almost always available, and the discharge planner is a real expert. However, the planner can help only if you share your concerns.

An attorney specializing in elder law should be on your list for helping you set your financial affairs in order—to preserve your assets, to prepare a proper will, and perhaps to execute a durable power of attorney for both health care and financial management. If finances are a concern, ask your local senior center for the names of attorneys who offer free or low-cost services to seniors. Your local bar association chapter can also refer you to a list of attorneys who are competent in this area. These attorneys are generally familiar with the laws applying to younger persons with disabilities as well. Even if you are not a senior, your legal needs are much the same as those of the older person.

Finding In-Home Help

If you find that you cannot manage alone, the first option is usually to hire somebody to help. Most people just need a person called a home aide or something similar. These are people who provide no medically related services that require special licensing but do help with bathing, dressing, meal preparation, and household chores.

There are a number of ways to find somebody. The easiest, but most expensive, is to hire someone through one of the home care agencies, usually listed under "home care" or "home nursing" in the Yellow Pages. These are usually (but not always) private, for-profit businesses that supply caregiver staff to individuals at home. The fees charged vary with the skill and license of the caregiver and will include an amount for Social Security, insurance, bonding, and profit for the agency. The fees are usually about double what you would expect to pay for someone you hire directly. The advantage, if you can afford it, is that the agency assumes all payroll responsibilities, including Social Security and federal and state taxes, as well as responsibility for the skill and integrity of the attendant, and can replace an ill or no-show attendant right away. The agency pays the staff directly. The client pays the agency and has no involvement with paying the attendant.

Registered nurses (RNs) hired this way are very expensive, but it is rare that home care for a chronically ill person requires a registered nurse. Licensed vocational nurses (LVNs) cost somewhat less but are still expensive and are usually not needed unless nursing services (such as dressing changes, injections, or ventilator management) are required. Certified nursing assistants (CNAs) have some basic training in nursing, are much less expensive, and can provide satisfactory care for all but the most critically ill person at home.

Most of these agencies supply home aides as well as licensed staff. Unless you are bedridden or require some procedure that must be done by someone with a certain category of license, a home aide will most likely be the most appropriate choice for your needs.

The agencies maintain registries or lists of prescreened attendants or caregivers from which you select the one you wish to hire. The agency will charge a "placement fee," usually equal to one month's pay of the person hired. The agency will assume no liability for the skill or honesty of these people, and it will be necessary to check references and to interview carefully, just as you would for someone from any other source. This type of resource can be found in the Yellow Pages under the listing for "home nursing agencies" or "registries." Some agencies provide both their own staff and registries of staff for you to select from.

Other resources that may provide help at home include senior centers and centers serving the disabled. They often have listings of people who have called them to say they want work as a home attendant or who have posted a notice on a bulletin board there. These job seekers are not screened and need to be interviewed carefully and to have references checked before they start on the job.

Many experienced home care attendants use the local newspaper's classified "employment wanted" section to find new jobs. They may also advertise online such as on Craigslist. Home attendant jobs tend to be temporary because one's patient usually progresses to a need for more or sometimes less care than the attendant provides, so the attendant must then look for a new job. Again, one can find a competent helper through the newspaper or on the Internet, but the advice to interview carefully is valid here too.

Probably the best source of help is word of mouth, a recommendation from someone who has employed a person or knows of a person who has worked for a friend or relative. Putting the word out through your family and social network may lead you to a jewel.

Home sharing may be a solution for the person who has space and could offer a home to someone in exchange for help. This works best if the help needed consists mainly of household and garden chores. Some people may be willing to provide personal care, such as help with dressing, bathing, and meal preparation. Some communities have agencies or government bureaus that help match up home sharers and home seekers.

Note, finally, that every county in the United States has an Area Agency on Aging. You can find yours in the phone book or online. These are excellent agencies to call when you are looking for resources.

Finding Out-of-Home Care

As noted earlier, you have several options when considering to move out of your home to find the lifestyle and level of care you need.

Retirement communities

The person who needs very little personal care but recognizes the need to live in a more protected setting, with security, emergency response services, and so on, and who is older (usually over 50) may wish to consider a retirement community. These may be owned units, rental units, or so-called life care facilities. The life care facility requires a substantial advance payment (called an endowment, an accommodation fee, or something similar), plus a monthly charge that covers living space, services, and in some cases personal or nursing care when or if the need for that arises. Other such facilities are subsidized by the federal government for low-income applicants. The criteria for what constitutes "low income" are set by the rules governing the federal subsidy that finances the organization.

There are almost always waiting lists for retirement communities, even before they are built and ready for occupancy. If you think such a place would be right for you, you should get on the waiting list right away, or at least a couple of years before you think you want to move. You can always change your mind or decline if you are not ready when a space is offered. To locate a facility in your area, call your senior center or go to the library or the internet, and consult the directory of the Association of Homes for the Aged. Your reference librarian should be able to help you find this publication. YIf you have friends living in nearby retirement communities, ask to be invited for a visit and a meal. In this way you can get an inside view. Some communities have guest accommodations where you can arrange to stay for a night or two before you commit to a lease or contract.

Residential care homes

Residential care homes, also known as board-and-care homes, are licensed by the state or county social services agency. They provide nonmedical care and supervision for individuals who cannot live alone. These homes fall into two categories, large and small. The small ones have about six residents, who live in a family-like setting in a neighborhood residence. The large ones have more residents, sometimes hundreds, who live in a boardinghouse or hotel-like setting. They take meals in a central dining room and have individual or shared rooms, with activities conducted in large common rooms.

In either type of facility, the services to the residents are the same: all meals, assistance with bathing and dressing as needed, laundry, housekeeping, transportation to medical appointments, supervision, and assistance with taking medications. The larger facilities usually have professional activities directors. Residents of the larger facilities usually need to be more independent because they will not receive as much personal attention as in the smaller homes.

These homes are licensed in most states for either "elderly" (over 62) or "adult" (under 62). The adult category is further divided into facilities for the mentally ill, the developmentally delayed, and the physically disabled.

It is important when considering a residential care home to evaluate the type of residents already living there to make sure you will fit in. For example, some of these facilities may cater to individuals who are mentally confused. If you are mentally clear, you would not find much companionship there. If everybody is hard of hearing, you might have trouble finding somebody to talk to.

Although all homes are by law required to provide wholesome meals, you should make sure the cuisine is to your liking and can meet your dietary needs. If you need a salt-free or diabetic diet, for instance, be sure the operator is willing to prepare your special diet.

The monthly fees for residential care homes vary, depending on whether they are spartan or luxurious. The most spartan facilities cost about the same as the government Supplemental Security Income (SSI) benefit and will accept SSI beneficiaries, billing the government directly. The more luxurious the home is with respect to furnishings, neighborhood, services, and so on, the greater the cost. However, even the nicest of these will probably cost less than full-time, 24-hour, 7-days-a-week at-home care.

Skilled nursing facilities

Sometimes called a "nursing home" or "convalescent hospital," the skilled nursing facility provides the most comprehensive care for severely ill or disabled people. Typically, a person who has had a stroke or a hip or knee replacement will be transferred from the acute care hospital to a skilled nursing facility for a period of rehabilitation before going home. Recent studies have shown that almost half of all people over 65 will spend some time in a nursing home, many of them only for a short time.

No care situation seems to inspire more fear than the prospect of having to go to a nursing home. Horror stories in the news media help foster anxiety about the awful fate that will befall anyone who has the misfortune to have to go there.

Public scrutiny is valuable in helping ensure that standards of care and humane and competent treatment are provided. It must be remembered that nursing homes serve a critical need. When one really needs a nursing home, usually no other care situation will meet this need.

Skilled nursing facilities provide medically related care for people who can no longer function without such care. This means that there may be medications to be administered by injection or intravenously or monitored by professional nursing staff. A nursing home patient is usually very physically limited, needing help getting in and out of bed, eating, bathing, or dealing with bladder or bowel control. Skilled nursing facilities can also manage the care of feeding tubes, respirators, and other high-tech equipment.

For people who are partially or temporarily disabled, the skilled nursing facility also provides physical, occupational, and speech therapy, wound care, and other services.

Not all nursing homes provide all types of care. Some specialize in rehabilitation and therapies, and others specialize in long-term custodial care. Some are able to provide high-tech nursing services, and others do not.

In selecting a nursing home, you should seek out the help of the hospital discharge planner or social worker or a similar professional from a home care agency or center for seniors or the disabled. There are organizations to monitor local nursing homes. Each nursing home is required by law to post in a prominent place the name and phone number of the "ombudsman," a person assigned by the state licensing agency to assist patients and their families with problems related to their nursing home care. The agencies that can help you with this are listed in the Yellow Pages under "social service organizations." You may also want to have family or friends visit several facilities and make recommendations.

Will I Have Enough Money to Pay for My Care?

Next to the fear of physical dependence, many people fear not having enough money to pay for their needs. Being sick often requires expensive care and treatment. If you are too ill or disabled to work, the loss of income, and especially the loss of your health insurance coverage, may present an overwhelming financial problem. You can, however, avoid some of the risks by planning ahead and knowing your resources.

Health insurance and Medicare may meet only a part of the ultimate cost of your care. There are many needs that Medicare does not meet at all, and most private "Medigap" insurance

policies cover only the 20% that Medicare does not cover.

However, supplemental insurance policies offer the kind of coverage that provides for care needs that Medicare and Medigap insurance do not pay for. If you plan to buy such insurance for yourself, carefully read the sections on limitations and exclusions. Be sure the policy covers nursing home care at a daily rate that is realistic for your community. Check that it will cover treatments or care for preexisting conditions. Some policies have a waiting period for such preexisting conditions, usually 3 to 6 months.

Others won't cover you at all for any condition that was diagnosed before the start date of the policy. Health care reform has brought many changes in both Medicare and private insurance, some of which may be difficult to understand. We suggest that you talk to people at your local senior center or Area Agency on Aging to find trustworthy sources of information.

If you are too sick to work—either permanently or for some extended period—you may be entitled to draw Social Security on the basis of your disability. If you have dependent children, they would also receive benefits. If you have been disabled for a specified period (as of this writing, it is 2 years), you may be entitled to Medicare coverage for your medical treatment needs. Disability payments are based only on disability, not on need.

If you have minimal savings and little or no income, the federal Medicaid program can pay for medical treatment and long-term skilled or custodial care. The eligibility rules on assets and income differ from state to state. You should consult your local social services department to see if you are entitled to benefits. An elder care attorney may also be able to help.

If Social Security benefits are unavailable or insufficient, the Supplemental Security Income (SSI) program is available to individuals who meet the eligibility criteria for Medicaid.

The social services department in the hospital where you have obtained treatment can advise you about your own situation and the probability of your being eligible for these programs. The local agency serving the disabled usually has advisers who can refer you to programs and resources for which you may be eligible. Senior centers often have counselors knowledgeable about the ins and outs of health care insurance.

If you own a home, you may be able to get a reverse mortgage, whereby the bank pays you a monthly amount based on the value of your home. The nice thing is that no matter how long you live, you can never be thrown out of your home.

I Need Help but Don't Want Help—Now What?

Let's talk about the emotional aspects of needing help. Every human being emerges from childhood reaching for and cherishing every possible sign of independence—the driver's license, the first job, the first credit card, the first time we go out and don't have to tell anybody where we are going or when we will be back, and so on. In these and many other ways, we demonstrate to ourselves as well as to others that we are "grown up"—in charge of our lives and able to take care of ourselves without any help from parents.

If a time comes when we must face the realization that we can no longer manage completely on our own, it may seem like a return to childhood and having to let somebody else be in charge of our lives. This can be very painful and embarrassing.

Some people in this situation become extremely depressed and can no longer find any joy in life. Others fight off the recognition of their need for help, thus placing themselves in possible danger and making life difficult and frustrating for those who would like to be helpful. Still others give up completely and expect others to take total responsibility for their lives, demanding attention and services from their children or other family members. If you are having one or more of these reactions, you can help yourself feel better and develop a more positive response.

The concept of "changing the things I can change, accepting the things I cannot change, and being able to know the difference" is really fundamental to being able to stay in charge of our lives. You must be able to evaluate your situation accurately. You must identify the activities that require the help of somebody else (going shopping and cleaning house, for instance) and those that you can still do on your own (getting dressed, paying bills, writing letters). Another way to look at this is to get help from others for the things you least like to do, giving you the time and energy to do the things you want to do.

This means making decisions, and as long as you are making the decisions, you are in charge. It is important to make a decision and take action while you are still able to do so, before circumstances intervene and the decision gets made for you. That means being realistic and honest with yourself. Decision-making tools can be found on pages 322-325.

Some people find that talking with a sympathetic listener, either a professional counselor or a sensible close friend or family member, is comforting and helpful. An objective listener can often point out alternatives and options you may have overlooked or were not aware of. The person can provide information or contribute another point of view or interpretation of a situation that you would not have come upon

yourself. This can be an important part of the self-management process.

Be very careful, however, in evaluating advice from somebody who has something to sell you. There are many people whose solution to your problem just happens to be whatever it is they are selling—health or burial insurance policies, annuities, special and expensive furniture, "sunshine cruises," special magazines, or health foods with magical curative properties.

In talking with family members or friends who offer to be helpful, be as open and reasonable as you can be and, at the same time, try to make them understand that you will reserve for yourself the right to decide how much and what kind of help you will accept. They will probably be more cooperative and understanding if you can say, "Yes, I do need some help with . . . , but I still want to do . . . myself." More tips on asking for help can be found in Chapter 9.

Insist on being consulted. Lay the ground rules with your helpers early on. Ask to be presented with choices so that you can decide what is best for you as you see it. If you try to objectively weigh the suggestions made to you and not dismiss every option out of hand, people will consider you able to make reasonable decisions and will continue to give you the opportunity to do so.

Be appreciative. Recognize the goodwill and efforts of people who want to help. Even though you may be embarrassed, you will maintain your dignity by accepting with grace the help that is offered, if you need it. If you are truly convinced that you are being offered help you don't need, you can decline it with tact and appreciation. For example, you can say, "I appreciate your offer to have Thanksgiving at your house, but I'd like to continue having it here. I could really use some help, though—maybe with the cleanup after dinner."

If you reach the point of being unable to come to terms with your increasing dependence on others, you should consult a professional counselor. This should be someone who has experience with the emotional and social issues of people with disabling health problems.

Your local agency providing services to the disabled can refer you to the right kind of counselor. The local or national organization dedicated to serving people with your specific health condition (American Lung Association, American Heart Association, American Diabetes Association, etc.) can also direct you to support groups and classes to help you in dealing with your condition. You should be able to locate the agency you need through the telephone book Yellow Pages under the listing "social service organizations." You can also do research on the Internet.

Akin to the fear and embarrassment of becoming physically dependent is the fear of being abandoned by family members who would be expected to provide needed help. Tales of being "dumped" in a nursing home by children who never come to visit haunt many people, who worry that this may happen to them.

We need to be sure that we do reach out to family and friends and ask for the help we need when we recognize that we can't go on alone. It sometimes happens that in expectation of rejection, people fail to ask for help. Some people try to hide their need in fear that their need will cause loved ones to withdraw. Families often complain, "If we'd only known . . . ," when it is revealed that a loved one had needs for help that were unmet. If you really cannot turn to close family or friends because they are unable or unwilling to become involved in your care, there are agencies dedicated to providing for such situations. Through your local social services department's "adult protective services" program or Family Services Association, you should be able to locate a "case manager" who will be able to organize the resources in your community to provide the help you need. The social services department in your local hospital can also put you in touch with the right agency.

Grieving: A Normal Reaction to Bad News

When we experience any kind of a loss—small ones (such as losing one's car keys) or big ones (such as losing a life partner or facing a disabling or terminal illness)—we go through an emotional process of grieving and coming to terms with the loss.

A person with a chronic, disabling health problem experiences a variety of losses. These include loss of confidence, loss of self-esteem, loss of independence, loss of the lifestyle we knew and cherished, and perhaps the most painful of all, loss of a positive self-image if our condition has an effect on appearance (such as rheumatoid arthritis or the residual paralysis from a stroke).

Elizabeth Kübler-Ross, who has written extensively about this process, describes the stages of grief:

- **Shock**, when one feels both a mental and a physical reaction to the initial recognition of the loss

- **Denial**, when the person thinks, "No, it can't be true," and proceeds to act for a time as if it were not true

- **Anger**, when we fume "Why me?" and search for someone or something to blame (if the doctor had diagnosed it earlier, the job caused me too much stress, etc.)

- **Bargaining**, when we promise, "I'll never smoke again," or "I'll follow my treatment regimen absolutely to the letter," or "I'll go to church every Sunday, if only I can get over this."

- **Depression**, when awareness sets in, we confront the truth about the situation, and experience deep feelings of sadness and hopelessness

- **Acceptance**, when we recognize that we must deal with what has happened and make up our minds to do what we have to do

We do not pass through these stages in a linear fashion. We are more apt to flip-flop between them. Don't be discouraged if you find yourself angry or depressed again when you thought you had reached acceptance.

I'm Afraid of Death

Fear of death is something most of us begin to experience only when something happens to bring us face to face with the possibility of our own death. Losing someone close, having an accident that might have been fatal, or learning we have a health condition that may shorten our lives usually causes us to consider the inevitability of our own eventual passing. Many people, even then, try to avoid facing the future because they are afraid to think about it.

Our attitudes about death are shaped by our own central attitudes about life. This is the product of our culture, our family's influences, perhaps our religion, and certainly our life experiences.

If you are ready to think about your own future—about the near or distant prospect that your life will most certainly end at some time—then the ideas that follow will be useful to you.

If you are not ready to think about it just yet, put this aside and come back to it later.

As with depression, the most useful way to come to terms with your eventual death is to take positive steps to prepare for it. This means to get your house in order by attending to all the necessary details, large and small. If you continue to avoid dealing with these details, you will create problems for yourself and for those involved with your situation.

There are several components to getting your house in order:

- **Decide and then convey to others** your wishes about how and where you want to be during your last days and hours. Do you want to be in a hospital or at home? When do you want procedures to prolong your life stopped? At what point do you want to let nature take its course when it is determined that death is inevitable? Who should be with you—only the few people who are nearest and dearest or all the people you care about and want to see one last time?

- **Make a will.** Even if your estate is a small one, you may have definite preferences about who should inherit what. If you have a large estate, the tax implications of a proper will may be significant. A will also ensures that your belongings go where you would like them to go. Without a will, some distant or "long-lost" relative may end up with your estate.

- **Plan your funeral.** Write down your wishes or actually make arrangements for your funeral and burial. Your grieving family will be very relieved not to have to decide what you would want and how much to spend. Prepaid funeral plans are available, and you can purchase your burial space in the location and of the type you prefer.

- **Draw up a durable power of attorney** for health care and also one for managing your financial affairs. (These are discussed later in this chapter.) You should also discuss your wishes with your personal physician, even if he or she doesn't seem interested. (Your physician may also have trouble facing the prospect of losing you.) Have some kind of document or notation included in your medical records that indicates your wishes in case you can't communicate them when the time comes.

Be sure that the persons you want to handle things after your death are aware of all that they need to know about your wishes, your plans and arrangements, and the location of necessary documents. You will need to talk to them, or at least prepare a detailed letter of instructions and give it to someone who can be counted on to deliver it to the proper person at the appropriate time. This should be a person close enough to you to know when that time is at hand. You may not want your spouse to have to take on these responsibilities, for example, but your spouse may be the best person to keep your letter and know when to give it to your designated agent.

You can purchase at any well-stocked stationery store a kit in which you place a copy of your will, your durable powers of attorney, important papers, and information about your financial and personal affairs. Another useful source to help organize this information is "My Life in a Box", which is noted in the reading and resources lists at the end of this chapter. There are forms that you fill out about bank and charge accounts, insurance policies, the location of important documents, your safe deposit box and where the key is kept, and so on. This is a handy, concise way of getting everything together that anyone might need to know about. Some of us keep these documents on our computers. If this is the case, be sure others can find your passwords and accounts.

Finish your dealings with the world around you. Mend your relationships. Pay your debts, both financial and personal. Say what needs to be said to those who need to hear it. Do what needs to be done. Forgive yourself. Forgive others.

Talk about your feelings about your death. Most family and close friends are reluctant to initiate such a conversation but will appreciate it if you bring it up. You may find that there is much to say to and to hear from your loved ones. If you find that they are unwilling to listen to you talk about your death and the feelings that you are experiencing, find someone who will be comfortable and empathetic in listening to you. Your family and friends may be able to listen to you later on. Remember, those who love you will also go through the stages of grieving when they have to think about the prospect of losing you.

A large component in the fear of death is fear of the unknown: "What will it be like?" "Will it be painful?" "What will happen to me after I die?"

Most people who die of a disease are ready to die when the time comes. Painkillers and the disease process itself weaken body and mind, and the awareness of self diminishes without the realization that this is happening. Most people just "slip away," with the transition between the state of living and that of no longer living hardly identifiable. Reports from people who have been brought back to life after being in a state of clinical death indicate they experienced a sense of peacefulness and clarity and were not frightened.

A dying person may sometimes feel lonely and abandoned. Regrettably, many people cannot deal with their own emotions when they are around a person they know to be dying and so deliberately avoid his or her company, or they may engage in superficial chitchat, broken by long, awkward silences. This is often puzzling and hurtful to those who are dying, who need companionship and solace from the people they counted on.

You can sometimes help by telling your family and friends what you want and need from them—attention, entertainment, comfort, practical help, and so on. Again, a person who has something positive to do is more able to cope with difficult emotions. If you can engage your family and loved ones in specific activities, they can feel needed and can relate to you around the activity. This will give you something to talk about, to occupy time, or at least provide a definition of the situation for them and for you.

Palliative Care and Hospice Care

In most parts of the United States, as well as in many other parts of the world, both palliative care and hospice care are available. In everyone's life there comes a time when regular medical care is no longer helpful and we need to prepare for death. This preparation means that medical and other care is aimed at making the patient as comfortable as possible and providing a good quality of life. Recently we have learned that at least for some diseases, people who receive hospice care actually live longer than those who receive more aggressive treatment. Today we

often have several weeks or months, and sometimes years, to make these preparations. This is when hospice care is so very useful. The aim of hospice care is to provide the terminally ill patient (someone who is expected to die within months) with the highest quality of life possible. Palliative care is available for those expected to live more than 6 months. At the same time, hospice professionals help both the patient and the family prepare for death with dignity and also help the surviving family members. Today most hospices are "in-home" programs. This means that the patient stays in his or her own home and the services come to them. In some places there are also residential hospices where people can go for their last days.

One of the problems with hospice care is that often people wait until the last few days before death to ask for this care. They somehow see asking for hospice care as "giving up." By refusing hospice care, they often put an unnecessary burden on themselves, friends, and family. The reverse is also often true. Families say they can cope without help. This may be true, but the patient's life and dying may be much better if hospice cares for all the medical things so that family and friends are free to give love and support.

Hospice care can be most useful in the months before death. Most hospices only accept people who are expected to die within 6 months. This does not mean that you will be thrown out if you live longer. It is important that you recognize that if you, a family member, or a friend is in the end stage of illness, you should find and make use of your local hospice. It is a wonderful final gift.

Making Your Wishes Official: Advance Directives for Health Care

Although none of us can have absolute control over our own death, this, like the rest of our lives, is something we can help manage. That is, we can have input, make decisions, and probably add a great deal to the quality of our death. Proper management can lessen the negative impact of our death on our family and friends. An advance directive can help you manage some of the medical and legal issues concerning death as well as help you plan for both expected and unexpected end-of-life situations.

What Are Advance Directives?

Advance directives are written instructions that tell your doctor what kind of care you would like to receive if and when you are not able to make medical decisions for yourself—for example, if you are unconscious, in a coma, or mentally incompetent. Usually an advance directive describes both the types of treatments you want and those you do not want. There are different types of advance directives.

A living will is a document that states the kind of medical or life-sustaining treatments you would want if you were seriously or terminally ill. A living will, however, does not let you appoint someone to make those decisions for you.

A durable power of attorney (DPA) for health care allows you to name someone to act for you as your agent but also gives guidelines to your agent about your health care wishes. If you want, you can let your agent make the decisions. Many people, however, prefer to give guidance to their agent. This guidance can indicate almost anything you want done for your care; it may range from the use of aggressive life-sustaining measures to the withholding of these measures. Whereas a living will is good only in the case of a terminal illness, a DPA can be used anytime you are unconscious or unable to make decisions due to any illness, accident, or injury. It is important to understand that a durable power of attorney for health care allows you to appoint someone else to act as your agent for only your health care; it does not give this person the right to act on your behalf in other ways, such as in handling your financial matters. In general, a DPA is more useful than a living will because it allows you to appoint someone to make decisions for you, and it can be activated at any time when you are unable to make decisions. The only time a DPA may not be the best choice is if there is no one you trust to act on your behalf.

A do not resuscitate (DNR) order is a request not to be given cardiopulmonary resuscitation (CPR) if your heart stops or if you stop breathing. A DNR can be included as part of a living will or durable power of attorney for health care; however, you do not need to have either of those in order to have a DNR order. Your doctor can put a DNR in your medical chart so that it may guide the actions of the hospital and any health care provider. You can also put a DNR on your refrigerator so that emergency personnel will know your wishes. Without a DNR order, hospital or emergency personnel will make every effort to resuscitate you. DNR orders are accepted in all states.

Although advance directives for health care are generally used for end-of-life situations, they may also be prepared to direct the type of mental health treatment one wishes to receive in the event a person with mental illness becomes incapacitated due to that illness. Under federal law, most states may combine advance directives for health care and mental health care in one document and allow you to appoint an agent to act on your behalf for both health and mental health issues. Some states, however, require separate documents, which also allow you to choose different agents, one for health care and another for mental health care. For more information on mental health advance directives and the specific practices in your state, check the Web site of the National Resource Center on Psychiatric Advance Directives given at the end of this chapter.

A power of attorney (POA) is a document that gives someone you appoint the power to make your financial or business decisions. If you are no longer able to make these decisions and you need to pay for care, your family or friends or even sometimes the state will have to go to court. This can be very expensive. You may want to talk to your lawyer about the advantages and disadvantages of a POA.

Preparing a Durable Power of Attorney for Health Care

Adults (anyone age 18 or older) should prepare a durable power of attorney for health care. Unexpected events can happen to anyone at any age. This is a different document from a regular power of attorney. The DPA for health care applies only to health care decisions. Here is what you need to do.

Choose your agent. Your agent can be a friend or family member. It cannot be the physician who is providing your care. Here are things to consider as you make this important choice. This person should probably live in your area. If the agent is not available on short notice to make decisions for you, he or she is not much help. Just to be on the safe side, you can also name a backup or secondary agent who would act for you if your primary agent were not available.

Be sure that your agent thinks like you or at least would be willing to carry out your wishes. You must be able to trust that this person has your interests at heart and truly understands and will respect your wishes.

The person should be someone who you feel would be able to carry out your wishes. He or she should be mature, composed, and comfortable with your wishes. Sometimes a spouse or child is not the best agent because this person is too close to you emotionally. For example, if you wished not to be resuscitated in the case of a severe heart attack, your agent has to be able to tell the doctor not to resuscitate. This could be very difficult or impossible for a family member to decide then and there. Be sure the person you choose as your agent is up to this task and would not say "do everything you can" at this critical time. You want your agent to be someone who will not find this job too much of an emotional burden. The person has to be comfortable with the role, as well as willing and able to carry out your wishes. In review, look for the following characteristics in an agent:

- Someone who is likely to be available should they need to act for you

- Someone who understands your wishes and is willing to carry them out

- Someone who is emotionally prepared, able to carry out your wishes, and will not feel burdened by doing so

Finding the right agent is a very important task. This may mean talking to several people. These may be the most important interviews that you will ever conduct. We will talk more about discussing your wishes with family, friends, and doctor later.

Determine what you want. In other words, what are your directions to your agent? What you want will be guided by your beliefs and values. Some DPA forms give several general statements of desires concerning medical treatment. These can help you decide on your wishes. Here are some examples:

- *I do not want my life to be prolonged and I do not want life-sustaining treatment to be provided or continued (1) if I am in an irreversible coma or persistent vegetative state or (2) if I am terminally ill and the application of life-sustaining procedures would serve only to artificially delay the moment of my death or (3) under any other circumstances where the burdens of the treatment outweigh the expected benefits. I want my agent to consider the relief of suffering and the quality as well as the extent of the possible extension of my life in making decisions concerning life-sustaining treatment.*

- *I want my life to be prolonged, and I want life-sustaining treatment to be provided unless I am in a coma or vegetative state that my doctor reasonably believes to be irreversible. Once my doctor has reasonably concluded that I will remain unconscious for the rest of my life, I do not want life-sustaining treatment to be provided or continued.*

- *I want my life to be prolonged to the greatest extent possible without regard to my condition, the chances I have for recovery, or the cost of the procedures.*

If you use a form containing such suggested general statements, all you need to do is initial the statement that applies to you.

Other forms make a "general statement of granted authority," in which you give your agent the power to make decisions. However, you do not write out the details of what these decisions should be. In this case, you are trusting that your agent will follow your wishes. Since these wishes are not explicitly written, it is very important that you have discussed them in detail with your agent.

All forms also have a space in which you can write out any specific wishes. You are not required to give specific details but may wish to do so.

Knowing what details to write is a little complicated. None of us can predict the future or knows the exact circumstances in which the agent will have to act. You can get some idea by asking your doctor what he or she thinks are the most likely developments for someone with your condition. Then you can direct your agent on how to act. Your directions can discuss outcomes, specific circumstances, or both. If you discuss outcomes, the statement should focus on which types of outcomes would be acceptable and which would not—for example, "resuscitate if I can continue to fully function mentally." The following are some of the more common specific circumstances encountered with major chronic diseases.

■ **You have been diagnosed with Alzheimer's disease and other neurologic problems that may eventually leave you with little or no mental function.** As noted earlier, these are generally not life-threatening, at least not for many years. However, things

happen to these patients that can be life-threatening, such as pneumonia and heart attacks. What you need to do is decide how much treatment you want. For example, do you want antibiotics if you get pneumonia? Do you want to be resuscitated if your heart stops? Do you want a feeding tube if you are unable to feed yourself? Remember, it is your choice as to how you answer each of these questions. You may not want to be resuscitated but may want a feeding tube. If you want aggressive treatment, you may want to use all means possible to sustain life; alternatively, you may not want any special means to be used to sustain life. For example, you may want to be fed but may not want to be placed on life-support equipment.

■ **You have very bad lung function that will not improve.** Should you become unable to breathe on your own, do you want to be placed in an intensive care unit on a mechanical ventilator (a breathing machine)? Remember, in this case you will not improve. To say that you never want ventilation is very different from saying that you don't want it if it is used to sustain life when no improvement is likely. Obviously, mechanical ventilation can be lifesaving in cases such as a severe asthma attack when it is used for a short time until the body can regain its normal function. Here the issue is not whether to use mechanical ventilation ever but rather when or under what circumstances you wish it to be used.

■ **You have a heart condition that cannot be improved with surgery.** You are in the cardiac intensive care unit. If your heart stops functioning, do you want to be resuscitated? As with artificial ventilation, the question is not "Do you ever want to be resuscitated?" but rather "Under what conditions do you or do you not want resuscitation?"

From these examples you can begin to identify some of the directions that you might want to give in your advance directive or durable power of attorney for health care. Again, to understand these better or to make them more personal to your own condition, you might want to talk with your physician about what the common problems and decisions are for people with your condition.

In summary, there are several decisions you need to make in directing your agent on how to act in your behalf:

- Generally, how much treatment do you want? This can range from the very aggressive—that is, doing many things to sustain life—to the very conservative—which is doing almost nothing to sustain life, except to keep you clean and comfortable.

- Given the types of life-threatening events that are likely to happen to people with your condition, what sorts of treatment do you want and under what conditions?

- If you become mentally incapacitated, what sorts of treatment do you want for other illnesses, such as pneumonia?

Although each state has different regulations and forms for advance directives, the information presented here should be useful wherever you live. Check out some of the Web sites at the end of this chapter for forms you can download. You can also find them at the local health department, Area Agency on Aging, hospitals, or even the offices of your health care providers. For information about advance directives in other countries, go to http://www.growthhouse.org/.

Note that many states recognize durable powers of attorney for health care that are created in another state. However, this is not always the case. As of now, this is an unclear legal issue. To be on the safe side, if you move or spend a lot of time in another state, it is best to check with a lawyer in that state to see if your document is legally binding there.

Sharing Your Wishes with Others

Writing down your wishes and having a durable power of attorney is not the end of the job. A good manager has to do more than just write a memo. He or she has to see that the memo gets delivered. If you really want your wishes carried out, it is important that you share them fully with your agent, your family, and your doctor. This is often not an easy task.

Before you can have this conversation, though, everyone involved needs to have copies of your DPA for health care. Once you have completed the documents, have them witnessed and signed. In some places you can have your DPA notarized instead of having it witnessed. Make several copies at a copy center. You will need copies for your agents, family members, and doctors. Also, it does not hurt to give one to your lawyer.

Now you are ready to talk about your wishes. People don't like to discuss their own death or that of a loved one. Therefore, it is not surprising that when you bring up this subject, the response is often "Oh, don't think about that," or "That's a long time off," or "Don't be so morbid; you're not that sick." Unfortunately, this is usually enough to end the conversation. Your job as a good self-manager is to keep the conversation open. There are several ways to do this. First, plan on how you will have this discussion. Here are some suggestions.

Prepare your durable power of attorney, and then give copies to the appropriate family members or friends. Ask them to read it and then set a specific time to discuss it. If they give you one of the avoidance responses, explain that you understand that this is a difficult topic but that it is important to you that you discuss it with them. This is a good time to practice the "I" messages discussed in Chapter 9—for example, "I understand that death is a difficult thing to talk about. However, it is very important to me that we have this discussion."

Another strategy might be to get blank copies of the DPA form for all your family members and suggest that you all fill them out and share them. This could even be part of a family get-together. Present this as an important aspect of being a mature adult and family member. Making this a family project involving everyone may make it easier to discuss. Besides, it will help clarify everyone's values about death and dying.

If these two suggestions seem too difficult or for some reason are impossible to carry out, you might write a letter or e-mail or prepare a video or CD that can then be sent to family members. Talk about why you feel your death is an important topic to discuss and that you want them to know your wishes. Then state your wishes, providing reasons for your choices. At the same time, send them a copy of your DPA for health care. Ask that

they respond in some way or that you set aside some time to talk in person or on the phone.

Of course, as mentioned previously, when deciding on your agent, it is important that you choose someone with whom you can talk freely and exchange ideas. If your chosen agent is not willing to or is unable to talk to you about your wishes, you have probably chosen the wrong agent. Remember, the fact that someone is very close to you does not mean that he or she really understands your wishes or would be able to carry them out. This topic should not be left to an unspoken understanding unless you don't mind if your agent decides differently from what you wish. For this reason, choosing someone who is not as close to you emotionally and then talking things out with your agent are essential. This is especially true if you have not written out the details of your wishes.

Talking with Your Doctor

From our research, we have learned that people often have a more difficult time talking to their doctors about their wishes surrounding death than to their families. In fact, only a very small percentage of people who have written DPAs for health care or other advance directives ever share these with their physician.

Even though it is hard, it is important to talk with your doctor. You need to be sure that your doctor's values are similar to yours. If you and your doctor do not have the same values, it may be difficult for him or her to carry out your wishes. Second, your doctor needs to know what you want. This allows him or her to take appropriate actions such as writing orders to resuscitate or not to use mechanical resuscitation. Third, your doctor needs to know who your agent is and how to contact this person. If an important decision has to be made and your wishes are to be followed, the doctor must talk with your agent.

Be sure to give your doctor a copy of your DPA for health care so that it can become a permanent part of your medical record.

As surprising as it may seem, many physicians also find it hard to talk to their patients about their end-of-life wishes. After all, doctors are in the business of keeping people alive and well; they don't like to think about their patients dying. On the other hand, most doctors want their patients to have durable powers of attorney for health care. These documents relieve both you and your doctor from pressure and worry.

If you wish, plan a time with your doctor when you can discuss your wishes. This should not be a side conversation at the end of a regular visit. Rather, start a visit by saying, "I want a few minutes to discuss my wishes in the event of a serious problem or impending death." When put this way, most doctors will make time to talk with you. If the doctor says that he or she does not have enough time, ask when you can make another appointment to talk with him or her. This is a situation where you may need to be a little assertive. Sometimes a doctor, like your family members or friends, might say, "Oh, you don't have to worry about that; let me do it," or "We'll worry about that when the time comes." Again, you will have to take the initiative, using an "I" message to communicate that this is important to you and that you do not want to put off the discussion.

Sometimes doctors do not want to worry you. They think they are doing you a favor by not describing all the unpleasant things that might happen to you or the potential treatments in case of serious problems. You can help your doctor by telling him or her that having control and making some decisions about your future will ease your mind. Not knowing or not being clear on what will happen is more worrisome than being faced with the facts, unpleasant as they may be, and dealing with them.

Even knowing all that's been said so far, it is still sometimes hard to talk with your doctor. Therefore, it might also be helpful to bring your agent with you when you have this discussion. The agent can facilitate the discussion and at the same time make your doctor's acquaintance. This also gives everyone a chance to clarify any misunderstandings. It opens the lines of communication so that if your agent and physician have to act to carry out your wishes, they can do so with few problems. If you aren't able to talk with your doctor, it is still important that he or she receive a copy of your DPA for health care for your medical record.

When you go the hospital, be sure the hospital has a copy of your DPA. If you cannot bring it, be sure your agent knows to give a copy to the hospital. This is important, as your doctor may not be in charge of your care in the hospital.

There is one thing not to do. Do not put your durable power of attorney in your safe deposit box—no one will be able to get it when it is needed. And by the way, you do not need to see a lawyer to draw up a durable power of attorney. You can do this by yourself with no legal assistance.

Now that you have done all the important things, the hard work is over. However, remember that you can change your mind at any time. Your agent may no longer be available, or your wishes might change. Be sure to keep your DPA for health care updated. Like any legal document, it can be revoked or changed at any time. The decisions you make today are not forever.

Making your wishes known about how you want to be treated in case of serious or life-threatening illness is one of the most important tasks of self-management. The best way to do this is to prepare a durable power of attorney for health care and share this with your family, close friends, and physician.

Suggested Further Reading

Atkinson, Jacqueline M. *Advance Directives in Mental Health: Theory, Practice and Ethics.* London: Jessica Kingsley Publishers, 2007.

Burkman, Kip. *The Stroke Recovery Book: A Guide for Patients and Families.* Omaha, Neb.: Addicus Books, 1998.

Callahan, Maggie, and Patricia Kelley. *Final Gifts: Understanding the Special Awareness, Needs, and Communications of the Dying.* New York: Bantam Books, 1997.

Doukas, David John, and William Reichel. *Planning for Uncertainty: Living Wills and Other Advance Directives for You and Your Family,* 2nd ed. Baltimore: John Hopkins University Press, 2007.

Godkin, M. Dianne. *Living Will, Living Well: Reflections on Preparing an Advance Directive.* Edmonton: University of Alberta Press, 2008.

Kübler-Ross, Elizabeth. *On Death and Dying.* New York: Scribner Classics, 1997.

Kurz, Gary. *Cold Noses at the Pearly Gates: A Book of Hope for Those Who Have Lost a Pet.* New York: Citadel Press, 2008.

Lewinson, Peter M., Rebecca Forster, and Mary A. Youngsen. *Control Your Depression.* New York: Simon & Schuster, 1992.

Long, Laurie Ecklund. *My Life in a Box: A Life Organizer: How to Build an Emergency Tool Box,* 4th ed. Fresno, Calif.: AGL, 2010.

Olick, Robert S. *Taking Advance Directives Seriously: Prospective Autonomy and Decisions Near the End of Life.* Washington, D.C.: Georgetown University Press, 2001.

Pettus, Mark C. *The Savvy Patient: The Ultimate Advocate for Quality Health Care.* Sterling, Va.: Capital Books, 2004.

Sitarz, Daniel. *Advance Health Care Directives Simplified.* Carbondale, Ill.: Nova, 2007.

Stolp, Hans. *When a Loved One Dies: How to Go On After Saying Goodbye.* Hampshire, England: O Books, 2005.

Wilkinson, James A. *A Family Caregiver's Guide to Planning and Decision Making for the Elderly.* Minneapolis, Minn.: Fairview, 1999.

Other Resources

☐ AARP, http://www.aarp.org/Advance-Directive

☐ National Hospice and Palliative Care Organization, http://www.caringinfo.org/

☐ National Resource Center on Psychiatric Advance Directives, http://www.nrc-pad.org/

☐   Benefits Check Up: http://www.benefitscheckup.org/

☐   Five Wishes (Aging with Dignity): http://www.agingwithdignity.org/

☐   Growth House, Improving Care for Dying: http://www.growthhouse.org/

☐   Leading Age (homes for the aged): http://www.leadingage.org/

☐   My Life in A Box: A Life Organizer: http://mylifeinabox.com/

☐   National Council on Aging: http://www.ncoa.org

Index